Dermatology
for Clinicians

Dermatology for Clinicians

A practical guide to common skin conditions

Massad Gregory Joseph, MD

Assistant Clinical Professor of Medicine/Dermatology
UCLA School of Medicine, Los Angeles, California

The Parthenon Publishing Group
International Publishers in Medicine, Science & Technology

A CRC PRESS COMPANY
BOCA RATON   LONDON   NEW YORK   WASHINGTON, D.C.

Published in the UK and Europe by
The Parthenon Publishing Group
23–25 Blades Court
Deodar Road
London SW15 2NU, UK

Published in the USA by
The Parthenon Publishing Group
345 Park Avenue South, 10th Floor
New York, NY 10010, USA

British Library Cataloguing in Publication Data
Joseph, Massad Gregory
  Dermatology for clinicians
  1. Dermatology 2. Skin - Diseases
  I.Title
  616.5

  ISBN 1842141260

Library of Congress Cataloging-in-Publication Data
Joseph, Massad Gregory
  Dermatology for clinicians / by Massad Gregory Joseph
     p.;cm.
  Includes bibliographical references and index.
  ISBN 1-84214-126-0 (alk. paper)
    1. Dermatology--Handbook, manuals etc. 2. Skin–Diseases--Handbooks, manuals,
  etc. I. Title
    [DNLM: 1. Skin Diseases--diagnosis. 2. Skin Diseases--therapy. 3. Primary
  Health Care-methods. WR 140 J829d 2002]
  RL74 J674 2002
  616.3–dc21   2002025104

Typeset by Siva Math Setters, Chennai, India
Printed and bound in Great Britain by Butler &Tanner Ltd, Frome and London

Notice: Our knowledge in clinical sciences is constantly changing. As new information becomes available, changes in treatment and in the use of drugs become necessary. The author and publisher of this volume have taken care to make certain that the doses of drugs and schedules of treatment are correct and compatible with the standards generally accepted at the time of publication. The reader is advised to consult carefully the instruction and information material included in the package insert of each drug or therapeutic agent before administration. This advice is especially important when using new or infrequently used drugs.

Contents

Preface

Dermatological conditions are among the most common ailments with which patients present to primary care physicians, many of whom are not comfortable using more advanced dermatological options when treating these patients. However, there are more advanced dermatological approaches (used by dermatologists and not typically used by primary care physicians) with which primary care physicians can become familiar and utilize when dealing with common dermatological conditions. My intent in this book is to discuss these more advanced approaches, as well as basic approaches, to common dermatological conditions in a clear, simple, detailed, orderly, non-intimidating, step-by-step, 'how to' fashion such that primary care physicians can easily understand and use these approaches comfortably and confidently.

In addition, I have included useful information – including unique, not well known, or not previously described so-called 'pearls' – regarding common dermatological conditions and the approaches related to them.

Although aimed at primary care physicians, the nature of this book also makes it useful for physicians in dermatology residency training, for nurse practitioners and physician's assistants as well as medical students.

However, there are two important caveats to this book; as with all medications, before prescribing any medication mentioned in this book, the physician should be appropriately familiar with the information provided in the medication's package insert and labeling. Also, patients with any dermatological condition that is persisting or not being controlled well or for which the diagnosis is in any doubt should be referred to a dermatologist for consultation.

Acknowledgements

I would like to thank William V. R. Shellow, MD, Marc D. Chalet, MD, A. Bernard Ackerman, MD, Richard G. Bennett, MD, William E. Freije, MD, William A. Freije, MD, Nancy P. Lee, Pharm D, Theresa A. Freije, MA, and William M. Freije, Pharm D, for their professional assistance. I would also like to thank Cathy Clark-Joseph for her astute judgement.

About the author

College Education: BA (Magna Cum Laude, Phi Beta Kappa) in Biochemistry, Occidental College, Los Angeles, California

Medical School Education: MD, Harvard Medical School, Boston, Massachusetts

Internship: Internal Medicine, Hospital of the Good Samaritan, Los Angeles, California

Residency: Dermatology, Combined UCLA/Wadsworth VA Dermatology Residency Program, Los Angeles, California

Board Certification: Diplomate, American Board of Dermatology

Faculty Appointment: Assistant Clinical Professor of Medicine/Dermatology, UCLA School of Medicine, Los Angeles, California

Professional Organizations: Fellow and Life Member, American Academy of Dermatology

Fellow, Los Angeles Metropolitan Dermatological Society

Professional Clinical Experience: 18 years in the clinical practice of dermatology

To Cathy Clark-Joseph, Lillian Freije Joseph, Julia Veronica Freije, William Elias Freije, MD, and Virgil Massad Freije

1

Understanding and using topical corticosteroids and non-steroidal topical immunomodulator substitutes for topical corticosteroids

OVERVIEW

Because topical corticosteroids (topical steroids) are used so frequently in treating dermatological conditions, I would like to start off discussing them in a separate section as their own specific topic.

Non-steroidal topical immunomodulator (TIM) substitutes for topical steroids will also be discussed in this chapter. (A non-steroidal TIM substitute for topical steroids has been approved for the treatment of atopic dermatitis in appropriate patients; see Chapter 2).

TOPICAL STEROIDS

Topical steroid potency

Topical steroids come in a range of potency classes. A pocket-size copy for easy reference of a table showing all of the potency classes and the various brand names and generic names of the topical steroids within the classes can be readily obtained from the drug representative of the manufacturer of any of these topical steroids. These potency classes range from the most potent class, class I, which contains the so-called super-potent topical steroids, to class VII, which contains the least potent topical steroids. Arbitrarily, topical steroids in class I are called super-potent topical steroids, those in class II can be called high-potency topical steroids, those in class III can be considered to be high mid-potency topical steroids, those in class IV can be called mid-potency topical steroids, those in class V can be considered to be low mid-potency topical steroids, those in class VI can be considered to be high low-potency topical steroids, and those in class VII can be called low-potency topical steroids. A topical steroid from class II, one from class IV and/or one from class VII will take care of most patients with most dermatological conditions requiring topical steroid therapy. (Elaboration of this is presented later in this chapter.)

In my experience, different topical steroid preparations that are rated as having the same potency also generally have, for a given site, the same level of clinical efficacy as well as the same level of potential risk for the development of adverse effects (excluding adverse effects that are due to an allergic or irritant reaction to a topical steroid preparation). Hence, for a given site, switching from the use of one topical steroid preparation to the use of another that is rated as having the same potency as the original topical steroid preparation generally makes no difference in these regards (unless you are dealing with an allergic or irritant reaction to a topical steroid preparation). This is because the level of clinical efficacy as well as the level of the potential risk for the development of adverse effects (excluding allergic or irritant reactions) for topical steroid preparations for a given site is generally directly linked to topical steroid potency. (The adverse effects of and susceptibility to topical steroids and allergic and irritant reactions to topical steroid preparations are discussed later in this chapter.)

Occlusion regarding topical steroids

If you look at a topical steroid potency class table, as described above, you will notice that the ointment preparation of a specific concentration of a specific topical steroid is frequently more potent than is the corresponding cream preparation. The reason for this is that an ointment provides greater occlusion (i.e. greater inhibition of evaporation of water from the skin surface), which results in greater hydration of the stratum corneum, thus greater absorption and penetration of the steroid chemical from the skin surface into the skin. There is a resulting greater concentration of the steroid chemical present in the skin, thus a greater steroid effect than that which occurs when the corresponding topical steroid cream preparation is applied to the skin surface. (The stratum corneum is the dead, horny, most superficial layer of the epidermis and consists of the protein keratin. The epidermis is the superficial cutaneous layer that is located immediately above the dermis. Ointments, creams and other topical steroid vehicles are discussed below.)

An even greater occlusive effect (producing an even greater steroid effect – i.e. producing even greater steroid potency) can be achieved when the area of application of a topical steroid cream is subsequently occluded by covering with plastic clingfilm, plastic or latex gloves, or other occlusive material that prevents evaporation of water from the skin surface. I feel that ointment vehicles should generally not be used under such occlusion, which may be more likely to produce such problems as folliculitis (inflammation of hair follicles) when an ointment vehicle is being occluded. Also, super-potent, class I topical steroids (see above) should not be used under such occlusion. Generally, when I use topical steroids, I do not use them under such occlusion, regardless of their vehicle, mainly because I have found it unnecessary to do so in the vast majority of cases.

Adverse effects of topical steroids and susceptibility to topical steroid effects

Overview

As topical steroids become more potent (and they become even more potent under occlusion, as described above), they become more efficacious, but they likewise generally have greater potential for steroid-induced adverse effects. In general, the more potent a topical steroid is, the greater is its potential for steroid-induced adverse effects.

Also, another independent variable is that certain areas of the body are more susceptible to the beneficial effects of topical steroids but are also more susceptible to the adverse effects of topical steroids; this variable is to a large extent based on stratum corneum thickness: the thinner a body area's stratum corneum is, the greater is that area's susceptibility to the effects of topical steroids. Also, it is impotant to note that topical steroid use on the eyelids or periorbital region can lead to glaucoma and cataracts involving the ipsilateral eye. If normal skin thickness is present, the areas that have a 'high' topical steroid susceptibility include the face, ears, area around the ears, genitals and skin folds – I generally use the low-potency topical steroid hydrocortisone (e.g. Hytone®) 1% for involvement in these areas, excluding the eyelids and periorbital regions, in adults, and I gener-ally use hydrocortisone (e.g. Delcort®) 0.5% for involvement on the eyelids and periorbital regions in adults; the areas that have a 'mid-level' topical steroid susceptibility include the scalp, neck, trunk, arms and legs – I gen-erally use a mid-potency topical steroid such as triamcinolone (e.g. Kenalog® or Aristocort®) 0.1% for involvement in these areas in adults; and the areas that have a 'low' topical steroid susceptibility include the hands and feet – I generally use a high-potency topical steroid such as fluocinon-ide (e.g. Lidex®) for involvement in these areas in adults.

Skin thickness that is less than normal for an area can be considered to result in further increase of the topical steroid susceptibility of the area. Elderly patients, for example, commonly have thin skin. Therefore, particular caution should be exercised when topical steroids are used on areas of thinned or atrophic skin or in elderly patients.

I consider pediatric patients to be more susceptible to the adverse effects of topical steroids than are adults, so I use topical steroids with particular caution in pediatric patients, for whom I generally use the following low-potency topical steroids: hydrocortisone 0.5% for involvement on the face, ears, area around the ears, genitals and skin folds (bearing in mind that the nominally higher potency topical steroid hydrocortisone 1% may sometimes be needed) and hydrocortisone 1% for involvement on the scalp, neck, trunk, arms, legs, hands and feet (bearing in mind that the nominally higher potency topical steroid hydrocortisone 2.5% may sometimes be needed).

Local adverse effects of topical steroids

The steroid-induced local adverse effects that can occur at the site of topical steroid application include atrophy (thinning) of the skin such that the skin appears thin, somewhat shiny and somewhat transparent, so that there may be increased visibility of underlying structures such as blood vessels, with the skin surface sometimes showing fine, cigarette paper-like wrinkling, striae (stretch marks), telangiectases (fine, red, blood vessels which appear to be on the skin surface), hypopigmentation (decreased pigmentation), and persistent erythema (blanchable redness).

It should again be emphasized that the more potent a topical steroid is (and topical steroids become even more potent under occlusion, as discussed above), the greater is its efficacy, but also the greater in general is its potential for the development of the above-described local adverse effects at the site of application of the topical steroid. Likewise, in general, the longer a topical steroid is used or the higher its application frequency is, the greater is its efficacy, but also the greater is the risk for development of the above-described local adverse effects.

Systemic adverse effects of topical steroids

Topical steroids can also be systemically absorbed through the skin surface and lead to systemic adverse effects, which can include hypothalamic–pituitary–adrenal axis suppression as well as the clinical manifestations of Cushing's syndrome, which can include 'moon' (full, rounded) facies, central obesity, violaceous striae (stretch marks), 'buffalo hump' (deposition of fat at the base of the posterior aspect of the neck), hypertension, hyperglycemia proximal muscle weakness and 'brittle bones'.

Generally, it can be said that the more potent a topical steroid is, or the larger the area of application of a topical steroid is, or the greater the amount of topical steroid that is used, or the longer a topical steroid is used, or the greater the use of topical steroid occlusion is, or the more frequent the application of the topical steroid is, the greater is the risk for the development of the above-described systemic adverse effects.

Recommendations regarding topical steroid selection

In general, when I need a low-potency topical steroid, I use hydrocortisone (e.g. Hytone) 1%. When I need a topical steroid that is nominally lower in potency than hydrocortisone 1%, I use hydrocortisone (e.g. Delcort) 0.5%, and when I need a topical steroid that is nominally higher in potency than hydrocortisone 1%, I use hydrocortisone (e.g. Hytone) 2.5%. When I need a mid-potency topical steroid, I use triamcinolone (e.g. Kenalog or Aristocort) 0.1%, and when I need a high-potency topical steroid, I use fluocinonide (e.g. Lidex). I very seldom, if ever, use super-potent topical steroids, which include clobetasol propionate (e.g. Temovate®) and halobetasol propionate (e.g. Ultravate®), among others, because they generally have additional package insert restrictions on their use. These additional restrictions include not using these products continuously for longer than a certain period of time and not using more than a certain number of grams of these products per week.

For adults, as discussed previously, I generally use the low-potency topical steroid hydrocortisone (e.g. Delcort) 0.5% for involvement on the eyelids and the periorbital regions; the low-potency topical steroid hydrocortisone (e.g. Hytone) 1% for involvement on the face (excluding the eyelids and the periorbital regions), ears, area around the ears, genitals and skin folds; a mid-potency topical steroid such as triamcinolone (e.g. Kenalog or Aristocort) 0.1% for involvement on the scalp, neck, trunk, arms and legs; and a high-potency topical steroid such as fluocinonide (e.g. Lidex) for involvement on the hands and feet. As discussed above, particular caution should be exercised when topical steroids are used on areas of thinned or atrophic skin or in elderly patients.

As discussed previously, I consider pediatric patients to be more susceptible to the adverse effects of topical steroids than are adults, so I use topical steroids with particular caution in pediatric patients, for whom I generally use the following low-potency topical steroids: hydrocortisone 0.5% for involvement on the face, ears, area around the ears, genitals and skin folds (bearing in mind that the nominally higher potency topical steroid hydrocortisone 1% may sometimes be needed) and hydrocortisone 1% for involvement on the scalp, neck, trunk, arms, legs, hands and feet (bearing in mind that the nominally higher potency topical steroid hydrocortisone 2.5% may sometimes be needed).

I generally do not use topical steroids in a pregnant or breast-feeding patient unless their use is approved by the patient's obstetrician or breast-fed baby's pediatrician, respectively.

Tachyphylaxis regarding topical steroids

Topical steroids exhibit the phenomenon known as tachyphylaxis: if topical steroids are used for a given condition in a given patient continuously, the topical steroids over time become less and less effective to the point where they no longer have any beneficial effect on the condition being treated. If the topical steroids are stopped, after a while they again become effective when restarted, but for the time during which they are withheld, it is generally the case that the condition that was being treated worsens and flares.

Topical steroid vehicles

Topical steroids can be dispersed in a spectrum of vehicles: ointments, creams, gels, lotions and solutions. Vehicles are made up of inactive ingredients.

In general, ointment vehicles (ointments) tend to be used when treating skin conditions associated with dryness and scaling, because ointments tend to have a moisturizing (hydrating) effect, as described above (i.e. they tend to have an occlusive effect, which results in inhibition of evaporation of water from the skin surface, and this results in increased hydration of the stratum corneum).

Gels, lotions and solutions tend to be used when treating skin conditions associated with oozing, vesicles (small blisters) and/or bullae (large blisters), because these vehicles tend to have a drying, non-occlusive, non-hydrating effect. In addition, gels, lotions and solutions tend to be used when treating hairy areas such as the scalp, because these vehicles are easier and cosmetically more acceptable for the patient to use in these areas and are less likely to occlude hair follicles, the occlusion of which can result in folliculitis (inflammation of hair follicles).

Creams, being midway in the spectrum between occluding/hydrating and drying, can generally be used in almost any situation, and the cream vehicle is the vehicle that I use most often.

Allergic and irritant reactions to topical steroid preparations

Overview

The inactive ingredients described above can include preservatives, fragrances and other chemicals that can be important when treating skin conditions, because they can sometimes cause allergic or irritant reactions that can cause inflammation or exacerbation or lack of improvement of the condition being treated. Specific inactive ingredients that can cause such reactions include parabens, propylene glycol, benzyl alcohol, sodium laurel sulfate, lanolin, ethylenediamine hydrochloride, isopropyl palmitate, polysorbate 60, stearyl alcohol, chlorocresol and fragrance. Allergic reactions can also be caused by the steroid chemical itself.

If a condition undergoing treatment with a topical steroid preparation is being exacerbated, if the patient is experiencing new or increased burning or itching or new or increased signs of inflammation (e.g. erythema, blisters, scaling, etc.) at the sites of treatment with a topical steroid preparation, or if a condition is not improving as expected with treatment with a topical steroid preparation, an irritant or allergic reaction to the topical steroid preparation should be considered. It should be remembered that the reaction could be due to the topical steroid chemical itself or to an inactive ingredient in the vehicle in which the topical steroid chemical is dispersed, as described above. The situation in which a condition is not improving as expected with treatment with a topical steroid preparation can be thought of as occurring sometimes because the added inflammation of an allergic or irritant reaction resulting from the topical steroid preparation can be negated by the anti-inflammatory effect of the topical steroid preparation, such that the patient's clinical status stays the same without improvement or worsening.

How to deal with suspected allergic and irritant reactions
to topical steroid preparations

If an allergic or irritant reaction to a topical steroid preparation seems to be occurring, the topical steroid preparation being used should be discontinued, and a different preparation should be tried. In my experience, when such a reaction occurs, it is usually due to an inactive ingredient in the vehicle. When such a reaction occurs and if, for example, I am using a mid-potency topical steroid preparation such as generic triamcinolone cream 0.1%, I will switch to Aristocort A cream 0.1%, which is a specific brand of triamcinolone cream 0.1%. This does not contain parabens, propylene glycol, sodium laurel sulfate, lanolin, ethylenediamine hydrochloride, polysorbate 60, stearyl alcohol, chlorocresol, or fragrance, and is usually well tolerated. If the problem continues with this different preparation, I will switch again, this time to a preparation that has a steroid chemical that is different from triamcinolone, in case the reaction is to the active ingredient triamcinolone itself.

In my experience, I have found that, when a generic preparation seems to be causing a reaction, the problem frequently seems to disappear when I switch to the brand name. For example, if it seems that the generic low-potency topical steroid preparation hydrocortisone cream or ointment 1% or 2.5% is causing a reaction, switching to Hytone cream or ointment 1% or 2.5%, which is a specific brand of hydrocortisone, frequently takes care of the problem. Likewise, if it seems that the the generic high-potency topical steroid preparation fluocinonide cream or ointment is causing a reaction, switching to Lidex cream or ointment, which is a specific brand of fluocinonide, frequently takes care of the problem. Again, if the generic mid-potency topical steroid preparation triamcinolone cream or ointment 0.1% seems to be causing a reaction, switching to Aristocort A cream or ointment 0.1%, which is a specific brand of triamcinolone, frequently takes care of the problem.

In summary, if an allergic or irritant reaction to a topical steroid preparation is suspected, remember that the reaction can be due either to inactive ingredients in the preparation or to the active ingredient, which is the steroid chemical itself. When such a reaction seems to be occurring, consider switching from generic preparations to the name brand of the medication; consider switching to a preparation that does not contain such inactive ingredients as parabens, propylene glycol, benzyl alcohol, sodium laurel sulfate, lanolin, ethylenediamine hydrochloride, isopropyl palmitate, polysorbate 60, stearyl alcohol, chlorocresol, or fragrance; and/or consider switching to a different steroid chemical. When switching, remember to switch to a preparation that has the same potency as that of the preparation from which you are switching.

Lastly, in my experience, when one is dealing with suspected allergic or irritant reactions to topical steroid preparations, the low-potency Hytone brand of hydrocortisone cream or ointment 1% or 2.5%, the generally mid-potency Aristocort A brand of triamcinolone cream or ointment 0.1%

and the high-potency Lidex brand of fluocinonide cream or ointment frequently seem to be well tolerated.

Non-steroidal topical immunomodulator substitutes for topical steroids

As the name implies, non-steroidal TIM substitutes for topical steroids are TIMs that have immunosuppressant/anti-inflammatory-type effects and are not based on steroids. Such TIMs can be potentially useful in the treatment of skin disorders currently treated with topical steroids and have so far not been shown to exhibit tachyphylaxis (which was discussed previously in this chapter) or adverse effects that are typical for topical steroids (such adverse effects were discussed previously in this chapter).

One such agent, tacrolimus ointment, has been approved by the Food and Drug Administration (FDA) for the treatment of atopic dermatitis (see Chapter 2) in appropriate patients and is marketed under the brand name Protopic Ointment®. Systemic tacrolimus is approved for prophylaxis for the rejection of a transplanted allogeneic kidney or liver. Protopic ointment is the first non-steroidal TIM substitute for topical steroids to be released in the USA. Tacrolimus ointment has been shown to be safe and effective for the treatment of atopic dermatitis in adults and children as young as 2 years of age. The only significant adverse effect of tacrolimus ointment is that, in the first week of treatment, it can produce increased skin burning and pruritus. Topically applied tacrolimus ointment is not associated with significant systemic absorption or a significant increase in infections.

2

Dermatitis/eczema/eczematous dermatitis and lichen simplex chronicus/prurigo nodularis

OVERVIEW

In current common usage, for all intents and purposes, dermatitis is synonymous with eczema, which is synonymous with eczematous dermatitis. All of these names can be considered to refer to a general condition in which the following primary lesions can be observed: erythematous macules, which, if they coalesce, form erythematous patches that may be edematous; erythematous papules, which, if they coalesce, form erythematous plaques; and vesicles and bullae. (Erythematous refers to blanchable redness, which is erythema. Macules are small, non-raised, non-palpable lesions. Patches are large, non-raised, non-palpable lesions. Papules are bumps. Plaques are broad, raised lesions. Vesicles are small blisters. Bullae are large blisters.) The secondary changes that can be seen include oozing and crusting, scaling, lichenification, and fissuring. (Scaling is flaking. Lichenification is thickening of the skin, with increased prominence of skin lines, due to frequent scratching, rubbing and/or picking. Fissuring is cracking.) In dermatitis/eczema/eczematous dermatitis there tends to be a poorly demarcated border between abnormal and normal skin (i.e. the border is indistinct). There are different types of dermatitis (see below), and not all of the lesions and changes described above are seen in each type of dermatitis. Also, vesicles and bullae are seen only in acute involvement, whereas lichenification is seen only in chronic involvement. Symptomatically, pruritus is typically present, and burning can sometimes be present.

Specific types of dermatitis include autosensitization dermatitis; contact dermatitis, a variant of which can be considered to be so-called 'hand dermatitis' or 'hand eczema' and another variant of which can be considered to be so-called 'diaper dermatitis'; nummular dermatitis; seborrheic dermatitis; stasis dermatitis; atopic dermatitis; and dyshidrotic dermatitis. (For discussion of so-called 'diaper candidiasis' as opposed to so-called 'diaper dermatitis', see Chapter 18). Sometimes cases of dermatitis are such that they cannot be classified as a definite type of dermatitis as described above, so I assign the diagnosis of non-specific dermatitis to such cases.

I feel that lichen simplex chronicus/prurigo nodularis (which some dermatologists have called neurodermatitis) can be considered to be a condition related to dermatitis.

All of these above-described conditions and their treatment are discussed below.

NON-SPECIFIC DERMATITIS

Overview

When dermatitis is non-specific and, therefore, the specific type is unclear, I feel that the condition can be referred to as 'non-specific dermatitis' or 'dermatitis'. In my experience the patient tends to present with sometimes itchy erythematous macules, erythematous patches, erythematous papules and/or erythematous plaques, with scaling frequently being present.

Special considerations regarding non-specific dermatitis

Common differential diagnosis of limited/localized non-specific dermatitis

The common differential diagnosis of limited/localized non-specific dermatitis can include such conditions as: psoriasis (see Chapter 4); bacterial folliculitis (see Chapter 17); acne (see Chapter 9); rosacea, perioral dermatitis, (which is not typically classified among the 'true' dermatitides that are discussed in this chapter), steroid dependent facial dermatosis, and acne keloidalis nuchae (see Chapter 10). Squamous cell carcinoma in-situ, invasive squamous cell carcinoma and superficial basal cell carcinoma (see Chapter 26). Mammary Paget's disease and extramammary Paget's disease; mammary Paget's disease consists of a dermatitic-appearing, neoplastic lesion that usually involves the nipple and/or areola and which is indicative of ductal carcinoma involving the underlying breast, and extramammary Paget's disease consists of a dermatitic-appearing, neoplastic lesion that most commonly involves the anogenital skin but can instead involve other areas and which may be associated with an underlying local or distant malignancy. Shave biopsy (as described in Chapter 26) that includes the epidermis can be done to confirm the diagnoses of mammary Paget's disease and extramammary Paget's disease, which can be taken care of by a dermatologist and other specialists as appropriate. Tinea and superficial cutaneous candidal infection (see Chapter 18). Pseudofolliculitis barbae (or pili incarnati), if involvement is limited to shaved hairy areas, such as the bearded region in men, pseudofolliculitis barbae (pili incarnati), which is not due to infection but is an inflammatory reaction to ingrown hairs resulting from shaving, should be considered in the differential diagnosis (see Chapter 19). Scabies should also be considered in limited/localized non-specific dermatitis (see Chapter 16).

Common differential diagnosis of extensive/generalized non-specific dermatitis

When non-specific dermatitis involvement is generalized, drug eruption (see Chapter 3) and secondary syphilis (see Chapter 27) should be considered in the differential diagnosis, if the associated circumstances are appropriate for such diagnoses. This is because drug eruptions and secondary syphilis are 'the great mimickers'; they can look like virtually any skin condition. Other conditions such as psoriasis (see Chapter 4), pityriasis rosea (see Chapter 6) and extensive bacterial folliculitis (see Chapter 17) might also be considered in the differential diagnosis. If the clinical situation is appropriate, viral eruption should also be considered in the differential diagnosis. In my experience, there are viruses that can produce non-specific eruptions (see Chapter 6).

A negative Venereal Disease Research Laboratories (VDRL) or rapid plasma reagin (RPR) test will rule out secondary syphilis; a complete blood count (CBC) showing lymphocytosis would be suggestive of a viral eruption, which may have associated constitutional symptoms and/or signs and typically presents as erythematous macules that may coalesce, erythematous papules, vesicles, and/or pustules (viral culture of vesicle and/or pustule contents might reveal a virus); and a CBC showing eosinophilia might be suggestive of a drug eruption. Severe, serious drug eruptions may show lymphocytosis with atypical lymphocytes and may have associated constitutional symptoms and/or signs along with other findings. Current evidence is that eosinophilia on CBC is an uncommon finding for common drug reactions and is a parameter that is of little value in diagnosing common drug reactions, but an eosinophil count greater than 1000/μl may be seen with severe, serious drug eruptions.

The untreated rash of secondary syphilis would resolve spontaneously (at which time the patient would be said to have latent syphilis). If the diagnosis of secondary syphilis is made, this obviously should be evaluated, treated and followed accordingly, and if the patient is pregnant, her obstetrician should be notified because of the potential effect of syphilis on the fetus. Viral eruption generally needs only symptomatic treatment, since it is generally self-limited, but if the patient is pregnant, and viral eruption is considered, the patient's obstetrician should be notified regarding the possibility of associated harm to the fetus. If the diagnosis of a viral eruption is made, appropriate precautions need to be taken to prevent transmission of the condition to other individuals.

The common differential diagnosis of extensive/generalized nonspecific dermatitis can also include such conditions as: parapsoriasis, a scaly patchy condition that is similar in appearance to but is distinct from dermatitis and psoriasis. Referral to a dermatologist must be done to confirm the diagnosis and treatment of parapsoriasis. Early cutaneous T-cell lymphoma, which again must be referred to a dermatologist to confirm the diagnosis of early cutaneous T-cell lymphoma (a type of which is called mycosis fungoides), should then be taken care of by a dermatologist and/or an oncologist. Erythema multiforme, a condition that has been considered to be a characteristic type of hypersensitivity reaction to such factors as infectious agents and drugs, is characterized by the presence of so-called target lesions (which are lesions with concentric zones of varying color), and should be taken care of by a dermatologist. Vasculitis (which is inflammation of vasculature walls) characteristically has purpuric lesions, although purpuric lesions can also be seen in viral eruptions. Purpuric refers to purpura, which refers to cutaneous extravasated red blood cells that produce a reddish or purplish coloration of the skin which does not blanch when pressure is applied. Vasculitis should be taken care of by a dermatologist. Urticaria (see Chapter 21). Papular acrodermatitis of childhood (Gianotti-Crosti Syndrome), this is characterized by an eruption of small papules on the face and extremities in children 2 to 6 years of age, lasts about 3 weeks, and is associated with viral infections (e.g. hepatitis B virus, coxsackievirus, parainfluenza virus, Epstein-Barr virus, enterovirus, cytomegalovirus and adenovirus). While papular acrodermatitis of childhood is self-limited and classically non-pruritic, the associated viral infection can be taken care of by the patient's pediatrician. Cutaneous manifestations of HIV disease such as severe seborrheic dermatitis (discussed later in this chapter), eosinophilic folliculitis (which is clinically characterized by pink-to-red follicular papules and histologically characterized by follicular inflammation containing eosinophils predominantly), and pruritic papular eruption of HIV disease (which has been reported to appear to be the same entity as eosinophilic folliculitis) or so-called 'itchy red bump disease' (not all cases of which turn out to be eosinophilic folliculitis on biopsy) might be considered in the differential diagnosis. The diagnosis of cutaneous manifestations of HIV disease would be supported by a positive HIV test. Cutaneous manifestations of HIV disease should be treated by a dermatologist. Cutaneous graft-versus-host reaction, occurs most commonly in the setting of bone marrow transplantation and would be treated by the patient's transplant physicians. Rashes associated with the viral hepatitides might also be considered in the differential diagnosis; the diagnosis would be supported by abnormal liver function tests and positive viral hepatitis serology and managed in conjunction with a dermatologist. Numerous squamous cell carcinomas in situ, invasive squamous cell carcinomas and/or superficial basal cell carcinoma are described in Chapter 26. See Chapter 9 for discussion of extensive acne; Chapter 18 for extensive tinea and superficial cutaneous candidal infection, and Chapter 16 for scabies.

Primary treatment of non-specific dermatitis

Primary treatment of limited/localized non-specific dermatitis

When the area of involvement of non-specific dermatitis is relatively limited, the primary treatment of choice is the use of topical steroids (see Chapter 1). If the involvement is on a particularly hairy area such as the scalp, I would use a solution or lotion vehicle; otherwise, I would use a cream vehicle, but if the involvement is particularly dry and scaly, I might consider using an ointment vehicle rather than a cream vehicle. If the involvement is on the eyelids or periorbital regions, I would in general use the low-potency topical steroid hydrocortisone (e.g. Delcort®) 0.5% to the involvement 2–4 times daily as circumstances may require for inflammation in adults. If the involvement is on the face (excluding the eyelids and the periorbital regions), ears, area around the ears, genitals or skin folds, I would in general use the low-potency topical steroid hydrocortisone (e.g. Hytone®) 1% to the involvement 2–4 times daily as circumstances may require for inflammation in adults. If the involvement is on the scalp, neck, truck, arms, or legs, I would in general use a mid-potency topical steroid such as triamcinolone (e.g. Kenalog® or Aristocort®) 0.1% to the involvement 2–4 times daily as circumstances may require for inflammation in adults. If the involvement is on the hands or feet, I would in general use a high-potency topical steroid such as fluocinonide (e.g. Lidex®) to the involvement 2–4 times daily as circumstances may require for inflammation in adults.

I generally do not use topical steroids in pregnant or breast-feeding patients unless their use is approved by the patient's obstetrician or breast-fed baby's pediatrician, respectively.

For pediatric patients, I would be particularly cautious with regard to topical steroid use, and I would in general use the following low-potency topical steroids: hydrocortisone 0.5% for involvement on the face, ears, area around the ears, genitals and skin folds (bearing in mind that the nominally higher potency topical steroid hydrocortisone 1% may sometimes be needed) and hydrocortisone 1% for involvement on the scalp, neck, trunk, arms, legs, hands and feet (bearing in mind that the nominally higher potency topical steroid hydrocortisone 2.5% may sometimes be needed), as discussed in Chapter 1.

Patients with persistent non-specific dermatitis should be referred to a dermatologist for consultation.

Primary treatment of extensive/generalized non-specific dermatitis

If secondary syphilis, viral eruption, pityriasis rosea (which may be caused by an infectious agent, possibly a virus; see Chapter 6), bacterial folliculitis, tinea, superficial cutaneous candidal infection, erythema multiforme (which may be triggered by an infectious agent and for which the use of systemic steroids is otherwise controversial), papular acrodermatitis of childhood (which is associated with viral infections), cutaneous manifestations of HIV disease, rashes associated with the viral hepatitides, and psoriasis, including eruptive or guttate psoriasis (see Chapter 4), are not being considered or have been ruled out and if the non-specific dermatitis involvement is particularly extensive and bothersome to the patient, I would consider using a course of a systemic steroid, if not otherwise unadvisable. Psoriasis (as well as secondary syphilis, viral eruption, pityriasis rosea, bacterial folliculitis, tinea, superficial cutaneous candidal infection, papular acrodermatitis of childhood, cutaneous manifestations of HIV disease, rashes associated with the viral hepatitides, and, for all intents and purposes, erythema multiforme) should not be treated with systemic steroids (see Chapter 4). If a patient has hypertension, diabetes mellitus, peptic ulcer disease, osteoporosis, immunosuppression, tuberculosis, other infection, etc., I would consider not using a systemic steroid, or I would be very cautious and would take appropriate additional precautions when using it, depending on the situation. If the patient is pregnant or breast-feeding, I would not use a systemic steroid unless it is clearly needed and unless its use is approved by the patient's obstetrician or breast-fed baby's pediatrician, respectively.

If it is not otherwise unadvisable and if it is decided to put the patient on a course of a systemic steroid, I usually got good results with the following regimen for adults: prednisone 40 mg orally every morning for 1 week, then

20 mg orally every morning for 1 week, then 10 mg orally every morning for 1 week, and then finally 5 mg orally every morning for 1 week. Alternatively, the adult patient can be given an injection of triamcinolone 40 mg intramuscularly in the hip, and this will provide systemic steroid coverage for 1 month. However, I tend not to use this, because if for some reason the patient needs to be taken off the systemic steroid, this obviously cannot be done after the patient has been given the intramuscular injection of triamcinolone, the effects of which last for about 1 month, whereas if the patient is on a course of prednisone, the prednisone can be stopped, if required, because the prednisone is taken daily.

Shorter-acting systemic steroids can be injected intramuscularly, but I have not found them to be particularly useful in the situations in which I use systemic steroids. The use of systemic steroids in 'dose packs' (which contain steroid pills for oral use in pre-packaged tapering doses) can be considered, but I do not use these, because I do not find any particularly outstanding advantage to their use. For an otherwise healthy patient, while the patient is on the systemic steroid, I have the patient take Tums® as circumstances may require for stomach symptoms, and I have the patient notify me right away if he or she develops any stomach symptoms; I also have the patient take Citracal® with D (calcium with vitamin D).

I have very rarely needed to use systemic steroids in children or infants; if it was felt that such treatment was necessary, I consulted with the patient's pediatrician, and he or she and I, together, decided on the dosage and duration of treatment, with the dosage basically being the pediatric equivalent of the adult dosage described above, scaled down accordingly to correspond to the child's age and weight.

It is important to remember that excessive use of systemic corticosteroids in adult or pediatric patients can result in hypothalamic–pituitary–adrenal axis suppression as well as the clinical manifestations of Cushing's syndrome, as is the case with all forms of corticosteroid use.

If extensive/generalized non-specific dermatitis does not respond to treatment within two weeks, the patient needs to be seen by a dermatologist; the same applies if the condition is persistent.

Adjunctive treatment modalities that can be used in the treatment of non-specific dermatitis

Open wet compresses

Cool, plain water, open wet compresses can be soothing and are performed as follows: gauze is soaked in cool, plain water and then applied to the involvement for 20 min (the gauze is re-soaked every 10 min to prevent it from drying out) 2–4 times daily (before application of the topical steroid if a topical steroid is being used).

Tub soaks

If the dermatitis involvement is extensive and particularly uncomfortable (e.g. itchy), tub soaks using plain tepid water for about 15 min 1–2 times daily can be soothing. Alternatively, tub soaks using Plain Aveeno Bath Powder® or Aveeno-Oilated Bath Powder® mixed in tepid water can be used. (Plain Aveeno Bath Powder and Aveeno-Oilated Bath Powder are oatmeal-based powders that can be obtained, with instructions on how to use them, over the counter at virtually any pharmacy. Aveeno-Oilated Bath Powder is more moisturizing than is plain Aveeno Bath Powder, which is slightly more drying. Both powders, but especially the oilated powder, can make the bath tub more slippery, so appropriate precautions should be taken accordingly, especially with elderly patients.)

Bland emollients

If there is involvement that is particularly dry, frequent use of a bland emollient can be helpful and soothing. Bland emollients are basically mois-turizers such as Nutraderm Lotion®, Cetaphil Moisturizer Lotion® (which is to be distinguished from Cetaphil Cleanser Lotion®), Lubriderm Seriously Sensitive Lotion® (which, in my experience, has one of the lowest risks for producing an allergic or irritant reaction), Eucerin Lotion®, Cetaphil Cream®, Eucerin Cream®, or Aquaphor Ointment®. It should be noted that going from lotion to cream to ointment, in general, results in increasing moisturization but also results in increasing greasiness and sensation of occlusiveness.

Oral antihistamines

If itching is particularly bothersome, use of an oral H1-type antihista-mine may be beneficial. Sedating H1-type antihistamines are generally more effective in this regard than are non-sedating H1-type antihista-mines, in that the sedation that the former type of antihistamine can pro-duce can be used to take the edge off the itching and can aid in sleeping at night.

I usually first try the sedating H1-type antihistamine hydroxyzine (Atarax®) 10 mg one to three pills every 4–6 h as required for itching in adults. I have the patient start out at the lowest dose and frequency and have the patient adjust the dose and frequency according to response and adverse effects. I warn the patient regarding the medication's potential for sedation (excessive drowsiness can be transitory and may disappear in a few days of continued therapy or upon dosage reduction) and its potential for increasing the effects of alcohol. The prescriber should take into consideration that hydroxyzine potentiates the effect of other central nervous system depressants, and the patient should be warned about this. Because of hydroxyzine's potential for sedation, patients taking hydroxyzine should be warned regarding driving vehicles or operating dangerous machinery. Dosage for pediatric patients is as described in the package insert. Hydroxyzine is contraindicated in early pregnancy and should not be given to breast-feeding patients.

If the patient is not having a problem with excessive sedation, but the hydroxyzine is not producing a satisfactory beneficial effect in terms of the itching, I then switch to a trial of the sedating H1-type anthihistamine diphenhydramine (Benadryl®) 25 mg one to two pills every 4–6 h as may be required for itching in adults. I have the patient start out at the lowest dose and frequency and have the patient adjust the dose and frequency according to response and adverse effects. I warn the patient regarding diphenhydramine's potential for sedation and its additive effect with alcohol. The prescriber should take into consideration that diphenhydramine has an additive effect with other central nervous system depressants, and the patient should be warned about this. Because of diphenhydramine's potential for sedation, patients taking diphenhydramine should be warned regarding activities requiring mental alertness, such as driving vehicles, operating machinery, etc. When prescribing diphenhydramine, the prescriber should be aware that monoamine oxidase inhibitors prolong and intensify the anticholinergic effects of diphenhydramine. Dosage for pediatric patients is as described in the package insert (particularly in young pediatric patients, diphenhydramine, like other antihistamines, may cause excitation). In elderly patients (e.g. 60 years of age or older), diphenhydramine, like other antihistamines, is more likely to cause dizziness, sedation and hypotension. Diphenhydramine is contraindicated in neonates, premature infants and breast-feeding patients. It is not contraindicated in pregnant patients, in whom it should be used only if clearly needed. Diphenhydramine, like other antihistamines, should be used with particular caution in patients with narrow-angle glaucoma, stenosing peptic ulcer, pyloroduodenal obstruction, symptomatic prostatic hypertrophy or bladder-neck obstruction.

Diphenhydramine should also be used with caution in patients with asthma, increased intraocular pressure, hyperthyroidism, cardiovascular disease, hypertension, or lower respiratory disease.

I have not found cetirizine (Zyrtec®), which is a human metabolite of hydroxyzine, to be particularly superior to hydroxyzine.

If a patient is having a problem with antihistamine-associated sedation, I try switching the antihistamine to the non-sedating H1-type antihistamine loratadine (Claritin®) 10 mg once daily for patients 6 years of age and older. For children 2 to 5 years of age, the recommended dose is Claritin® Syrup 5 mg (one teaspoonful) once daily. In patients 6 years of age and older with liver failure or renal insufficiency (glomerular filtration rate less than 30 ml/min), the starting dose should be 10 mg every other day. In children 2 to 5 years of age with liver failure or renal insufficiency, the starting dose should be Claritin® Syrup 5 mg (one teaspoonful) every other day. Loratadine should be used during pregnancy only if clearly needed, and should not be administered to a breast-feeding patient.

I have not found the non-sedating H1-type antihistamine fexofenadine (Allegra®) to be superior to loratadine.

Secondary bacterial infection of non-specific dermatitis involvement

Evidence of secondary bacterial infection includes the presence of excessive oozing and/or crusting, swelling, tenderness, pain, increased erythema and/or purulence. 'Honey colored' crusting is suggestive of impetigo (see Chapter 17) and impetiginization (which is impetigo secondarily involving another cutaneous condition).

If there is concern that the non-specific dermatitis involvement might be secondarily infected, I obtain a bacterial culture and sensitivities (C&S) of the suspected involvement and empirically start the patient on a course of cephalexin (Keflex®), usually 250 mg to 500 mg every 6 h for 10 days for adults, if not otherwise unadvisable. If the patient is allergic to cephalosporins or penicillin (there is evidence of partial cross-allergenicity of the penicillins and the cephalosporins), I would instead use erythromycin, usually 250 mg to 500 mg every 6 h for 10 days for adults, if not otherwise unadvisable. For children or infants, I consult the package insert for its dosage recommendations, which are generally based on age and weight. I subsequently modify the treatment according to the patient's response to therapy and the results of the bacterial C&S (bearing in mind that bacterial C&S results can be falsely negative).

AUTOSENSITIZATION DERMATITIS

Overview

According to Donald V. Belsito in *Fitzpatrick's Dermatology in General Medicine,* 5th edn., 'Autosensitization dermatitis refers to a phenomenon in which an acute dermatitis develops at cutaneous sites distant from an inflammatory focus and where the secondary acute dermatitis is not explained by the inciting cause of the primary inflammation.' The secondary acute dermatitis can be considered to be autosensitization dermatitis.

Treatment of autosensitization dermatitis

The primary inflammation is treated accordingly. The treatment of the secondary dermatitis (i.e. the autosensitization dermatitis) would include the use of topical steroids; systemic steroids; bland emollients; cool, plain water open wet compresses; tub soaks; and/or oral antihistamines as discussed for non-specific dermatitis previously in this chapter. If there are blisters and/or oozing, a solution or lotion vehicle for the topical steroids would generally be the preferred vehicle, and plain Domeboro® solution open wet compresses can be used as an alternative to cool, pain water, open wet compresses. (Plain Domeboro solution is a brand of modified Burow's solution, which contains the active ingredient aluminum acetate.) Plain Domeboro solution open wet compresses provide a drying and cleansing effect, have a slight anti-microbial effect, and are performed as follows: gauze is soaked in plain Domeboro solution at a dilution of 1 : 40 and then applied to the involvement for 20 min (the gauze is re-soaked every 10 min to prevent it from drying out and to prevent an increase in the concentration of the Domeboro solution in the gauze compresses as a result of water evaporating from the Domeboro solution-soaked gauze compresses) 2–4 times daily (before application of the topical steroid if a topical steroid is being used). Plain Domeboro powder with directions on how to make a 1 : 40 diluted solution with water can be obtained over the counter at virtually any pharmacy.

CONTACT DERMATITIS

Overview

Contact dermatitis is due to an allergic reaction or a primary irritant reaction resulting from the contact of an antigenic substance or a primary irritant substance, respectively, with the skin, thereby resulting in allergic contact dermatitis or primary irritant contact dermatitis, respectively. Allergic contact dermatitis results from an allergic/hypersensitivity-type immune system reaction to an antigenic substance contacting the skin, whereas primary irritant contact dermatitis results from a chemically induced, primary destructive-type, non-allergic/non-hypersensitivity-type reaction to a primary irritant substance contacting the skin.

Allergic contact dermatitis will be considered here, as will irritant contact dermatitis due to mild irritants. However, severe contact dermatitis representing chemical burns due to potent irritants such as potent acids and alkalis is beyond the scope of this guide and will not be considered here.

Clinically, pruritic erythema; erythematous papules; erythematous, edematous plaques; vesicles; and/or bullae along with oozing and crusting are typically present in cases of acute allergic contact dermatitis. Pruritic, erythematous, scaling lichenification is typically present in cases of chronic allergic contact dermatitis, in which papulovesiculation may or may not be present. It is important to note that the scalp, palms and soles tend to be resistant to allergic contact dermatitis; there may be little involvement at these sites despite their exposure to the causative antigenic substance. Also, autosensitization may occur; involvement representing autosensitization dermatitis may develop at sites other than the primary site of contact dermatitis, even though there has been no known exposure of these other sites to the causative antigenic substance. (Autosensitization and autosensitization dermatitis are discussed previously in this chapter.)

As noted above, severe, acute, primary irritant contact dermatitis due to potent irritants is beyond the scope of this guide and is not discussed here. Chronic, repeated, primary irritant contact dermatitis due to relatively mild irritants is typically characterized by itchy, burning, erythematous, scaling patches, sometimes with tiny vesicles.

Evaluation and treatment of contact dermatitis in general

The most important aspect of the treatment of contact dermatitis is withdrawal of the offending substance causing the contact dermatitis. Additionally, treatment that is geared more specifically toward the patient's symptoms and signs is provided.

In my experience, the offending substance causing the contact dermatitis is in most cases readily apparent to the patient and his or her physician as a result of the patient's history and the pattern and distribution of the skin involvement. For the few cases in which the offending substance is not obvious and in which the problem persists, consultation with a dermatologist would be useful, because the dermatologist can arrange to do patch testing to try to determine the identity of the offending substance if the condition is allergic contact dermatitis. In addition, the dermatologist can provide assistance with regard to deducing the identity of the offending contactant.

Treatment geared more specifically toward the patient's symptoms and signs of contact dermatitis would include the use of topical steroids; systemic steroids; bland emollients; cool, plain water, open wet compresses; tub soaks; and/or oral antihistamines as discussed for non-specific dermatitis previously in this chapter. If there are blisters and/or oozing, a solution or lotion vehicle for the topical steroids would generally be the preferred vehicle, and plain Domeboro solution open wet compresses can be used as an alternative to cool, plain water open wet compresses. (Plain Domeboro solution is a brand of modified Burow's solution, which contains the active ingredient aluminum acetate.) Plain Domeboro solution open wet compresses provide a drying and cleansing effect, have a slight anti-microbial effect, and are performed as follows: gauze is soaked in plain Domeboro solution at a dilution of 1 : 40 and then applied to the involvement for 20 min (the gauze is re-soaked every 10 min to prevent it from drying out and to prevent an increase in the concentration of the Domeboro solution in the gauze compresses as a result of water evaporating from the Domeboro solution-soaked gauze compresses) 2–4 times daily (before application of the topical steroid if a topical steroid is being used). Plain Domeboro powder with directions on how to make a 1 : 40 diluted solution with water can be obtained over the counter at virtually any pharmacy.

Evaluation and treatment of contact dermatitis due to poison oak/poison ivy/poison sumac

The somewhat special situation regarding contact dermatitis due to poison oak/poison ivy/poison sumac should be discussed. Typically, after having been in a wild, wooded, or verdant environment, the patient presents with itchy erythema; erythematous papules; erythematous, edematous plaques; vesicles; and/or bullae. Oozing and crusting are also frequently present. The involvement is typically somewhat linear, presumably as a result of the offending foliage 'brushing' against the skin in a linear fashion, thereby resulting in this linear pattern of contact dermatitis.

When treating contact dermatitis due to poison oak/poison ivy/poison sumac, it should be taken into account that the cutaneous allergic reaction due to the cutaneous contact of the poison oak/poison ivy/poison sumac oleoresin at the sites of involvement can continue to occur for up to 4 weeks (presumably as a result of persistence of antigen binding in the skin).

If the involvement is not extensive, I generally treat the problem with an appropriate topical steroid as discussed for non-specific dermatitis previously in this chapter (for involvement in which there are blisters and/or oozing, a solution or lotion vehicle for the topical steroid is generally the preferred vehicle). If the involvement is severe, I generally treat the problem, if not otherwise unadvisable, with a 4-week course of a systemic corticosteroid as discussed for non-specific dermatitis previously in this chapter. When treating contact dermatitis due to poison oak/poison ivy/poison sumac with systemic steroids, the treatment should be continued for about 4 weeks, even if before then the involvement appears to have resolved due to the systemic steroid treatment. As indicated previously, the hypersensitivity reaction to the offending antigens can continue to occur for up to 4 weeks, presumably because of the persistence of antigen binding in the skin; if systemic steroid treatment is stopped before then, the reaction can relapse and flare.

If needed for itching, I will also use an oral antihistamine, and for additional soothing symptomatic relief, I might also use cool, plain water open wet compresses or tub soaks as discussed for non-specific dermatitis previously in this chapter. If blisters and oozing are significant, plain Domeboro solution open wet compresses, as an alternative to cool, plain water open wet compresses, can be used as discussed for the treatment of contact dermatitis in general previously in this chapter.

Also, since the oleoresin containing the offending antigens can stick to clothing, fur and inanimate objects such as fishing rods, golf clubs, baseball bats and tools and since this can result in the patient later coming into contact with the offending antigens again, thereby resulting in continuing relapse of the contact dermatitis, I have the patient carefully wash with water and soap or detergent all clothing that he or she was wearing and all inanimate objects that were with the patient when he or she initially came into contact with the offending foliage, and, likewise, I have the patient carefully bathe the fur of any pet that was with the patient at that time.

Evaluation and treatment of so-called 'hand dermatitis' or 'hand eczema'

Another special situation regarding contact dermatitis involves a relatively specific condition that has been called 'hand dermatitis' or 'hand eczema'.

(I have heard the terms 'dishwater hands' and 'housewives' hands' used to refer to this particular condition.) Hand dermatitis in this situation can be thought of as a type of primary irritant contact dermatitis due to irritation typically resulting from frequent exposure of the hands to water. It generally presents as typically itchy or burning erythema, scaling and dryness involving the dorsal aspects of the hands (which are more sensitive than are the palms). (Compare this clinical presentation to that of dyshidrotic dermatitis, which, when it involves the hands, typically presents as itchy recurrent vesicles, erythema and scaling involving the sides of the fingers and/or the palms, as discussed later in this chapter.)

Treatment of this specific type of hand dermatitis involves having patients avoid exposing their hands to water excessively and avoid washing their hands excessively. Patients should be told to wear white cotton gloves under plastic (i.e. vinyl) gloves whenever their hands are exposed to water for prolonged periods of time (e.g. when washing dishes, washing cars, etc.) and whenever they are doing activities that would otherwise require them to wash their hands afterward. White cotton gloves and plastic (i.e. vinyl) gloves can be obtained through pharmacies. The white cotton gloves are worn to absorb the excessive sweat that would otherwise accumulate as a result of the plastic gloves being worn. The presence of the excessive sweat that would otherwise accumulate would make it as though the patients' hands were immersed in water. More specific treatment involves the use of soothing bland emollients (i.e. moisturizers) frequently and topical steroids as described for non-specific dermatitis previously in this chapter.

Evaluation and treatment of so-called 'diaper dermatitis'

Mention should be made of so-called 'diaper dermatitis', which I consider to be a form of primary irritant contact dermatitis (due, for example, to urine and moisture) and which typically presents as erythema involving the diaper area. (For discussion of so-called 'diaper candidiasis', see Chapter 18).

Secondary fungal (typically candidal) and/or bacterial infection may or may not be present. Potassium hydroxide (KOH) preparation and fungal culture of skin scrapings from affected areas can be performed to test for the presence of fungi, and bacterial C&S of affected areas can be done to test for the presence of bacteria. (For discussion of KOH preps, fungal cultures and fungal infections, see Chapter 18.)

Since fungal testing can be falsely negative, the broad-spectrum, topical, over-the-counter, imidazole-type antifungal agent clotrimazole (Lotrimin-AF®) lotion or, if the patient is allergic to imidazole-type antifungal agents, the broad-spectrum, topical, prescription-requiring, ethanolamine-type antifungal agent ciclopirox olamine (Loprox®) lotion can be empirically used twice daily to the involvement in addition to hydrocortisone lotion 1% twice daily until clearing, in order to treat active disease. If bacterial C&S reveal pathogenic bacteria, a coarse of an appropriate oral antibiotic should also be prescribed.

To hasten the resolution of active disease and to prevent recurrence of the problem once it has resolved, the involved areas should be kept meticulously dry. This can be facilitated by changing diapers as soon as they become soiled, by avoiding the use of occlusive (e.g. plastic) coverings over the diapers, and by the use of an absorbent powder such as Zeasorb® powder. (When an absorbent powder such as Zeasorb powder is applied, it should always be applied to a clean, dry surface, because it otherwise builds up and becomes doughy and 'caked on'.)

Contact dermatitis due to nail polish

Another special situation regarding contact dermatitis deserves mentioning. Dermatitis involving the eyelids can be due to contact dermatitis due to nail polish (people inadvertently touch their eyelids frequently throughout the day), so this diagnosis should be considered in addition to contact dermatitis due to eye makeup and in addition to seborrheic dermatitis (which is discussed later in this chapter) in patients who present with eyelid dermatitis.

Secondary bacterial infection of contact dermatitis involvement

Possible secondary bacterial infection of contact dermatitis involvement in general can be approached as described for possible secondarily infected non-specific dermatitis previously in this chapter.

NUMMULAR DERMATITIS

Overview

Nummular dermatitis is a type of dermatitis that is typically characterized acutely by usually itchy, nummular (i.e. coin-shaped), erythematous lesions that are macular, patch-type, and/or plaque-type with tiny, associated vesicles, papules, oozing and crusting. Initially, there are tiny vesicles and erythematous papules that become confluent. Involvement is usually on the extremities and/or trunk. Chronically, scaling and lichenification rather than vesicles and oozing are present, and in some patients the involvement from the beginning is chronic-appearing with erythematous scaling patches. The number and size of lesions can vary, and sometimes central clearing within lesions occurs, resulting in an annular configuration resembling tinea corporis (see Chapter 18).

Special considerations regarding nummular dermatitis

If the clinical situation is appropriate, the 'great mimickers' secondary syphilis (see Chapter 27) and drug eruption (see Chapter 3) should be considered in the differential diagnosis of nummular dermatitis. In addition, pityriasis rosea (see Chapter 6) and psoriasis, including eruptive or guttate psoriasis (see Chapter 4) should also be considered in the differential diagnosis.

A negative VDRL or RPR test will rule out secondary syphilis. A CBC showing eosinophilia might be suggestive of a drug eruption. Severe, serious drug eruptions may show lymphocytosis with atypical lymphocytes and may have associated constitutional symptoms and/or signs along with other findings. Current evidence is that eosinophilia on CBC is an uncommon finding for common drug reactions and is a parameter that is of little value in diagnosing common drug reactions, but an eosinophil count greater than 1000/µl may be seen with severe, serious drug eruptions.

The untreated rash of secondary syphilis would resolve spontaneously (at which time the patient would be said to have latent syphilis). If the diagnosis of secondary syphilis is made, this obviously should be evaluated, treated and followed accordingly, and if the patient is pregnant, her obstetrician should be notified because of the potential effect of syphilis on the fetus.

Other conditions that may be considered in the differential diagnosis are: tinea, especially tinea corporis (see Chapter 18). Squamous cell carcinoma in-situ, invasive squamous cell carcinoma and superficial basal cell carcinoma (see Chapter 26). Mammary Paget's disease and extramammary Paget's disease (see Chapter 26). Urticaria (see Chapter 21). For brief discussion of parapsoriasis; early cutaneous T-cell lymphoma; erythema multiforme, and papulosquamous cutaneous manifestations of HIV disease see page 12: *Common differential diagnosis of non-specific dermatitis.*

Treatment of nummular dermatitis

The treatment of nummular dermatitis generally consists of the use of topical steroids as discussed for non-specific dermatitis previously in this chapter. Adjunctively, oral antihistamines can be used for itching, and bland emollients (i.e. moisturizers) and tub soaks can be used for their soothing effect, as discussed for non-specific dermatitis previously in this chapter.

If a patient is uncomfortable and suffering from extensive nummular dermatitis and if it is not otherwise unadvisable, a course of a systemic steroid can be considered, as discussed and described for non-specific dermatitis previously in this chapter. Nummular dermatitis can be a chronic condition, so one must be careful to avoid excessive use of systemic steroids, as discussed for atopic dermatitis later in this chapter.

If the nummular dermatitis problem persists or is not being controlled well, or if there is any doubt regarding the diagnosis, the patient should be referred to a dermatologist for consultation.

Secondary bacterial infection of nummular dermatitis involvement

Possible secondary bacterial infection of nummular dermatitis involvement can be approached as described for possible secondarily infected non-specific dermatitis previously in this chapter.

SEBORRHEIC DERMATITIS

Overview

Seborrheic dermatitis is characterized by generally asymptomatic but occasionally itchy erythematous flaking involving the so-called 'seborrheic areas', which typically include the nasolabial folds, the glabella, the alar grooves, the eyelids, the eyelids margins, the ears, the areas around the ears (particularly the retroauricular areas), the external ear canals and the scalp (where frequently flaking and no erythema may be present, in which case the involvement has been referred to as 'dandruff'). The nasolabial folds are the bilateral creases that extend between the sides of the nose and the sides of the mouth. The glabella is the area between the eyebrows. The alar grooves are the creases on both sides of the nose. The retroauricular areas are the areas behind the ears. Seborrheic dermatitis of the eyelid margins has been called 'seborrheic blepharitis'. Also, involvement can occur on the sternal region, the interscapular area, the genital region, the axillae, the inframammary regions, the umbilicus, the groins and the intergluteal cleft. The interscapular area is the area on the back between the shoulder blades. The inframammary regions are the areas below the breasts. The intergluteal cleft is the area between the buttocks. It should be noted that one or more of any of these areas may be involved.

Seborrheic dermatitis can occur in newborns, adolescents and adults. Seborrheic dermatitis in newborns is possibly connected to the influence of transiently elevated hormone levels present in newborns. I have not seen seborrheic dermatitis in pediatric patients other than newborns and adolescents.

It should be noted that it is not uncommon for seborrheic dermatitis and psoriasis (see Chapter 4) to be present simultaneously in the same patient, and the term sebopsoriasis has been used to describe involvement that has features suggestive of both seborrheic dermatitis and psoriasis. In my experience, this type of involvement usually occurs on the scalp and sometimes on the face, ears, area around the ears, genitals, or intertriginous (skin-fold) areas.

Seborrheic dermatitis is a common manifestation of HIV infection, and there seems to be an increased frequency of seborrheic dermatitis in patients with parkinsonism.

Treatment of seborrheic dermatitis

Standard treatment modalities for seborrheic dermatitis

Seborrheic dermatitis is perhaps the only type of dermatitis for which the primary treatment does not involve the use of topical steroids. It has been felt that seborrheic dermatitis might be an allergic reaction to non-pathogenic yeasts that are normally found on the skin in the seborrheic areas (see above).

The treatment of choice for areas of involvement other than the eyelid margins consists of the topical, broad-spectrum, imidazole-type antifungal agent Nizoral® (ketoconazole 2%) cream, which I have the patient apply to the involvement twice daily until clearing. For scalp involvement, the patient can use Nizoral (ketoconazole 2%) shampoo, with which the patient shampoos twice a week for 4 weeks (with at least 3 days between each shampooing) and then intermittently as needed to maintain control. Nizoral (ketoconazole 2%) cream and Nizoral (ketoconazole 2%) shampoo require prescriptions, but Nizoral AD (ketoconazole 1%) shampoo is available over the counter.

Although Nizoral cream is the only antifungal medication that is approved by the FDA for the treatment of seborrheic dermatitis [other than Loprox® (ciclopirox olamine) gel for seborrheic dermatitis of the scalp],

I have found that any topical, broad-spectrum antifungal medication is equally effective. Such medications include Lotrimin-AF® (clotrimazole) cream, lotion, or solution (which is available without a prescription and which I have the patient apply to the involvement twice daily until clearing) or Loprox (ciclopirox olamine) cream, lotion, or gel (which requires a prescription and which I have the patient apply twice daily to the involvement until clearing). Nizoral and Lotrimin-AF are imidazole-type antifungal agents, and Loprox is an ethanolamine-type antifungal agent, so if a patient is allergic to or cannot use Nizoral, Lotrimin-AF or other imidazole-type antifungal agents, he or she should be able to use Loprox.

For scalp involvement, other shampoos that contain tar (e.g. DHS Tar® shampoo or DHS Tar Gel® shampoo, both of which are available over the counter), zinc pyrithione (e.g. DHS Zinc® shampoo or Head and Shoulders® shampoo, both of which are available over the counter), or selenium sulfide [e.g. Selsun® (selenium sulfide 2.5%) shampoo/lotion, which requires a prescription, or Selsun Blue® (selenium sulfide 1%) shampoo/lotion, which is available over the counter] can be used in place of Nizoral shampoo, although I do not consider that they are as effective as Nizoral shampoo.

Seborrheic dermatitis of the eyelid margins (i.e. seborrheic blepharitis) is usually first treated by trying daily cleansing of the eyelid margins with water and Johnson & Johnson's No More Tears Baby Shampoo®.

In general, depending on what I am prescribing to treat seborrheic dermatitis, if the patient is pregnant, breast feeding, or a newborn, I have the patient or the patient's parent accordingly check with the patient's obstetrician, breast-fed baby's pediatrician, or pediatrician, accordingly, before using the medication.

Off-label use of itraconazole (Sproranox®) capsules for the treatment of seborrheic dermatitis

Mention should be made of the systemic triazole-type antifungal medication itraconazole (Sporanox) capsules with regard to the treatment of seborrheic dermatitis. (For additional discussion of itraconazole (Sporanox) capsules, see Chapter 18.) Although this medication is not FDA approved for the treatment of seborrheic dermatitis, some dermatologists have used Sporanox capsules 200 mg orally once daily with meals for 1 week for adults for treatment of this condition. (Meals enhance the absorption of Sporanox.)

Sporanox is contraindicated for the treatment of seborrheic dermatitis in patients with evidence (or history) of ventricular dysfunction such as congestive heart failure (CHF). Also, Sporanox should not be used for the treatment of seborrheic dermatitis in patients with risk factors for CHF. Sporanox therapy should be stopped immediately if signs or symptoms of CHF develop (all patients taking Sporanox should be instructed as to the signs and symptoms of CHF).

Sporanox is contraindicated for the treatment of seborrheic dermatitis in pregnant patients and in women contemplating pregnancy. Sporanox should not be given to women of child-bearing potential for the treatment of seborrheic dermatitis unless they are taking effective measures to prevent pregnancy and unless they begin Sporanox therapy on the second or third day following the onset of menses. Effective contraception should be continued throughout Sporanox therapy and for 2 months following the end of treatment.

The use of Sporanox with cisapride, oral midazolam, pimozide, quinidine, dofetilide and triazolam is contraindicated, as is use of Sporanox with HMG CoA reductase inhibitors metabolized by CYP3A4, such as lovastatin and simvastatin. Since Sporanox has the potential for drug interactions with many other drugs, it is especially important that the package insert for Sporanox be consulted for potential drug interactions before Sporanox is prescribed for a patient taking any other medication(s). Also, patients on Sporanox should be instructed to contact their health care provider before taking any medications concomitantly with Sporanox, so that potential drug interactions with Sporanox can be avoided.

Sporanox has been associated with rare cases of serious hepatotoxicity, including hepatic failure and death, and in some of these cases there were no pre-existing liver disease and no serious underlying medical condition. Some cases of serious hepatotoxicity occurred within the first week of treatment. Sporanox should not be initiated for the treatment of seborrheic dermatitis in patients who have elevated liver enzymes or active liver disease or who have had liver toxicity with other medications. Monitoring of liver function tests should be considered for all patients receiving Sporanox. I recommend obtaining liver function tests at baseline and then monthly while the patient is on Sporanox therapy. Also, Sporanox therapy should be stopped immediately and liver function testing should be performed if signs or symptoms suggestive of liver dysfunction develop (all patients taking Sporanox should be instructed to report any unusual fatigue, anorexia, nausea and/or vomiting, jaundice, dark urine or pale stools).

Sporanox therapy should not be used for the treatment of seborrheic dermatitis in breast-feeding patients.

The safety and efficacy of Sporanox have not been established in pediatric patients.

Secondary bacterial infection of seborrheic dermatitis involvement

Possible secondary bacterial infection of seborrheic dermatitis involvement can be approached as described for possible secondarily infected non-specific dermatitis previously in this chapter.

STASIS DERMATITIS

Overview

Stasis dermatitis results from venous insufficiency in the lower legs and presents as usually itchy erythematous flaking, frequently associated with brown discoloration and frequently associated with edema, involving one or both distal lower extremities. The brown discoloration is most commonly due to hemosiderin deposition in the skin, but can also be due to a component of post-inflammatory hyperpigmentation, in which there is increased melanin pigmentation of the skin. Post-inflammatory hyperpigmentation is discussed in Chapter 7. Melanin is a pigment that is normally found in the epidermis, which is the superficial cutaneous layer that is located immediately above the dermis.

Treatment of stasis dermatitis

Stasis dermatitis is generally treated with a topical steroid such as triamcinolone (e.g. Kenalog or Aristocort) cream 0.025% or 0.1% as described for non-specific dermatitis previously in this chapter, leg elevation (if there is no arterial insufficiency) and bland emollients such as Lubriderm Seriously Sensitive Lotion®, Eucerin Cream®, or Aquaphor Ointment®.

It should be noted that patients with stasis dermatitis tend to have an increased susceptibility to contact dermatitis at the sites of the stasis dermatitis, so one should be aware of this, and topical preparations that have an increased tendency to cause contact dermatitis (such as topical antibiotics containing neomycin and topical anti-itch preparations containing 'caine' derivatives) should be avoided.

Support hose extending from the foot to the top of the thigh can be used if the patient does not have arterial insufficiency. Because the use of support hose in patients who have active stasis dermatitis can be irritating and/or uncomfortable, I generally use support hose solely for the prevention of stasis dermatitis (i.e. I generally use support hose only in patients who have venous insufficiency but no active stasis dermatitis).

Secondary bacterial infection of stasis dermatitis involvement

Possible secondary bacterial infection can be approached as described for possible secondarily infected non-specific dermatitis previously in this chapter.

ATOPIC DERMATITIS

Overview

Atopic dermatitis is a component of atopy. Atopy is a condition in which there is a personal and/or family history of atopic dermatitis, asthma and/or hay fever. Atopic dermatitis generally presents in childhood and frequently improves or remits by adulthood. It has been thought of as a condition in which the patient has a decreased 'itch threshold' (it has been called 'the itch that rashes'), and it is known to be exacerbated by extremes in humidity (high and low humidity), extremes in temperature (high and low temperature), woolly, 'scratchy' fabrics and stress. It can be said that patients with atopic dermatitis have exquisitely sensitive skin that has an increased reactivity to stimuli.

Patients with atopic dermatitis not uncommonly have *Staphylococcus aureus* colonizing their skin and have anti-staphylococcal IgE. Also, *S. aureus* can cause the release of mediators from keratinocytes, thereby ultimately resulting in an inflammatory response. Keratinocytes are the cells that make up the bulk of the epidermis and produce the protein keratin. The epidermis is the superficial cutaneous layer that is located immediately above the dermis. Keratin is the substance of which hair, nails and the stratum corneum are composed. The stratum corneum is the dead, horny, most superficial layer of the epidermis. The above may possibly be factors contributing to the etiology and pathogenesis of atopic dermatitis.

Patients with atopic dermatitis have a tendency to have allergen sensitivities, but these sensitivities tend not to be related to the clinical cutaneous manifestations of atopic dermatitis.

Atopic dermatitis is generally characterized by itching and dryness of the skin, the scratching of which typically results in erythematous, flaky, lichenified patches, plaques and sometimes papules (black patients tend to have papular atopic dermatitis) along with excoriations. Involvement typically occurs on the antecubital fossae, popliteal fossae, hands, face, ears, neck and trunk. The antecubital fossae are the flexural areas on the anterior arms at the level of the elbows. The popliteal fossae are the areas behind the knees. Some or all of these areas may be involved at various times. For unclear reasons, it is unusual to see atopic dermatitis involving the diaper area, which tends to be spared in patients with atopic dermatitis (this is the so-called 'diaper sign' of atopic dermatitis), and this is useful in making the diagnosis of atopic dermatitis in unclear cases. Also, the areas over the scapulae (shoulder blades) are relatively spared in patients with atopic dermatitis (this is the so-called 'butterfly sign' of atopic dermatitis), presumably because it is difficult for patients to reach these areas for scratching.

Patients with atopic dermatitis can be highly susceptible to mollusca contagiosa (see Chapter 23) and herpes simplex (see Chapter 5) and can develop extensive involvement of mollusca contagiosa and of herpes simplex. Therefore, such conditions should be kept in mind when evaluating, treating and following patients with atopic dermatitis.

Atopic dermatitis can cause psychological and social disturbances and can interfere with social development. Also, psychological disturbances caused by atopic dermatitis can in turn exacerbate atopic dermatitis.

Treatment of atopic dermatitis

Traditional, conventional treatment of atopic dermatitis

Traditionally and conventionally, treatment of atopic dermatitis consists of the avoidance of the above-described exacerbating factors, frequent use of moisturizers, the use of oral antihistamines as described for non-specific dermatitis previously in this chapter, and the use of topical steroids as described for non-specific dermatitis previously in this chapter. In terms of moisturizers and topical steroids, a lotion, cream, or ointment can be used, whichever the patient prefers. Regarding moisturizers, I typically recommend Cetaphil Moisturizer Lotion®, Lubriderm Seriously sensitive Lotion, Cetaphil Moisturizer Cream®, Eucerin Cream or Aquaphor Ointment. Sedating antihistamines are generally more effective than are non-sedating antihistamines; the sedation that the former can produce can be used to take the edge off of the itching and can aid in sleeping at night.

Some dermatologists feel that avoidance of soap and water contact is beneficial for patients with atopic dermatitis, and I have found that such avoidance is in fact beneficial for many of my patients with atopic dermatitis.

When I have a patient avoid soap and water contact, bathing is done using only Aquanil® cleanser or Cetaphil cleanser without soap or water. The cleanser is wiped on with a soft, white, cotton cloth and then wiped off with a fresh soft, white, cotton cloth without use of soap or water. So-called 'dirty' areas, such as the axillae (arm pits), groins and anogenital region, can be bathed using water and a gentle cleanser such as white, unscented Dove Bar®.

Other dermatologists feel that daily bathing with a mild soap and water (done properly) is not harmful and can be helpful in that it removes dead skin, removes skin bacteria and, for infants, provides good bonding with the parent doing the bathing. One should limit the time of the bathing and minimize the use of soap, which should be gentle (I generally recommend white, unscented Dove Bar) and which should be used only at the end of the bathing. Following bathing, a thick moisturizer, such as Aquaphor Ointment (white petrolatum in a water-miscible base), should be applied within minutes after completion of the bathing, when the skin is still hydrated from the bathing.

It is interesting to note that sometimes when a patient's atopic dermatitis involvement does not seem to be improving as expected with the above-described treatment modalities, a 10-day course of an oral antibiotic such as cephalexin (Keflex) or erythromycin seems to result in some improvement of the patient's atopic dermatitis even when no overt infection is noted. An explanation for this phenomenon may be that, in these patients for whom this phenomenon is observed, bacterial colonization of the skin may be in some way causing an inflammatory reaction (e.g. as discussed previously regarding *S. aureus* in the Overview section for atopic dermatitis), and suppression of these bacteria by the systemic antibiotic may be the cause of the observed improvement. Another explanation is that it has been noted that some oral antibiotics provide a non-specific anti-inflammatory effect unrelated to their antimicrobial properties.

When patients are uncomfortable and suffering from extensive atopic dermatitis involvement that is not responding adequately to the above-described treatment modalities, a period of relief can be provided, if not otherwise unadvisable, by a 4-week course of a systemic corticosteroid as described for non-specific dermatitis previously in this chapter. However, since atopic dermatitis is a chronic condition, one has to be careful to avoid excessive use of systemic corticosteroids, as is the case with all forms of corticosteroids, because of their potentially serious adverse effects (which include hypothalamic–pituitary–adrenal axis suppression as well as the clinical manifestations of Cushing's syndrome), the risk of which is obviously increased with increased use of the systemic steroids. For this reason I do not use courses of systemic steroids in these patients more often than about every 6 months, and I 'save' the use of a course of a systemic steroid for use as a 'last resort' when a patient is not responding to the other treatment modalities and is suffering and uncomfortable. I discuss the above-described reasons for this approach at length with the patient, who otherwise frequently does not understand why we cannot use the systemic steroids more extensively.

As noted above, patients with atopic dermatitis have a tendency to have allergen sensitivities, but these sensitivities tend not to be related to the clinical cutaneous manifestations of atopic dermatitis. Therefore, dietary manipulation on the whole is not helpful and not called for. In addition, for most children with atopic dermatitis, changing formulas is not beneficial and not necessary. Although food avoidance diets in pediatric patients with atopic dermatitis may sometimes help in otherwise unresponsive patients, such diets should be used only under the direction of an allergist and nutritionist. In general, most dermatologists refer atopic dermatitis patients to an allergist regarding allergen sensitivities only in selected cases in which the patient does not respond to standard atopic dermatitis treatment; in which the patient has a strong history of his or her atopic dermatitis reacting to allergens; or in which the patient has other, antigen-mediated diseases.

Atopic dermatitis patients and families should be referred for appropriate counseling when psychological and/or social disturbances are present.

Use of a non-steroidal topical immunomodulator substitute
for topical steroids in the treatment of atopic dermatitis

Non-steroidal topical immunomodulator (TIM) substitutes for topical steroids are discussed in general in Chapter 1.

One such agent, tacrolimus ointment, has been approved by the FDA for the treatment of atopic dermatitis in appropriate patients and is marketed under the brand name Protopic Ointment®. Systemic tacrolimus is approved for the prophylaxis of rejection of a transplanted allogeneic kidney or liver. Tacrolimus ointment is the first non-steroidal TIM substitute for topical steroids to be released in the USA. Tacrolimus ointment has been shown to be safe and effective for the treatment of atopic dermatitis in adults and children as young as 2 years of age and has so far not been shown to exhibit tachyphylaxis (see Chapter 1 for a discussion of tachyphylaxis).

Tacrolimus (Protopic) ointment, 0.03% and 0.1% for adults and only 0.03% for children aged 2–15 years, is indicated for short-term and intermittent long-term treatment of moderate to severe atopic dermatitis in patients for whom alternative, conventional therapies are unadvisable because of potential risks and in patients who are inadequately responsive to or are intolerant of alternative, conventional therapies.

Clinical infections at sites to be treated with tacrolimus ointment should be cleared before treatment with tacrolimus ointment is begun. Since treatment with tacrolimus ointment may be associated with an increased risk of varicella-zoster virus and herpes simplex virus infections, the risks and benefits of using tacrolimus ointment in the presence of these infections should be taken into consideration. Patients using tacrolimus ointment should minimize or avoid natural and artificial sunlight exposure, because an animal photocarcinogenicity study showed an enhancement of ultraviolet carcinogenicity with tacrolimus ointment. Application of tacrolimus ointment may cause a localized burning sensation or pruritus, which is most common during the first few days of treatment and typically subsequently improves as the atopic dermatitis lesions heal. Because of the potential for increased systemic absorption of tacrolimus, the use of tacrolimus ointment is not recommended for patients with Netherton's syndrome. The safety of Protopic Ointment in patients with generalized erythroderma has not been established. Tacrolimus ointment should not be used in breastfeeding patients and should be used in pregnant patients only if the potential benefit to the mother justifies a potential risk to the fetus.

Since transplant patients on immunosuppressive therapy (e.g. systemic tacrolimus) have an increased risk for developing lymphoma, patients who receive Protopic Ointment therapy and who develop lymphadenopathy should be investigated regarding the etiology of the lymphadenopathy. If there is no clear etiology for the lymphadenopathy or if acute infectious mononucleosis is present, discontinuation of the Protopic Ointment should be considered. In addition, patients who develop lymphadenopathy should be followed to be sure that the lymphadenopathy resolves.

Tacrolimus ointment is applied to the affected areas twice daily until 1 week after clearing of the symptoms and signs of atopic dermatitis. Tacrolimus ointment should not be used under occlusive dressings.

Secondary bacterial infection of atopic dermatitis involvement

Sometimes the atopic dermatitis involvement can be secondarily infected with bacteria. Secondary bacterial infection can manifest itself as increased erythema, swelling, oozing, crusting, purulence, pain and/or tenderness. 'Honey colored' crusting is suggestive of impetigo (see Chapter 17) and impetiginization (with is impetigo secondarily involving another cutaneous condition).

If secondary bacterial infection is suspected, I obtain a bacterial C&S of the affected areas; place the patient on a 10-day coarse of an appropriate oral antibiotic, such as cephalexin (Keflex) if not otherwise unadvisable (if the patient cannot take cephalexin, I generally use erythromycin instead, if not otherwise unadvisable); and modify the antibiotic according to patient response and the results of the bacterial C&S, as described for possible secondarily infected non-specific dermatitis previously in this chapter.

DYSHIDROTIC DERMATITIS

Overview

Dyshidrotic dermatitis is characterized by sometimes itchy recurrent vesicles, scaling and erythema typically involving the sides of the fingers, palms, sides of the toes and/or the soles. The vesicles contain serum, which is a clear and colorless or yellow fluid. This is in comparison to pustules, which contain pus, which is a cloudy and yellow or whitish fluid. Vesicles are typically seen in dyshidrotic dermatitis whereas pustules are seen in pustular psoriasis (see Chapter 4), which can sometimes be limited to the palms and/or soles.

Special considerations regarding dyshidrotic dermatitis

The clinical presentation of dyshidrotic dermatitis is similar to that of inflammatory tinea, which should be ruled out by KOH preparation and/or fungal culture of scrapings of scaling and/or vesicle roofs. (Tinea, KOH preparations and fungal cultures are discussed further in Chapter 18). If the result of the testing indicates tinea, the patient is treated accordingly for tinea, as described in Chapter 18. If the testing is negative for tinea, the patient is treated for dyshidrotic dermatitis, as described below.

It should be noted that when testing for tinea, particularly inflammatory tinea, one can obtain false-negative KOH preparation and fungal culture test results. If false-negative fungal test results are suspected, the patient can be treated with the topical steroid that is described below for the treatment of dyshidrotic dermatitis, in which case the fungal testing should be repeated a week or two later, at which time the use of the topical steroid in the interval will make the fungal testing more likely to show the presence of tinea, if tinea is indeed present, and therefore less likely to result in false-negative test results for tinea. It should be noted that, if tinea is still strongly suspected despite negative test results for tinea, I treat the patient for tinea empirically.

The differential diagnosis of dyhsidrotic dermatitis also includes a dermatophytid (or 'id') reaction, in which the patient has tinea (usually inflammatory tinea) on, for example, the feet and a sterile inflammatory reaction similar to dyshidrotic dermatitis on, for example, the hands. A dermatophytid reaction can be thought of as a localized hypersensitivity reaction to the presence of tinea elsewhere or as a manifestion of autosensitization resulting in autosensitization dermatitis. Autosensitization and autosensitization dermatitis are discussed previously in this chapter. In the above example of a dermatophytid reaction, KOH preparation and/or fungal culture of scrapings of involvement on the feet should show tinea, and KOH preparation and/or fungal culture of scrapings of involvement on the hands should be negative. In this case, the treatment of the tinea on the feet would be the same as that described for tinea in Chapter 18, and the treatment of the dermatophytid reaction on the hands would be the same as that described below for dyshidrotic dermatitis.

Treatment of dyshidrotic dermatitis

Since some patients with dyshidrotic dermatitis report that their involvement is exacerbated by exposure to water, patients with dyshidrotic dermatitis should avoid excessive water exposure. In the case of dyshidrotic dermatitis involving the hands, patients should be advised to avoid excessive hand washing and should be told to wear white cotton gloves under plastic (i.e. vinyl) gloves whenever their hands are exposed to water for prolonged periods of time (e.g. when washing dishes, washing cars, etc.) and whenever they are doing activities that would otherwise require them to wash their hands afterwards. White cotton gloves and plastic (i.e. vinyl) gloves can be obtained through pharmacies. The white cotton gloves are worn to absorb the excessive sweat that would otherwise accumulate as a result of the plastic gloves being worn. The presence of the excessive sweat that would otherwise accumulate would make it as though the patient's hands were immersed in water.

More specific treatment of dyshidrotic dermatitis involves the use of topical steroids as described for non-specific dermatitis previously in this chapter (for involvement in which there are blisters and/or oozing, a solution or lotion vehicle for the topical steroids is generally the preferred vehicle).

If a patient is suffering from severe disabling dyshidrotic dermatitis and if it is not otherwise unadvisable, one can consider using a course of a systemic steroid as described for non-specific dermatitis previously in this chapter. Dyshidrotic dermatitis can be a chronic condition, so one must be careful to avoid excessive use of systemic steroids, as discussed for atopic dermatitis previously in this chapter.

Secondary bacterial infection of dyshidrotic dermatitis involvement

Possible secondary bacterial infection of dyshidrotic dermatitis can be approached as described for possible secondarily infected non-specific dermatitis previously in this chapter.

Dyshidrotic dermatitis that is persistent or poorly controlled or for which the diagnosis is in doubt

If the dyshidrotic dermatitis problem persists or is not being controlled well, or if the diagnosis remains in doubt, the patient should be referred to a dermatologist for consultation.

LICHEN SIMPLEX CHRONICUS/PRURIGO NODULARIS

Overview

As noted at the beginning of this chapter, I feel that lichen simplex chronicus (LSC)/prurigo nodularis (which some dermatologists have called neurodermatitis) can be considered to be a condition related to dermatitis. This condition is characterized by skin thickening, with increased prominence of skin lines, due to frequent scratching, rubbing and/or picking to the point of the development of plaques (generally due to frequent scratching and/or rubbing and generally called LSC) and sometimes to the point of the development of papules or nodules (generally due to frequent picking and generally called prurigo nodularis). It should be noted that, underlying the LSC/prurigo nodularis, there can sometimes be another, separate skin condition that causes the patient to scratch, rub and/or pick, thereby resulting in the development of LSC/prurigo nodularis 'overlying' the primary skin condition.

It has been said that the pathogenesis of LSC/prurigo nodularis can be characterized by a 'vicious cycle' in which scratching, rubbing and/or picking of the skin results in skin thickening, which results in increased skin itching, which results in continued scratching, rubbing and/or picking, which results in continued skin thickening, which continues the above-described cycle.

Treatment of lichen simplex chronicus/prurigo nodularis

The treatment of LSC/prurigo nodularis is geared toward breaking the above-described itch–scratch cycle. This is done by discussing this cycle with the patient (thereby providing the patient with insight regarding his or her problem); using topical steroids as described for non-specific dermatitis previously in this chapter; and, for additional control of itching, using oral antihistamines as described for non-specific dermatitis previously in this chapter.

A topical steroid preparation that is particularly useful for this condition is Cordran® (flurandrenolide) tape. This medication consists of tape permeated with the topical steroid flurandrenolide (Cordran). Cordran tape is an effective, very potent topical steroid that has been classified as a superpotent, class I topical steroid (see Chapter 1) and is administered by applying the medicated tape to the LSC/prurigo nodularis lesions as described in the medication's package insert. This medication is particularly effective for LSC/prurigo nodularis lesions, not only because it is very potent but also because the lesions are covered by tape, and the fact that the lesions are covered by tape reminds the patient not to scratch and discourages the patient from scratching. Because Cordran tape is so potent, topical steroid-induced adverse effects, which are discussed in Chapter 1, are more likely to occur when this medication is used. I generally do not recommend using Cordran tape on the face, ears, area around the ears, genitals, or skin folds, which, as discussed in Chapter 1, are areas that are highly susceptible to the adverse as well as the beneficial effects of topical steroids. Likewise, I would use Cordran tape in pediatric patients with great caution, if at all, because pediatric patients can be considered to be especially susceptible to its adverse effects, as discussed in Chapter 1. Because of its very high potency, I would not use Cordran tape in a pregnant or breast-feeding patient unless its use is approved by the patient's obstetrician or breast-fed baby's pediatrician, respectively.

Intralesional steroid injections for the treatment of papules and nodules of prurigo nodularis

For recalcitrant papules or nodules of prurigo nodularis, intralesional steroid injections (billed as 'intralesional injections') can be considered. It should be noted that this treatment modality is particularly potent and effective, but it also carries with it particular risk of steroid-induced adverse effects (steroid-induced adverse effects are discussed in Chapter 1), especially steroid atrophy at the site of treatment (i.e. at the site of injection).

For this treatment modality, I generally use an injectable Kenalog (triamcinolone) suspension at a concentration of 2.5 mg/ml in a 3-ml syringe with a 30-gauge needle. I first take a bottle of injectable Kenalog 10 mg/ml suspension and shake it up well (since the Kenalog is in suspension, it needs to be shaken up well in order to be dispersed in the suspension adequately), and then, using a 3-ml syringe with a larger (e.g. 21-gauge) needle, I carefully draw up 0.25 ml of the Kenalog suspension into the 3-ml syringe. I then replace the 21-gauge needle on the 3-ml syringe with another 21-gauge needle. Without moving the syringe plunger, I then carefully insert the needle into a bottle of injectable 1% plain lidocaine solution or a bottle of injectable saline solution for medication dilution. (Injectable plain lidocaine solution causes a 'burning' sensation on injection, but provides an anesthetic effect after the injection, whereas injectable saline solution causes no such burning on injection, but provides no anesthetic effect after injection.) Without inadvertently injecting the Kenalog suspension that is in the syringe into the bottle of plain lidocaine or saline, I then carefully draw up 0.75 ml of the plain lidocaine or saline, and this produces 1 ml of a 2.5-mg/ml suspension of Kenalog in the 3-ml syringe. I then replace the 21-gauge needle that is on the syringe with a 30-gauge needle. I thoroughly mix the Kenalog suspension and plain lidocaine or saline solution in the syringe by drawing back the syringe plunger (thereby producing an air space in the syringe) and then vigorously and repeatedly turning the syringe upside down and right side up so that the Kenalog suspension and the plain lidocaine or saline solution in the syringe are thoroughly mixed in the air space that has been created in the syringe. I then remove this air space in the syringe by pushing the syringe plunger back in. (Different amounts of this suspension can be made by making appropriate adjustments in the amounts of Kenalog suspension and plain lidocaine or saline solution used.)

The lesion to be injected is cleaned with an alcohol swab and then dried with sterile gauze. I then inject the 2.5-mg/ml suspension of Kenalog into the dermis of the papule or nodule of prurigo nodularis being treated, ideally until the lesional area being injected blanches from the pressure of the intralesional intradermal injecting, but be aware that such blanching does not always occur, especially when the medication is being injected slowly. (Injecting slowly is less painful for the patient than is injecting more rapidly.) In order to prevent accidental intravascular injection of medication, aspiration (pulling back on the syringe's plunger) should be done immediately prior to the injection of the medication. This treatment can be carried out every 4–6 weeks until the lesion resolves. I do not use more than a total of 20 mg of intralesionally injected Kenalog every 4–6 weeks in adults. (I virtually never need to approach this limit even closely when intralesionally injecting papules and nodules of prurigo nodularis.) Excessive use of intralesionally injected corticosteroids can result in the clinical manifestations of Cushing's sydrome and hypothalamic–pituitary–adrenal axis suppression, as is the case with all forms of corticosteroid use.

I generally do not use intralesionally injected Kenalog, particularly large amounts, in pregnant or breast-feeding patients unless its use is approved by the patient's obstetrician or breast-fed baby's pediatrician, respectively. Likewise, I would use intralesionally injected Kenalog in pediatric patients with particular caution, if at all (pediatric patients can be considered to be especially susceptible to its adverse effects); in any case, pediatric patients are generally not compliant enough to undergo this treatment.

Secondary bacterial infection of lichen simplex chronicus/prurigo nodularis

Possible secondary bacterial infection of LSC/prurigo nodularis involvement can be approached as described for possible secondarily infected non-specific dermatitis previously in this chapter.

3

Drug eruptions

OVERVIEW

Drug eruptions are cutaneous adverse effects resulting from reactions to systemically administered medications. Although such reactions are stereotypically allergic in nature, this is not always the case. In fact, cutaneous drug reactions resulting from immunologic mechanisms are less common than those from non-immunologic mechanisms.

It is important to emphasize that drug eruption is one of the 'great mimickers' in that it can resemble virtually any kind of skin condition. The other 'great mimicker' is secondary syphilis – see Chapter 27 – which is ruled out by a negative rapid pasma reagin (RPR) or Venereal Disease Research Laboratories (VDRL) test.

EVALUATION OF DRUG ERUPTIONS

When confronted with a possible drug eruption, it is important to assess its potential seriousness. According to Robert Stern and Bruce Wintroub in *Fitzpatrick's Dermatology in General Medicine*, 5th edn., features of serious drug eruptions include the cutaneous clinical findings of confluent erythema, facial edema or central facial involvement, skin pain, palpable purpura, skin necrosis, blisters or epidermal detachment, positive Nikolsky's sign, mucous membrane erosions, urticaria (see Chapter 21) and tongue swelling; the general clinical findings of high fever (temperature higher than 40°C), enlarged lymph nodes, arthralgias or arthritis, shortness of breath, wheezing and hypotension; and the laboratory findings of eosinophil count greater than 1000/µl, lymphocytosis with atypical lymphocytes, and abnormal liver function tests. Purpura is cutaneous extravasated red blood cells (red blood cells outside blood vessels) that produce a reddish or purplish coloration of the skin. Areas of purpura do not blanch (i.e. the reddish or purplish coloration does not disappear) when pressure is applied to areas of purpura. The epidermis is the superficial cutaneous layer that is located immediately above the dermis. Nikolsky's sign is the easy ability to separate

Table 1   Clinical and laboratory findings associated with serious cutaneous drug eruptions

---

Clinical findings

Cutaneous

    Confluent erythema[1]

    Facial edema or central facial involvement

    Skin pain

    Palpable purpura[2]

    Skin necrosis

    Blisters or epidermal detachment[3]

    Positive Nikolsky's sign[4]

    Mucous membrane erosions

    Urticaria

    Swelling of tongue

General

    High fever (temperature 40 °C)

    Enlarged lymph nodes

    Arthralgias or arthritis

    Shortness of breath, wheezing, hypotension

Laboratory findings

Eosinophil count > 1000/microliter

Lymphocytosis with atypical lymphocytes

Abnormal results on liver function tests

1, Erythema is blanchable redness; 2, purpura is cutaneous extravasated red blood cells that produce a reddish or purplish coloration of the skin. Areas of purpura do not blanch when pressure is applied; 3, The epidermis is the superficial cutaneous layer that is located immediately above the derms; 4, The outer layer of the epidermis separates readily from the basal layer with lateral pressure. Table reproduced with permission from Freedberg I. *Fitzpatrick's Dermatology in General Medicine*, fifth edition. New York: The McGraw-Hill Co., 1999

the superficial portion of the epidermis from the lower portion by application of lateral pressure on the skin (See Table 1).

In determining whether or not an eruption is a drug eruption, and when attempting to identify the medication causing a drug eruption, it is important to consider the following: in most cases, cutaneous drug reactions occur within 1–2 weeks after initiation of therapy with the offending medication, but in some cases, particularly those manifested by the hypersensitivity syndrome (manifested by a rash that is associated with fever, lymphadenopathy and internal organ involvement), the onset may occur perhaps as long as 2 months after initiation of therapy with the offending medication. Particularly in the case of some more serious reactions, the onset is not likely to occur more than 2 months after initiation of therapy with the offending medication. However, I am aware of cases in which a drug eruption purportedly occurred after the patient had been on the

Table 2 Skin reactions to selected drugs received by at least 500 patients

Drug	Reaction rate per 1000 recipients
Amoxicillin	51
Trimethoprim-sulfamethoxazole	47
Ampicillin	42
Semisynthetic penicillins	29
Blood, whole human	28
Penicillin G	16
Cephalosporins	13
Quinidine	12
Gentamicin sulfate	10
Packed red blood cells	8.1
Mercurial diuretics	9.5
Dipyrone	8.0
Heparin	7.7
Trimethobenzamide hydrochloride	6.6
Nitrazepam	4.0
Barbiturates	4.0
Chlordiazepoxide	4.0
Diazepam	4.0
Propoxyphene	3.4
Isoniazid	3.0
Guaifenesin	2.9
Chlorothiazide	2.8
Furosemide	2.6
Isophane insulin suspension	1.3
Phenytoin	1.1
Phytonadione	0.9
Flurazepam hydrochloride	0.5
Chloral hydrate	0.2

Data are adapted from Arndt and Jick, and Bigby *et al*. If reactions are noted in both studies, the average rate is reported here. Table reproduced with permission from Freedberg I. *Fitzpatrick's Dermatology in General Medicine*, fifth edition. New York: The McGraw-Hill Co., 1999

offending medication for a longer period of time. I also know of cases in which a drug eruption purportedly occurred in a patient who had taken the offending medication on prior occasions without a problem.

A complete blood count (CBC) showing eosinophilia might be suggestive of a drug eruption. Current evidence is that eosinophilia on CBC is an uncommon finding for common drug reactions and is a parameter that is of little value in diagnosing common drug reactions, but an eosinophil count greater than 1000/μl may be seen with severe, serious drug eruptions.

Also, knowing the empirical statistical frequency with which various medications produce cutaneous reactions (i.e. knowing the likelihood of

Table 3 Selected drugs received by more than 500 patients with no skin reactions[1]

Digoxin	Prednisone/prednisolone
Meperidine hydrochloride	Codeine
Acetaminophen	Fetracycline
Diphenhydramine	Morphine
hydrochloride	Regular insulin
Aspirin	Warfarin
Ammophylline	Folic acid
Prochlorperazine	Methyldopa
Ferrous sulfate	Chlorpromazine

1, Rash rates must be 3 per 1000 or less. Data are adapted from Arndt and Jick, and Bigby *et al*. Table reproduced with permission from Freedberg I. *Fitzpatrick's Dermatology in General Medicine*, fifth edition. New York: The McGraw-Hill Co., 1999

various drugs to produce a drug eruption), and knowing the typical morphology that is characteristic of the eruptions that various medications tend to produce, can be useful in determining the identity of the medication (among the medications that a given patient is taking) that is causing a given patient's eruption (see Tables 2–4).

FIXED DRUG ERUPTIONS

A fixed drug eruption is typically characterized by a single or a few round, sharply demarcated, erythematous, edematous plaque(s) that may be surmounted by central blisters. The lesions of fixed drug eruptions can be burning or pruritic and typically involve the face, genitalia, or acral areas (i.e. peripheral areas such as the hands or distal arms). The inflammation resolves, with gray or brown pigmentation – which may be persistent – remaining at the sites. The lesions usually develop within 1–2 weeks after the initial exposure to the offending medication. Usually within a few days after re-exposure to the offending medication, the active inflammation re-develops at the same sites, although sometimes lesions can develop at additional sites.

Medications that have been classically associated with fixed drug eruptions include sulfonamides, barbiturates, salicylates, non-steroidal anti-inflammatory drugs, tetracyclines and phenolphthalein.

TREATMENT OF DRUG ERUPTIONS

The treatment of a drug eruption involves withdrawal of the offending medication, and an antigenically unrelated medication should be used in its place. Treatment can also include topical corticosteroids (if there are blisters

Table 4   Selected drugs associated with cutaneous eruption morphologies

Acneiform[1]
  Hormones (ACTH,
    glucocorticoids, oral
    contraceptives, androgens)
  Halogens
  Dilantin
  Isoniazid
  Amoxapin
  Trazodone
  Lithium
  Haloperidol

Alopecia[2]
  Chemotherapeutic agents
  Anticoagulants
  Hormones (oral
    contraceptives, androgens)
  Dilantin
  Retinoids[3]
  NSAIDs
  Tofranil
  Valproate-sodium
  Bromocriptine
  Piroxicam

Erythema multiforme[4]
  Penicillin
  Barbiturates
  Dilantin
  Sulfonamides
  Phenothiazines
  Griseofulvin
  Phenolphthalein
  Nitrogen mustard
  NSAIDs
  Codeine
  Tetracycline
  Minocycline
  Bactrim
  Glutethimide
  Cimetidine
  Methotrexate
  Prazosin
  Estinyl estradiol

Keroconazole
Sulfasalazine
Cefaclor
Allopurinol
Methazualone
Furosemide
Aminopenicillins
Streptomycin

Erythema nodosum[5]
  Oral contraceptives
  Sulfonamides
  Halogens
  Tetracycline
  Penicillin
  13-*cis*-Retinoic acid

Fixed drug eruptions[6]
  Oral contraceptives
  Barbiturates
  Phenolphthalein
  Phenacetin
  Salicylates
  Doriden
  Sulindac
  Naproxen
  Tolmetin
  Nystatin
  Quaalude
  Fiorinal
  Butazolidin-alka
  Tetracycline
  Minocycline
  Sulfonamides
  Maolate
  Metronidazole

Lichenoid[7]
  Gold
  Antimalarials
  Thiazides
  Levamisol
  Moban
  Tetracycline

Phenothiazines
Furosemide
Chlorpropamide
Nortlex
Diflunisal
Penicillamine
Propranolol
Captopril

Pholosensitivity[8]
  Griseofulvin
  Phenothiazines
  Thiazides
  Sulfonamides
  NSAIDs (benoxaprofen,
    piroxicam)
  Tetracyclines (including
    minocycline and
    doxycycline)
  DTIC
  Amiodarone
  Chloroquine
  Methotrexate
  Sulfonylureas
  Fluorouracil
  Vinblastine

Toxic epidermal necrolysis[4]
  Dilantin
  NSAIDs
  Allopurinol
  Sulfonamides
  Bactrim
  Minipress
  Thiabendazole
  Penicillin
  Mithramycin
  Fansidar
  Sulfasalazine
  L-Asparaginase
  Streptomycin
  Nitrofurantoin
  Amoxapin

Continued over

Vasculitis[10]	Quinidine	Mellaril
Allopurinol	Tetracycline	Dipyridamole
Thiazides	Penicillin	Chemotherapeutic
Gold	Cimetidine	agents
Sulfonamides		Amoxapin
Levamisole	*Vesiculobullous*[11]	Nalidixic acid
Hydralazine	NSAIDs	Penicillamine
NSAIDs	Griseofulvin	Captopril
Propylthiouracil	Thiazides	PUVA[12]
Dilantin	Barbiturates	Penicillin
Ketoconazole	Furosemide	Sulfonamides

1, Acneiform is acne-like; 2, alopecia is hair loss; 3, retinoids are vitamin A derivatives; 4, erythema multiforme is considered to be a characteristic type of hypersensitivity reaction to such factors as infectious agents and drugs; and it is characterized by the presence of so-called target lesions (lesions with concentric zones of varying color); 5, erythema nodosum is a reaction pattern typically characterized by deep-seated inflammatory raised areas on the extensor surfaces of the lower extremities; 6, a fixed drug eruption is typically characterized by a single or a few round, sharply demarcated, inflammatory lesions typically involving the face, genitalia, or acral areas (i.e., peripheral areas such as the hands or distal arms); 7, lichenoid is lichen planus-like. Lichen planus is a cutaneous condition typically consisting of pruritic, purplish, polygonal papules (the so-called '4 Ps') that are flat-topped; 8, photosensitivity is sensitivity to light, usually UV light; 9, toxic epidermal necrolysis is a reaction pattern characterized by extensive sloughing of the epidermis; 10, vasculitis characteristically has purpuric lesions; 11, vesiculobullous is blistering; 12, PUVA is a form of treatment tht consists of the topical or systemic use of the compound psoralen in conjunction with exposure to ultraviolet A light. Table reproduced with permission from Freedberg I. *Fitzpatrick's Dermatology in General Medicine*, fifth edition. New York: The McGraw Hill Co

and/or oozing, a solution or lotion vehicle for the topical corticosteroids would generally be the preferred vehicle); a course of a systemic corticosteroid; oral antihistamines, such as the sedating antihistamines hydroxyzine (Atarax®) or diphenhydramine (Benadryl®) or the non-sedating antihistamine loratadine (Claritin®) for itching; soothing bland emollients (i.e moisturizers); and/or soothing tub soaks using plain tepid water or using one of the oatmeal-based bath powders (i.e. Plain Aveeno Bath Powder® or Aveeno-Oilated Bath Powder®) mixed in tepid water as described for non-specific dermatitis in Chapter 2.

SECONDARY BACTERIAL INFECTION OF DRUG ERUPTION INVOLVEMENT

Possible secondary bacterial infection can be approached as described for possible secondarily infected non-specific dermatitis in Chapter 2.

4

Psoriasis

OVERVIEW

Clinically, psoriasis is typically characterized by sometimes itchy, erythematous, scaly plaques (broad raised lesions), typically involving the extensor surfaces of the extremities (particularly the elbows and knees), hands, feet, scalp, neck, trunk (particularly the sacrum) and/or buttocks. It can also involve the face, ears, area around the ears and genitals.

So-called inverse psoriasis can be seen both in conjunction with and not in conjunction with the above-described typical psoriasis involvement. Inverse psoriasis consists of sometimes itchy, erythematous, sometimes (but not commonly) scaly patches (non-raised, non-palpable lesions) and/or plaques involving intertriginous (skin-fold) areas such as the intergluteal cleft (the region between the buttocks), groins, axillae and/or, in females, the inframammary regions (under the breasts).

Typical fingernail and/or toenail changes are frequently seen in psoriasis patients, and these changes most commonly consist of pitting of the nails and/or onycholysis of the nails. Psoriatic nail pitting is characterized by small indentations (pits) on the surface of the nail plate; these pits are due to focal psoriatic involvement of the nail matrix, and this focal psoriatic nail matrix involvement results in the formation of a defective nail plate with pits on its surface. (The nail matrix is located under the proximal nail fold of the digit and produces the nail plate. The proximal nail fold is the skin fold that is located at the proximal edge of the nail plate.) Onycholysis is separation of the nail plate from the nail bed, and when it occurs in psoriasis, it is due to psoriatic involvement of the nail unit.

It should be noted that psoriasis exhibits the Koebner phenomenon, which means that lesions of psoriasis can develop at sites where trauma has occurred. Psoriasis can also develop at sites where inflammation from other causes has occurred. (For example, there are cases in which psoriasis developed at sites where there were lesions of drug eruption.)

It should also be noted that it is not uncommon for psoriasis and seborrheic dermatitis (see Chapter 2) to be present simultaneously in the same patient, and the term sebopsoriasis has been used to describe involvement that has features suggestive of both seborrheic dermatitis and psoriasis. In my experience, this type of involvement usually occurs on the scalp and sometimes on the face, ears, area around the ears, genitals, or intertriginous areas.

TREATMENT OF STABLE, LIMITED, PLAQUE-TYPE, NON-INVERSE PSORIASIS

Topical steroids and topical tar preparations

Overview

In terms of treatment of psoriasis, topical steroids are initially and rapidly effective, but provide short remissions. Because psoriasis is a chronic problem, tachyphylaxis (see Chapter 1) soon develops when topical steroids are used alone in treating psoriasis. Therefore, topical steroids should not be used alone in treating psoriasis.

Topical tar preparations are slowly effective in treating psoriasis, but provide longer remissions, and no tachyphylaxis is associated with their use.

A good initial treatment regimen using topical steroids
in conjunction with tar preparations

A good initial treatment regimen for stable, limited (non-extensive), plaque-type, non-inverse psoriasis consists of the use of topical steroids in conjunction with tar preparations.

For example, in adults one can use triamcinolone (e.g. Kenalog® or Aristocort®) cream 0.1% 1–2 times daily to involvement on the neck, trunk, arms, legs and buttocks (not between the buttocks); triamcinolone (e.g. Kenalog or Aristocort) lotion 0.1% 1–2 times daily to involvement on the scalp; fluocinonide (e.g. Lidex®) cream 1–2 times daily to involvement on the hands and feet; tar shampoo (e.g. DHS Tar Shampoo®, DHS Tar Gel Shampoo®, T-Gel Shampoo®, Doak Tar Shampoo®, or Ionil-T Plus Shampoo®) once daily (there is reportedly no risk of staining blond or silver hair when Ionil-T Plus Shampoo is used); a topical tar preparation (e.g. T-Derm Tar Emollient® or Doak Tar Lotion®) 1–2 times daily to involvement on the neck, trunk, arms, legs, buttocks, hands, feet and scalp; and once or twice daily tub soaks with Doak Tar Oil® or Balnetar® tar preparation for tub soaks mixed in tepid water. (The treatment regimen using topical steroids and tar preparations for psoriasis involvement on the face, ears, area around the ears and genitals as well as for inverse psoriasis is described later in this chapter.) I use this treatment regimen in pregnant or breast-feeding patients only if its use is approved by the patient's obstetrician or breast-fed baby's pediatrician, respectively. For pediatric patients, I would generally use for the topical steroid in this treatment regimen the low-potency topical steroid hydrocortisone 1% (bearing in mind that the nominally higher-potency topical steroid hydrocortisone 2.5% may sometimes be needed), as discussed and described in Chapter 1.

Anthralin

A treatment regimen using topical anthralin in conjunction with topical steroids and tar preparations

An alternative treatment regimen for stable, limited, plaque-type, non-inverse psoriasis involves the substitution of anthralin (e.g. Drithocreme®) in place of the topical tar preparation (i.e T-Derm Tar Emollient or Doak Tar Lotion) in the preceding regimen involving the use of topical steroids in conjunction with tar preparations. In this alternative regimen, the topical steroids, the tar shampoo and the tar tub soaks are used as described above, but anthralin is used in place of the above-described topical tar preparation. I do not use this anthralin regimen in pregnant, breast-feeding, or pediatric patients. Anthralin should not be used on the face, and I also do not use it on the ears, area around the ears, genitals, or skin folds. Anthralin should not be used for acute or actively inflamed psoriasis.

When anthralin is used, the patient should be advised that it can be irritating; it should be applied only to the psoriatic plaques and not to normal skin; it may transiently stain the surrounding normal skin a purplish color; it may temporarily stain fingernails and hair, especially white, silver or blond hair; and it may stain fabrics, plastics and the porcelain of bathroom fixtures. (To prevent staining of the porcelain of bathroom fixtures, the patient should be advised to wash off immediately with suitable cleanser any residual anthralin that may have got on to any bathroom porcelain.)

I feel that when anthralin is used to treat psoriasis, the best method of use is 'short contact anthralin therapy' ('SCAT'). When I prescribe this treatment regimen, I use the brand of anthralin called Drithocreme (which comes in 0.1%, 0.25%, 0.5% and 1.0% concentrations, with efficacy and potential for irritation increasing with increasing concentration), which can be used for psoriasis involvement on the skin (as well as for psoriasis involvement on the scalp). For anthralin treatment of psoriasis on the scalp, I use the brand of anthralin called Dritho-scalp® cream (which comes in 0.25% and 0.5% concentrations).

When I begin treatment with Drithocreme for psoriasis involvement on the skin, I start with the lowest concentration (0.1%), and I have the patient apply this daily to the psoriatic lesions on the skin and wash it off thoroughly by showering 30 min after the application. I have the patient do this for about 2 weeks, after which the concentration of the Drithocreme can be increased in a step-wise fashion, as tolerated, until the highest concentration that does not cause excessive irritation is reached, but I generally do not increase the concentration of Drithocreme above 0.5%. If the Drithocreme is causing excessive irritation, I decrease the frequency of its use and/or I decrease its concentration accordingly and, if necessary, discontinue its use. Once the excessive irritation has subsided satisfactorily, Drithocreme can be tried again, but at a lower frequency of use and/or a lower concentration, and, after a week or two, if tolerated, its frequency of use and/or its concentration can be increased in a step-wise fashion as tolerated, as described above.

I use Dritho-scalp cream for psoriatic lesions on the scalp exactly as described above regarding Drithocreme for psoriatic lesions on the skin, except that I start by using Dritho-scalp cream 0.25%.

When using this anthralin/topical steroid/tar regimen for psoriasis, the patient can be seen about every 2 weeks for monitoring, and if the treatment is being tolerated well, the treatment is stopped when the lesions being treated have entirely resolved, at which point nothing can be felt on touching with the fingers, and the skin surface at the sites feels normal.

Dovonex®

*A treatment regimen using Dovonex in conjunction
with a super-potent topical steroid*

An alternative path one can take in treating stable, limited, plaque-type, non-inverse psoriasis in adults consists of the use of a regimen involving the topical vitamin D derivative Dovonex (calcipotriene) in conjunction with the super-potent topical steroid Temovate® (clobetasol propionate). I do not use Dovonex in patients with liver insufficiency (Dovonex is cleared by the liver) or kidney insufficiency (Dovonex can cause hypercalcemia). Dovonex is contraindicated in patients with demonstrated hypercalcemia or evidence of vitamin D toxicity, and it should not be used on the face. I also do not use Dovonex on the ears, area around the ears, genitals, or skin folds.

This Dovonex–Temovate regimen is used as follows: Apply Dovonex Ointment or Cream to psoriasis lesions on the neck, trunk, arms, legs,

potential should have a negative pregnancy test having a sensitivity down to at least 50 mIU/ml for human chorionic gonadotropin (hCG) within 2 weeks before starting Tazorac therapy, which should be started during a normal menstrual period, and they should use adequate birth control measures when Tazorac is used. If the patient becomes pregnant while using Tazorac, treatment should be discontinued, and the patient should be informed of the potential hazard to the fetus. I generally do not use Tazorac in breast-feeding patients and Tazorac gel in patients under 12 years of age. Also, Tazorac can be very irritating, so it should be used cautiously and carefully, and it should not be used in skin folds except as described below. When Tazorac is prescribed, the patient should be informed of its significant potential for irritation, and it has been recommended that patients be seen by the prescribing health-care provider 7–14 days after initiation of Tazorac therapy so that, when the health-care provider sees the patient, he or she has the opportunity to take care of any problematic local irritation that may be present, so that the patient does not unnecessarily desist therapy with Tazorac. It should be noted that Tazorac gel should not be used on more than 20% of the patient's body surface area. (As a guide, I tell the patient that he or she can consider the palm of his or her hand to represent about 1% of his or her body surface area.) Tazorac can have a photosensitizing type of effect, so it should be used with caution in patients taking photo-sensitizing drugs; patients using Tazorac should accordingly avoid sunlight (including sunlamp) exposure, keep covered and use a sunscreen with sun protection factor 15 or greater when outdoors during the daytime. Patients with sunburn should not use Tazorac until they are fully recovered.

The regimen involving Tazorac gel in conjunction with Elocon cream is as follows. Apply Tazorac gel 0.1% (or 0.05% if 0.1% is too irritating) to psoriasis lesions on the neck, trunk, buttocks, scalp, arms, legs, hands and feet cautiously every evening at bedtime, and if this is too irritating (which it very well may be), the medication should be applied every other or every third evening at bedtime, accordingly, and, if possible and as tolerated, an attempt can be made to increase the frequency of application, in a step-wise fashion, to every evening at bedtime. When the Tazorac gel is applied, the patient should be sure that the sites where the medication is to be applied are dry before application of the medication, and the patient should be careful not to get any of the medication on the normal surrounding skin. After application of the Tazorac gel, it should be confirmed that the application sites are dry, so that there is no inadvertent spreading of the medication to unintended sites; the application sites are dry if no streaks are left behind when a finger is wiped through the application sites onto adja-cent skin. In addition, apply Elocon cream to psoriasis lesions on the neck, trunk, buttocks, scalp, arms, legs, hands and feet every morning. (The treatment regimen using Tazorac gel and a topical steroid for psoriasis involvement on the face, ears, area around the ears and genitals as well as for inverse psoriasis is described later in this chapter.)

It should be noted that, with this Tazorac gel–Elocon cream regimen, it can take as long as 8–12 weeks for improvement of the psoriatic involvement to be seen.

Tazorac cream 0.05% and 0.1% have recently become available and may be less irritating than Tazorac gel. The safety and efficacy of Tazorac cream in the treatment of psoriasis in patients less than 18 years of age have not been established.

Sun exposure

For more resistant, stable, plaque-type psoriasis involvement, one can add a trial of cautious, increasing sun exposure once daily to achieve a level of exposure that is just below that which produces sunburn (being very careful to avoid sunburn). Bear in mind that the use of tar preparations (as well as the use of Tazorac) increases the skin's sensitivity to sunlight, thereby increasing the risk of sunburn. I do not use sun exposure treatment when Tazorac is being used.

Softening and removing thick psoriatic scaling on the scalp

To soften and remove thick psoriatic scaling on the scalp, the following regimen is useful. The patient first wets the scalp thoroughly with water; then applies mineral oil to the areas of thick scaling; then wraps the scalp with a warm wet towel; and then, about 10–15 min later, using Johnson's No More Tears Baby Shampoo®, vigorously shampoos out the mineral oil with his or her fingers and tries to remove thick scaling with his or her fingers as he or she shampoos. This regimen is performed 1–2 times daily until the thick scaling is satisfactorily removed.

TREATMENT OF INVERSE PSORIASIS AND PSORIASIS INVOLVING THE FACE, EARS, AREA AROUND THE EARS AND GENITALS

Topical steroids and topical tar preparations

*A good initial treatment regimen using a topical
steroid in conjunction with tar preparations*

For inverse psoriasis and psoriasis involving the face, ears, area around the ears and genitals in adult and pediatric patients, the following regimen can be used. Apply T-Derm Tar Emollient or Doak Tar Lotion to psoriasis lesions involving the intertriginous areas, face, ears, area around the ears and genitals 1–2 times daily, cautiously because tar preparations can be more irritating in these areas. (If the tar preparation is too irritating when used at this frequency of application, it should be applied less frequently, and, if possible and as tolerated, an attempt can be made to increase the frequency of application, in a step-wise fashion, to 1–2 times daily.) In addition, apply hydrocortisone (e.g. Delcort®) cream 0.5% to eyelid/periorbital region involvement and hydrocortisone (e.g. Hytone®) cream 1% to the non-eyelid/non-periorbital region involvement 1–2 times daily for adult patients; for pediatric patients I would generally use hydrocortisone cream 0.5% in place of the hydrocortisone cream 1% (bearing in mind that the nominally higher-potency hydrocortisone cream 1% may sometimes be needed). Also, the patient should take once or twice daily tub soaks with Doak Tar Oil or Balnetar tar preparation mixed in tepid water. I use this treatment regimen in pregnant or breast-feeding patients only if its use is approved by the patient's obstetrician or breast-fed baby's pediatrician, respectively.

Tazorac®

A treatment regimen using Tazorac in conjunction with a topical steroid

Alternatively, inverse psoriasis and psoriasis involving the face, ears, area around the ears and genitals in adults can be treated with Tazorac gel and a topical steroid as described above for the treatment of stable, plaque-type, non-inverse psoriasis in adults, except that, for inverse psoriasis and psoriasis involving the face, ears, area around the ears and genitals, Tazorac gel 0.05% is used instead of 0.1%, and hydrocortisone cream 0.5% for eyelid/periorbital region involvement and hydrocortisone cream 1% for the non-eyelid/non-periorbital region involvement are used instead of Elocon cream. However, since Tazorac gel is likely to be more irritating when used in intertriginous areas and areas involving the face, ears, area around the ears and genitals, the patient in this situation should start using it every third or every other evening at bedtime, and then, if possible and as tolerated, the frequency of application can be increased, in a step-wise fashion, to every evening at bedtime. As noted above, it has been recommended that the patient be seen again by the prescribing health-care provider 7–14 days after initiation of Tazorac gel therapy (see above). Also, as previously noted, it may take as long as 8–12 weeks of treatment with this treatment regimen for improvement of the psoriatic involvement to be seen. In addition, Tazorac gel is contraindicated in pregnant patients, and appropriate measures to confirm that the patient is not pregnant and to prevent pregnancy should be taken, as discussed and described above. Also, I do not use Tazorac gel in patients under 12 years of age, and I generally do not use it in breast-feeding patients.

Tazorac cream 0.05% (and 0.1%) has recently become available and may be less irritating than the gel. However, the safety and efficacy of the cream has not yet been established in patients less than 18 years old.

Secondary candidiasis in association with inverse psoriasis

It should be noted that some dermatologists feel that a component of secondary candidiasis can frequently by associated with inverse psoriasis, so they empirically use a preparation such as the broad-spectrum, imidazole-type antifungal agent clotrimazole (Lotrimin-AF®) cream, lotion or solution two times daily in conjunction with specific treatment for inverse psoriasis. If the patient is allergic to imidazole-type antifungal agents, the broad-spectrum, ethanolamine-type antifungal agent ciclopirox olamine (Loprox®) lotion can be used instead.

USE OF ORAL ANTIHISTAMINES FOR THE SYMPTOMATIC TREATMENT OF PSORIATIC ITCHING

If a patient's psoriasis is itchy, an oral antihistamine [such as the sedating antihistamines hydoxyzine (Atarax®) or diphenhydramine (Benadryl®) or the non-sedating antihistamine loratadine (Claritin®)] can be prescribed as described for non-specific dermatitis in Chapter 2.

SECONDARY BACTERIAL INFECTION OF PSORIASIS INVOLVEMENT

Possible secondary bacterial infection can be approached as described for possible secondarily infected non-specific dermatitis in Chapter 2.

It should be noted that pathogenic bacteria not uncommonly colonize psoriatic skin (usually the scales) without causing infection. [In this situation, one could get a 'false-positive' bacterial culture and sensitivities (C&S) result, which would indicate pathogenic bacterial colonization and not true infection of the skin.]

It should also be noted that there is a type of psoriasis called pustular psoriasis, in which sterile pustules are present (see below).

EXTENSIVE, UNSTABLE, ERUPTIVE, ERYTHRODERMIC AND PUSTULAR PSORIASIS

Psoriasis can be extensive, unstable, eruptive, or erythrodermic. Eruptive psoriasis can be guttate (i.e. droplet-like), in which case small (0.5–1.5 cm) psoriatic lesions typically involve the upper trunk and proximal extremities and in which case frequently there is a preceding streptococcal throat infection or occasionally there is a preceding generalized macular drug eruption. Erythrodermic involvement consists of erythema and scaling involving the entire skin surface or nearly the entire skin surface. Macular lesions are non-raised and non-palpable. Also, sterile pustules can be associated with psoriasis, in which case the condition is called pustular psoriasis. A type of pustular psoriasis called generalized pustular psoriasis of von Zumbusch is a very serious condition that can be fatal. This condition is typically seen without other forms of psoriasis being present concurrently and is characterized by the sudden onset of a generalized eruption of sterile pustules on an erythematous background in association with fever and other systemic signs and symptoms.

Extensive, unstable, eruptive, erythrodermic and pustular psoriasis are more serious conditions that should be treated by a dermatologist, who may use methotrexate, the systemic retinoid acitretin (Soriatane®), cyclosporine, or phototherapy using ultraviolet B (UVB) light or the chemical psoralen in conjunction with ultraviolet A (UVA) light (PUVA).

PSORIATIC ARTHRITIS

Psoriasis can be associated with arthritis (i.e. psoriatic arthritis), for which the patient can be referred to a rheumatologist.

MISCELLANEOUS INFORMATION REGARDING PSORIASIS THERAPY

It is considered that the more complete the clearance of psoriasis is at the time of stopping therapy, the longer is the length of time that the clearance lasts. Informing the patient of this can be a motivating factor for the patient to continue therapy in order to try to achieve maximal clearance of psoriatic involvement.

Lastly, it should be noted that systemic steroids should never be used in the treatment of psoriasis, because their use in psoriasis can result in the development of generalized pustular psoriasis of von Zumbusch, which, as mentioned above, is a very serious condition that can be fatal.

5

Herpes simplex, varicella, herpes zoster, and aphthous stomatitis

HERPES SIMPLEX

Overview

Herpes simplex is a condition that is due to herpes simplex virus. In laymen's terms, the typical outbreaks, when they involve the lips, can be called 'cold sores' or 'fever blisters'. (Recurrences of herpes simplex outbreaks can be triggered by colds and other febrile illnesses as well as by menstruation and sun exposure.)

A herpes simplex outbreak typically consists of a usually painful and/or tender cluster of vesicles, frequently with a prodrome consisting of burning or tingling at the outbreak site shortly before the outbreak occurs. Each outbreak typically evolves to erosions and crusts and then to healing, usually over a period of about a week. If necessary, the diagnosis can be confirmed by obtaining a herpes simplex virus culture of blister fluid or of erosions/crusts. (Blister fluid is accessed by piercing the blister roof with a no. 11 scalpel or a 20-gauge needle. It needs to be remembered that one can obtain false-negative viral culture results.) It is not uncommon for patients to get outbreaks recurrently at the site of the initial outbreak. Outbreaks typically occur around the lips or involve the anogenital region, the former usually being non-sexually acquired and the latter usually being sexually acquired, but outbreaks can occur anywhere.

Special considerations regarding herpes simplex

Generally, depending on the degree of immunosuppression, immunosuppressed patients are at risk of developing severe, persistent herpes simplex lesions that can be manifested by persistent, deep ulcers and are also at risk of developing disseminated cutaneous herpes simplex infection with visceral involvement.

Herpes simplex is transmitted through contact with lesions, but transmission can also occur in the absence of lesions through asymptomatic viral shedding, although I have not personally seen clear-cut cases in which it can be documented that this latter form of transmission had occurred.

Patients should be counseled that they can transmit the disease when they have active lesions and contact is made with these active lesions, so such contact should be avoided, and in cases of genital herpes, intercourse should be avoided when lesions and/or symptoms are present. I also discuss with patients the fact that the disease can be transmitted through asymptomatic viral shedding.

Patients with anogenital herpes simplex should be checked for other sexually transmitted diseases, and this check should include, but is not limited to, obtaining a rapid plasma reagin (RPR) or Venereal Disease Research Laboratories (VDRL) test, and an HIV test.

Pregnant patients with a history of anogenital herpes simplex should notify their obstetricians of this early on, in order to prevent possible complications, particularly associated with parturition, regarding transmission to the baby.

Treatment of herpes simplex

Minor, infrequent outbreaks of herpes simplex that are not bothersome to the patient can go untreated.

Topical treatment of herpes simplex

Some patients use self-treatment of perioral herpes simplex with such over-the-counter, topical products as Cepacol Viractin® cold sore and fever blister treatment gel or cream; Orajel Covermed® fever blister/cold sore treatment cream; or Orajel Mouth-Aid® cold/canker sore medicine.

The only non-prescription cold sore medication that is approved by the FDA and that shortens cold sore healing time and duration of symptoms is docosanol (Abreva®) cream, which is approved for the treatment of cold sores in patients 12 years of age and older.

I feel that the best prescription topical treatment for simple herpes simplex outbreaks on the lips in adults is penciclovir (Denavir®) cream, which should be applied every 2 h during waking hours for a period of 4 days, and treatment should be started as early as possible (i.e. during the prodrome or when lesions appear). Safety and effectiveness of penciclovir cream in pediatric patients have not been established. I do not use penciclovir cream in breast-feeding patients.

I do not prescribe acyclovir (Zovirax®) ointment because I have not found it to be particularly effective.

Systemic treatment of herpes simplex

In my opinion, a good treatment for initial outbreaks of simple non-anogenital and anogenital herpes simplex in adults is oral acyclovir (Zovirax) 200 mg five times daily for 10 days, with the treatment being initiated at the earliest sign or symptom of involvement. Alternatively, valacyclovir (Valtrex®) 1 g twice daily for 10 days, with the treatment being initiated at the earliest sign or symptom of involvement, can be used.

A good intermittent treatment for recurrent outbreaks of simple non-anogenital and anogenital herpes simplex in adults is oral acyclovir (Zovirax) 200 mg five times daily for 5 days, with the treatment being initiated at the earliest sign or symptom (prodrome) of recurrence. Alternatively, valacyclovir (Valtrex) 500 mg twice daily for 3 days, with the treatment being initiated at the earliest sign or symptom (prodrome) of recurrence, can be used. Another treatment that can be used in immunocompetent adults is famciclovir (Famvir®) 125 mg twice daily for 5 days, with treatment being initiated at the earliest sign or symptom (prodrome) of recurrence; the dosage for HIV-infected adults is 500 mg twice daily for 7 days.

For chronic suppressive therapy of recurrent simple non-anogenital and anogenital herpes simplex in adults, I have found oral acyclovir (Zovirax) 400 mg twice daily for up to 12 months to be quite effective. After 12 months of therapy, the acyclovir should be discontinued, after which the frequency and severity of the patient's herpes outbreaks should be assessed in order to determine whether or not continued acyclovir therapy is needed. (Over time, the frequency and severity of herpes outbreaks can change.) Alternatively, valacyclovir (Valtrex) 1 g once daily can be used. (In patients with a history of nine or fewer recurrences per year, an alternative dose is 500 mg once daily.) It should be noted that the safety and efficacy of valacyclovir therapy continuing beyond 1 year have not been established. Another treatment that can be used in immunocompetent adults is famciclovir (Famvir) 250 mg twice daily for up to 1 year. The safety and efficacy of famciclovir therapy continuing beyond 1 year have not been established.

In patients with renal impairment, appropriate adjustments of the acyclovir, valacyclovir, and famciclovir dosages should be made in accordance with the recommendations in the corresponding package insert.

I generally do not use acyclovir, valacyclovir, or famciclovir in pregnant or breast-feeding patients unless its use is approved by the patient's obstetrician or breast-fed baby's pediatrician, respectively. I have generally not needed to use acyclovir for the treatment of simple 'cold sore' and 'fever blister' herpes simplex in children. The safety and effectiveness of oral acyclovir in pediatric patients under 2 years of age have not been established, and the safety and effectiveness of valacyclovir in pre-pubertal pediatric patients and of famciclovir in patients under 18 years of age have not been established.

It is important to note that there can be acyclovir, valacyclovir and famciclovir resistance (which can be manifested by poor clinical response during therapy), for which other antiviral treatment beyond the scope of this guide is indicated.

It is also important to note that immunocompromised patients receiving acyclovir therapy have developed thrombotic thrombocytopenic purpura/ hemolytic uremic syndrome (TTP/HUS), which has resulted in death. TTP/HUS, sometimes resulting in death, has also developed in patients with advanced HIV disease and also in allogeneic bone marrow transplant recipients and renal transplant recipients who were participating in clinical trials of valacyclovir at doses of 8 g/day.

VARICELLA

Overview

Varicella ('chickenpox') is a generally self-limited infectious disease due to varicella-zoster virus, which is a member of the herpesvirus family. Varicella is typically manifested by a characteristic, itchy, erythematous, papulovesi-culopustular eruption in which erythematous macules progress to papules, vesicles, pustules and then crusts. The pustules usually have characteristic umbilications (indentations) on their surfaces. Characteristically, lesions in all stages of development are present simultaneously. A prodrome and con-stitutional symptoms and/or signs occur variably. Generally, varicella tends to be the mildest in children; is more severe in non-pregnant adults; is even more severe in pregnant patients, in whom varicella is a threat to both the mother and the fetus; and is the most severe in immunocompromised patients. Although varicella generally tends to be the mildest in children, childhood varicella occurring in the perinatal period is more serious than is childhood varicella occurring later and is potentially very serious.

The diagnosis is generally easily made on clinical grounds, but it can be confirmed by obtaining a varicella-zoster virus culture of vesicle fluid or pustule contents, which are accessed by piercing the vesicle or pustule roof with a no. 11 scalpel or a 20-gauge needle. (Vesicles are much more likely to yield varicella-zoster virus on culture than are pustules, and varicella-zoster virus is almost never isolated from crusts.)

The attenuated Oka varicella-zoster virus vaccine has been approved for use in the USA.

Special considerations regarding varicella

If varicella is diagnosed in a pregnant patient, she should be followed in conjunction with her obstetrician because of the threat to both the mother and the fetus.

Regarding general transmission precautions, patients with varicella should be kept at home until all lesions have crusted. Exposure of susceptible adults to varicella patients should be avoided, and exposure of non-infected newborn infants, susceptible pregnant individuals and, especially, immunocompromised individuals to varicella patients should be strictly prevented.

In order to prevent or favorably modify potential subsequent varicella-zoster virus infection, products such as varicella-zoster immune globulin (VZIG), in conjunction with other measures as indicated, are used in high-risk individuals exposed to varicella-zoster virus.

Treatment of varicella

Simple varicella can be treated symptomatically with tub soaks using plain tepid water or using one of the oatmeal-based bath powders (Plain Aveeno Both Powder® or Aveeno-Oilated Bath Powder®) mixed in tepid water as described for non-specific dermatitis in Chapter 2. Also, an oral antihistamine [such as the sedating antihistamines hydroxyzine (Atarax®) or diphenhydramine (Benadryl®) or the non-sedating antihistamine loratadine (Claritin®)] can be used for itching, as described for non-specific dermatitis in Chapter 2. If needed, an antipyretic other than a salicylate can be used. Because of the association of salicylates with Reye's syndrome, salicylates must not be used.

Simple varicella in adults and children over 40 kg can also be treated with acyclovir (Zovirax) 800 mg orally four times daily for 5 days, with the treatment being initiated at the earliest sign or symptom of varicella. The acyclovir dosages for children 2 years of age and older and 40 kg and under and for patients with renal impairment are as recommended in the package insert. The safety and effectiveness of oral acyclovir in pediatric patients under 2 years of age have not been established. I use acyclovir in pregnant patients in conjunction with their obstetricians.

Intravenous acyclovir in suitable dosage is appropriate for the treatment of varicella in neonates, in patients whose varicella is severe, and in immunocompromised patients.

It is important to note that there can be acyclovir resistance (which can be manifested by poor clinical response during therapy), for which other antiviral treatment beyond the scope of this guide is indicated.

It is also important to note that immunocompromised patients receiving acyclovir therapy have developed TTP/HUS, which has resulted in death.

HERPES ZOSTER

Overview

Herpes zoster ('shingles') typically consists of a dermatomal, grouped outbreak consisting of erythematous macules and papules followed by vesicles, which evolve into pustules, which dry and form crusts, which generally resolve in about 2 to 3 weeks. The outbreak is usually painful, with the pain commonly preceding the outbreak. Herpes zoster occurs as a usually localized, generally self-limited outbreak caused by varicella-zoster virus generally acquired many years earlier as varicella.

The diagnosis of herpes zoster is usually readily made on clinical grounds, but it can be confirmed by obtaining a varicella-zoster virus culture of vesicle fluid or pustule contents, which are accessed by piercing the vesicle or pustule roof with a no. 11 scalpel or a 20-gauge needle. (Vesicles are much more likely to yield varicella-zoster virus on culture than are pustules, and varicella-zoster virus is almost never isolated from crusts.)

Special considerations regarding herpes zoster

Herpes zoster is more likely to occur, is more severe, and has an increased risk for dissemination in immunocompromised patients.

I consider herpes zoster involvement of the eye to be an ophthalmological emergency, and when this is suspected, I arrange for immediate ophthalmological consultation. Herpes zoster involvement of the tip and side of the nose has a relatively high association with herpes zoster involvement of the eye.

Mothers who have herpes zoster during pregnancy give birth to children who develop no evidence of intrauterine varicella-zoster virus infection serologically or clinically.

If a patient with herpes zoster is young (for example, middle-aged or younger) or if multiple dermatomes are involved, I consider the possibility of immunodeficiency. However, it should be noted that varicella infection acquired *in utero* can result in latent varicella-zoster virus being retained in sensory ganglia, thereby frequently resulting in the subsequent development of herpes zoster at an early age without the patient having had a preceding history of varicella.

Varicella may be transmitted to susceptible individuals by exposure to patients with herpes zoster. Therefore, susceptible individuals, especially those who are at increased risk for the development of severe varicella (as discussed above in the section on varicella), should not have direct contact with patients with localized herpes zoster, and patients with disseminated herpes zoster should be placed in respiratory isolation.

In order to prevent or favorably modify potential subsequent varicella-zoster virus infection, products such a VZIG, in conjuntion with other measures as indicated, are used in high-risk individuals exposed to varicella-zoster virus.

Patients with herpes zoster can have post-herpetic neuralgia, which can be considered to be herpes zoster herpetic pain that persists following the healing of the herpes zoster lesions. The presence of post-herpetic neuralgia increases in frequency with age. In general, it resolves spontaneously within 3 months in about 50% of patients and within a year in over 75% of patients.

Treatment of herpes zoster

Local care of simple herpes zoster can consist of open wet compresses with gauze soaked in plain water (as described for the treatment of non-specific dermatitis in Chapter 2) or in plain Domeboro® solution (as described for the treatment of contact dermatitis in general in Chapter 2). Domeboro solution has an enhanced drying effect in comparison to plain water and has an antimicrobial effect.

An appropriate oral analgesic can be prescribed for pain associated with herpes zoster, if needed and if not otherwise unadvisable.

In addition, one can treat simple herpes zoster with acyclovir (Zovirax) 800 mg orally five times daily for 7–10 days in adults. Alternatively, valacyclovir (Valtrex) 1 g three times daily for 7 days, with treatment being initiated at the earliest sign or symptom of herpes zoster, can be used. Another treatment that can be used is famciclovir (Famvir) 500 mg every 8 h for 7 days, with treatment being initiated at the earliest sign or symptom of herpes zoster.

In patients with renal impairment, appropriate adjustments of the acyclovir, valacyclovir and famciclovir dosages should be made in accordance with the recommendations in the corresponding package insert.

Intravenous acyclovir in suitable dosage is appropriate for the treatment of herpes zoster in immunocompromised patients, particularly those with severe immune system compromise.

I generally do not use acyclovir, valacyclovir, or famciclovir in pregnant or breast-feeding patients unless its use is approved by the patient's obstetrician or breast-fed baby's pediatrician, respectively. The safety and effectiveness of oral acyclovir in pediatric patients under 2 years of age have not been etablished, and the safety and effectiveness of valacyclovir in pre-pubertal pediatric patients and of famciclovir in patients under 18 years of age have not been established.

It is important to note that there can be acyclovir, valacyclovir and famciclovir resistance (which can be manifested by poor clinical response during therapy), for which other antiviral treatment beyond the scope of this guide is indicated.

It is also important to note that immunocompromised patients receiving acyclovir therapy have developed TTP/HUS, which has resulted in death. TTP/HUS, sometimes resulting in death, has also developed in patients with advanced HIV disease and also in allogeneic bone marrow transplant recipients and renal transplant recipients who were participating in clinical trials of valacyclovir at doses of 8 g/day.

In the past, particularly before the advent of acyclovir therapy for herpes zoster, some physicians have recommended the use of systemic steroids in the treatment of herpes zoster in order to reduce the likelihood of post-herpetic neuralgia (see above). I no longer find such treatment useful, and I therefore do not use systemic steroids in the treatment of herpes zoster.

Secondary bacterial infection of herpes simplex, varicella and herpes zoster involvement

Possible secondary bacterial infection, which might occur with herpes simplex, varicella, or herpes zoster, can be approached as described for possible secondarily infected non-specific dermatitis in Chapter 2.

APHTHOUS STOMATITIS

Overview

Apthous stomatitis ('canker sores', in layman's terms) is a condition consisting of recurrent erosions, which can be tender and/or painful, involving the mouth. Individual lesions generally resolve in about a week. The etiology is unclear.

Special considerations regarding aphthous stomatitis

Lesions that are not typical, do not resolve in a timely fashion with or without treatment, or are not of recent onset should be evaluated accordingly for other diagnoses, including carcinoma.

Treatment of aphthous stomatitis

Aphthous stomatitis involvement that is not bothersome to the patient can go untreated.

Some patients use self-treatment with such over-the-counter, topical products as Orajel Mouth-Aid for canker and cold sores or Zilactin Medicated Gel®. For more severe involvement, the following regimen is useful for the treatment of aphthous stomatitis lesions when present: tetracycline oral suspension 1 teaspoonful (250 mg) swish and spit four times daily along with Decadron Elixir® (dexamethasone) 1 teaspoonful swish and spit four times daily (swish and swallow the Decadron Elixir, if not otherwise unadvisable and if involvement is severe). This regimen should not be used in pregnant, breast-feeding, or pediatric patients.

Some patients respond to the topical steroid Kenalog in Orabase® (triamcinolone), which is applied to the aphthous stomatitis lesions, as described in the medication's package insert. Kenalog in Orabase is Kenalog (triamcinolone) in a vehicle specifically formulated for application to the mucosal surface of the mouth. An alternative to Kenalog in Orabase is Lidex® (fluocinonide) gel.

For symptomatic relief of discomfort, Benadryl Elixir (diphenhydramine) one teaspoonful swish and spit three times daily before meals can be used.

6

Pityriasis rosea and non-specific viral eruptions

PITYRIASIS ROSEA

Overview

Pityriasis rosea consists of an eruption that is typically characterized by sometimes itchy, erythematous, scaly plaques (broad, raised lesions) usually involving the trunk and proximal extremities, although there is an inverse type of pityriasis rosea in which the lesions have a primarily peripheral rather than central location on the body (i.e. involvement is mainly on the extremities rather than on the trunk). The onset of the eruption is sometimes preceded by a single, larger, erythematous, scaly plaque. This represents the so-called 'herald patch'. Individual lesions are typically oval and are typically oriented along skin lines with the long axes of the oval lesions being parallel to the direction of the corresponding skin lines such that the involvement on the back characteristically has what is called a 'Christmas tree' pattern. There is a papular variant (a papule is a bump) in which there may be rare scattered typical oval lesions. The eruption is self-limited and resolves spontaneously, usually in a few weeks.

The etiology of pityriasis rosea is unclear, but because of various characteristics of the condition, it has been speculated that pityriasis rosea may be due to an infectious agent, possibly a virus.

Special considerations regarding pityriasis rosea

Since secondary syphilis (see Chapter 27) can look like pityriasis rosea, a rapid plasma reagin (RPR) or Venereal Disease Research Laboratories (VDRL) test should be obtained in order to screen for secondary syphilis, if the clinical circumstances are appropriate, in all patients suspected of having pityriasis rosea. The other 'great mimicker', drug eruption (see Chapter 3), should also be considered in the differential diagnosis, if the clinical circumstances are appropriate. Also, psoriasis, especially eruptive or guttate psoriasis (see Chapter 4), and nummular dermatitis (see Chapter 2) should be considered in the differential diagnosis. Especially with regard to the papular variant of pityriasis rosea, extensive bacterial folliculitis (see Chapter 17) and, if the clinical circumstances are appropriate, viral eruption might also be considered in the differential diagnosis. In my experience, there are viruses that can produce non-specific eruptions (see below).

As alluded to above, a negative RPR or VDRL test would rule out secondary syphilis. A complete blood count (CBC) showing eosinophilia might be suggestive of a drug eruption. Severe, serious drug eruptions may show lymphocytosis with atypical lymphocytes and may have associated constitutional symptoms and/or signs along with other findings. Current evidence is that eosinophilia on CBC is an uncommon finding for common drug reactions and is a parameter that is of little value in diagnosing common drug reactions, but an eosinophil count greater than $1000/\mu l$ may be seen with severe, serious drug eruptions. A CBC showing lymphocytosis would be suggestive of a viral eruption, which may have associated constitutional symptoms and/or signs and typically presents as erythematous macules that may coalesce, erythematous papules, vesicles and/or pustules (a viral culture of vesicle/pustule contents, accessed by piercing the roof with a No 11 scapel or 20-gauge needle, may reveal a virus).

The untreated rash of secondary syphilis would resolve spontaneously (at which time the patient would be said to have latent syphilis). If the diagnosis of secondary syphilis is made, this obviously should be evaluated, treated and followed accordingly, and if the patient is pregnant, her obstetrician should be notified because of the potential effect of syphilis on the fetus. Viral eruption generally needs only symptomatic treatment since it is generally self-limited, but if the patient is pregnant, and viral eruption is considered, the patient's obstetrician should be notified regarding the possibility of associated harm to the fetus. If the diagnosis of a viral eruption is made, appropriate precautions need to be taken to prevent transmission of the condition to other individuals.

The common differential diagnosis of the typical type of pityriasis rosea can also include: extensive tinea corporis (see Chapter 18); papulosquamous cutaneous manifestations of HIV disease; erythema multiforme (see below); parapsoriasis; early cutaneous T-cell lymphoma. (For brief discussion of cutaneous manifestations of HIV disease, parapsoriasis, and T-cell lymphoma see page 13: *Common differential diagnosis of extensive/generalized non-specific dermatitis.*)

The common differential diagnosis of the papular type of pityriasis rosea can also include other entities. For example, papular cutaneous manifestations of HIV disease, such as eospinophilic folliculitis (which is clinically characterized by pink-to-red follicular papules and histologically characterized by follicular inflammation containing eosinophils predominantly) and so-called pruritic papular eruption of HIV disease (which has been reported to appear to be the same entity as eosinophilic folliculitis) or so-called 'itchy red bump disease' (not all cases of which turn out to be eosinophilic folliculitis on biopsy) might be considered in the differential diagnosis. The diagnosis of cutaneous manifestations of HIV disease would be supported by a positive HIV test and this condition should be treated by a dermatologist. The papular type of chronic cutaneous graft-versus-host reaction may occur if the patient has had a bone marrow transplantation and should be treated by the transplant physicians. Vasculitis (an inflammation of vasculature walls) characteristically has purpuric lesions, although purpuric lesions can also be seen in viral eruptions. Vasculitis should be taken care of by a dermatologist. Papular acrodermatitis of childhood (Gianotti-Crosti syndrome) is characterized by an eruption of small papules on the face and extremities in children 2 to 6 years of age, lasts about 3 weeks, and is associated with viral infections due to such viruses as hepatitis B virus, coxsackievirus, parainfluenza virus, Epstein-Barr virus, enterovirus, cytomegalovirus and adenovirus. While papular acrodermatitis of childhood is self-limited and classically non-pruritic, the associated viral infection can be taken care of by the patient's pediatrician. Erythema multiforme has been considered to be a characteristic type of hypersensitivity reaction to such factors as infectious agents and drugs, is characterized by the presence of so-called target lesions (which are lesions with concentric zones of varying color) and should be taken care of by a dermatologist. Scabies (see Chapter 16) might also be considered in the differential diagnosis of the papular type of pityriasis rosea.

Treatment of pityriasis rosea

Since pityriasis rosea is self-limited, it does not need to be treated, particularly if the involvement is not bothersome to the patient. Otherwise, the condition can be treated symptomatically with soothing bland emollients (i.e. moisturizers such as Lubriderm Seriously Sensitive Lotion®, Eucerin Cream®, or Aquaphor Ointment®) as well as topical steroids and, for itching, oral antihistamines [such as the sedating antihistamines hydroxyzine

(Atarax®) or diphenhydramine (Benadryl®) or the non-sedating antihistamine loratadine (Claritin®)] as described for non-specific dermatitis in
Chapter 2. Also, soothing tub soaks using plain tepid water or using one of
the oatmeal-based bath powders (Plain Aveeno Bath Powder® or Aveeno-
Oilated Bath Powder®) mixed in tepid water can be used as described for
non-specific dermatitis in Chapter 2.

For particularly bothersome, unresponsive involvement, a cautious trial
of sun exposure as described for psoriasis in Chapter 4 can be used, or the
patient can be referred to a dermatologist, who can arrange for therapy
with ultraviolet B (UVB) light, which can be beneficial.

NON-SPECIFIC VIRAL ERUPTIONS

Overview

In my experience, there are viruses that can produce non-specific eruptions,
and these non-specific viral eruptions can be described as usually self-
limited, typically fairly generalized eruptions typically consisting of sometimes itchy, erythematous macules that may coalesce, erythematous papules,
vesicles and/or pustules due to a viral infection to which no specific clinical
manifestations have been attributed. Constitutional symptoms and/or signs
may be present.

Special considerations regarding non-specific viral eruptions

When a non-specific viral eruption is considered, the 'great mimickers' drug
eruption (see Chapter 3) and secondary syphilis (see Chapter 27) should be
considered in the differential diagnosis, if the clinical situation is appropriate. A negative VDRL or RPR test will rule out secondary syphilis; a CBC
showing lymphocytosis would be suggestive of a viral eruption, which, as
noted above, may have associated constitutional symptoms and/or signs and
typically presents as erythematous macules that may coalesce, erythematous
papules, vesicles and/or pustules; and a CBC showing eosinophilia might be
suggestive of a drug eruption. Severe, serious drug eruptions may show
lymphocytosis with atypical lymphocytes and may have associated constitutional symptoms and/or signs along with other findings. Current evidence
is that eosinophilia on CBC is an uncommon finding for common drug
reactions and is a parameter that is of little value in diagnosing common
drug reactions, but an eosinophil count greater than 1000/μl may be seen with
severe, serious drug eruptions. Extensive bacterial folliculitis (see Chapter 17)

might also be considered in the differential diagnosis. Bacterial folliculitis would present as follicular, erythematous papules and/or pustules that may be pierced by hairs, as described in Chapter 17. In addition, the papular variant of pityriasis rosea, as described above, might be considered in the differential diagnosis.

If pustules are present, bacterial culture and sensitivities (C&S) of the pustule contents may confirm the diagnosis of bacterial folliculitis by growing out pathogenic bacteria, but be aware that false-negative bacterial culture results can occur. Pustule contents can be accessed by piercing pustule roofs with a no. 11 scalpel or a 20-gauge needle after cleaning the intact pustules with an alcohol swab and then drying the area with sterile gauze.

If vesicles or pustules are present, a viral culture of vesicle fluid or pustule contents can be obtained and can confirm the diagnosis of viral eruption if a virus is cultured out, but be aware that false-negative viral culture results can occur. Vesicle fluid or pustule contents can be accessed by piercing vesicle or pustule roofs with a no. 11 scalpel or a 20-gauge needle.

If a viral eruption is diagnosed or cannot be ruled out in a pregnant patient, the patient's obstetrician should be notified of the diagnosis, because of the possible effect that the viral infection might have on the patient's fetus.

If the diagnosis of a viral eruption is made, appropriate precautions should be taken to prevent transmission of the infection to other individuals.

The untreated rash of secondary syphilis would resolve spontaneously (at which time the patient would be said to have latent syphilis). If the diagnosis of secondary syphilis is made, this obviously should be evaluated, treated and followed accordingly, and if the patient is pregnant, her obstetrician should be notified, because of the potential effect of syphilis on the fetus.

The common differential diagnosis of non-specific viral eruptions might also include such conditions as: eruptive/guttate and pustular psoriasis (see Chapter 4); erythema multiforme; vasculitis; cutaneous graft-versus-host reaction; papular acrodermatitis of childhood (Gianotti-Crosti syndrome); scabies (see Chapter 16); rashes associated with the viral hepatitides; cutaneous manifestations of HIV disease. (For brief discussions of erythema multiforme, vasculitis, and papular acrodermatitis of childhood, see *Special considerations regarding pityriasis rosea* earlier in this chapter; for brief discussions of rashes associated with the viral hepatitides and cutaneous manifestations of HIV disease, see *Common differential diagnosis of extensive/generalized non-specific dermatitis* in Chapter 2.)

Treatment of non-specific viral eruptions

Since non-specific viral eruptions are generally self-limited, their treatment is basically symptomatic. Bland emollients, tub soaks and oral antihistamines can be used, as described above for pityriasis rosea.

Secondary bacterial infection of non-specific viral eruption involvement

Possible secondary bacterial infection can be approached as described for possible secondarily infected non-specific dermatitis in Chapter 2.

7

Common conditions consisting of pigmentary alteration

These conditions include melasma, post-inflammatory pigmentary alteration, pityriasis alba, idiopathic guttate hypomelanosis and vitiligo.

MELASMA

Overview

Melasma is a condition in which increased brownish pigmentation (i.e. hyperpigmentation) of the skin develops on the face, particularly on the central forehead, medial cheeks, nose bridge, skin of the upper lip and/or chin. It is not uncommon for this condition to be associated with pregnancy or with the use of birth control pills, and melasma has been associated with the use of combination estrogen/progestational agents in postmenopausal women. The use of phenytoin (Dilantin®) has also been associated with melasma-like hyperpigmentation. However, in many cases of melasma the etiology is unclear, and it should be noted that melasma can be seen in men.

The location of the hyperpigmentation in melasma can be in the epidermis, in which case the melasma tends to be brown in color; in the dermis, in which case the melasma tends to be blue-gray in color; or in both the epidermis and the dermis, in which case the melasma tends to be brown-gray in color. (The epidermis is the superficial cutaneous layer that is located immediately above the dermis.)

The location of the hyperpigmentation is important because only hyperpigmentation of the epidermis can be effectively treated. Except in patients with very dark normal skin color, epidermal hyperpigmentation can be distinguished from dermal hyperpigmentation in that epidermal hyperpigmentation is accentuated by exposure to the ultraviolet light of a Wood's lamp, whereas dermal hyperpigmentation is not accentuated by such exposure. This test does not work for patients with very dark normal skin color.

Treatment of melasma

In some cases of melasma, the involvement spontaneously resolves over time.

In treating this condition, the patient should avoid sunlamps and sun exposure (even on cloudy days), use a broad-spectrum sunscreen to the involvement, and wear a broad-brimmed hat when outdoors during the daytime. The sunscreen should provide protection from ultraviolet A (UVA) and ultraviolet B (UVB) light and have a sun protection factor (SPF) of 50 (e.g, sunscreen Solbar PF Cream SPF 50®).

The topical bleaching medication I use is Solaquin Forte®, which is applied to the involvement one to two times daily. Solaquin Forte is a prescription medication that contains the active ingredient hydro-quinone at a concentration of 4% in conjunction with sunscreen. A newer preparation is Lustra-AF®, a prescription medication that contains the active ingredient hydroquinone at a concentration of 4% in conjunction with sunscreen and an α-hydroxy acid in an antioxidant vehicle containing moisturizers.

When Solaquin Forte or Lustra-AF is used, the patient should first test it to see whether it causes irritation. This is done by applying a small amount of the medication to a patch of unbroken skin, which should be checked 24 h later. Minor redness is not a contraindication to the use of the medi-cation, but if there is itching, blister formation, or excessive inflammation, the medication should not be used.

The bleaching effect of Solaquin Forte and Lustra-AF can be augmented by the addition of tretinoin (e.g. Retin-A®) cream 0.025% to 0.1% every night at bedtime. Be aware that as the concentration of tretinoin increases, the potential for irritation and excessive dryness increases. If using tretinoin cream every night at bedtime is too irritating and/or drying, the tretinoin can be applied less often (e.g. every third or every other evening at bed-time), and, if possible and as tolerated, the frequency of application can be increased, in a step-wise fashion, to every night at bedtime. Also, a bland emollient, which can have a soothing and moisturizing effect, can be used if the tretinoin cream is irritating and/or drying. Such a bland emollient is Nutraderm Lotion®, which is non-comedogenic, i.e. it does not cause acne. Tretinoin makes the skin more sensitive to sunlight so patients with sunburn should not use tretinoin until they are fully recovered. Also, it has been recommended that wax epilation should not be performed on skin treated with tretinoin because of the potential for the development of erosions, and tretinoin should not be used on irritated or eczematous skin.

Improvement with this treatment regimen (Solaquin Forte or Lustra-AF in conjunction with tretinoin and sunscreen) is not always seen. If there is improvement, it can take weeks of treatment before it is seen. I generally do not use this treatment regimen in pregnant patients, breast-feeding patients, or patients below the age of 12 years.

Azelaic acid (e.g. Azelex®) cream alone or in conjunction with tretinoin cream or hydroquinone cream can also be used to treat melasma.

The use of lasers in the treatment of melasma is not generally recommended.

POST-INFLAMMATORY PIGMENTARY ALTERATION

Overview

Post-inflammatory pigmentary alteration is a term that includes the conditions post-inflammatory hyperpigmentation and post-inflammatory hypopigmentation/post-inflammatory depigmentation.

Post-inflammatory hyperpigmentation

Post-inflammatory hyperpigmentation is the increased brown pigmentation that can develop in the skin at sites where inflammatory lesions have healed. This condition tends to occur more commonly in dark-skinned individuals.

The location of the hyperpigmentation in post-inflammatory hyperpigmentation can be in the epidermis, in the dermis, or in both the epidermis and the dermis. (The epidermis is the superficial cutaneous layer that is located immediately above the dermis.)

The location of the hyperpigmentation is important because only hyperpigmentation of the epidermis can be effectively treated. Except in patients with very dark normal skin color, epidermal hyperpigmentation can be distinguished from dermal hyperpigmentation by the fact that epidermal hyperpigmentation is accentuated by exposure to the ultraviolet light of a Wood's lamp, whereas dermal hyperpigmentation is not accentuated by such exposure. This test does not work for patients with very dark normal skin color.

Post-inflammatory hyperpigmentation sometimes spontaneously fades over time, but if it does so, it can take years. It can be treated as described above for melasma, except that in treating post-inflammatory hyperpigmentation, the patient should in addition keep the involved areas covered with clothing and a hat as appropriate when outdoors during the daytime, and they should also be sure to avoid sun exposure (even on cloudy days), use a broad-spectrum sunscreen to exposed involvement and, for involvement on the face, wear a broad-brimmed hat when outdoors during the daytime. The broad-spectrum sunscreen should provide protection from UVA and UVB light and should have an SPF of 50. Such a sunscreen is Solbar PF Cream SPF 50 sunscreen.

The use of lasers in the treatment of post-inflammatory hyperpigmentation is not generally recommended.

Post-inflammatory hypopigmentation/post-inflammatory depigmentation

I use the term post-inflammatory hypopigmentation to refer to the decreased brown pigmentation (without total loss of brown pigmentation) that can develop in the skin at sites where inflammatory lesions have healed. I use the term post-inflammatory depigmentation to refer to total loss of brown pigmentation that can develop in the skin at sites where inflammatory lesions have healed. Post-inflammatory hypopigmentation/post-inflammatory depigmentation is generally more prominent in appearance in dark-skinned individuals, but it can occur in light-skinned individuals. Post-inflammatory hypopigmentation/post-inflammatory depigmentation sometimes improves spontaneously over time, but in my experience there is no really good treatment for this problem.

PITYRIASIS ALBA

Overview

Pityriasis alba generally affects pediatric patients with macules and/or patches that initially have slight erythema, which fades over a period of weeks, leaving behind slight hypopigmentation with poorly demarcated, indistinct borders and fine, powdery scaling. (Macules are small, non-raised, non-palpable lesions. Patches are large, non-raised, non-palpable lesions.) Pityriasis alba occurs in all races but is more noticeable in Blacks. Involvement typically occurs on the face and upper outer arms. Usually the lesions are asymptomatic, but occasionally burning or itching is present. The lesions typically disappear over time with age but occasionally persist into adulthood.

It has been thought that pityriasis alba is an eczematous-type dermatosis with post-inflammatory hypopigmentation.

Special considerations regarding pityriasis alba

Pityriasis alba is distinguished from the superficial cutaneous fungal infection pityriasis versicolor in that potassium hydroxide (KOH) preparations of scrapings from lesions of pityriasis alba are negative, which is not the case with pityriasis versicolor. (For discussions of KOH preparations and pityriasis versicolor, see Chapter 18).

The poorly demarcated, indistinct borders and the hypopigmentation as opposed to depigmentation of the lesions of pityriasis alba help distinguish pityriasis alba from vitiligo. (I use the term hypopigmentation to refer to a decrease in brown pigmentation without total absence of brown pigmentation, whereas I use the term depigmentation to refer to total absence of brown pigmentation. See below in this chapter for discussion of vitiligo.)

Treatment of pityriasis alba

Although some dermatologists recommend the use of a topical cortico-steroid (e.g. hydrocortisone cream 0.5% for involvement on the face and hydrocortisone 1% for involvement on the arms) in treating pityriasis alba, I have not found this to be particularly useful. Since pityriasis alba is self-limited, I generally prescribe no treatment for it other than a bland emol-lient such as Nutraderm Lotion or Lubriderm Seriously Sensitive Lotion®.

IDIOPATHIC GUTTATE HYPOMELANOSIS

Overview

Idiopathic guttate (i.e. droplet-like) hypomelanosis is a condition that typically occurs in adults, is more apparent in dark-skinned individuals and is manifested by typical small (usually about 5 mm in diameter), porcelain-white, asymptomatic macules with well-demarcated, well-circumscribed, very discrete borders. The lesions of idiopathic guttate hypomelanosis most commonly involve the extremities and generally do not occur on the face. The distinctive clinical appearance of idiopathic guttate hypomelanosis dis-tinguishes it from other conditions with decreased brown pigmentation.

Treatment of idiopathic guttate hypomelanosis

In my experience there is no really good treatment for this condition. However, virtually all of my patients with idiopathic guttate hypomelanosis have not desired treatment of the condition once they have been informed of the fact that it does not have the potential to evolve into the potentially large lesions that can occur with vitiligo (see below for discussion of vitiligo).

VITILIGO

Overview

Vitiligo is typically manifested by variously sized areas that are depigmented (as opposed to hypopigmented) with sharp, well-demarcated, frequently scalloped borders. (I use the term hypopigmentation to refer to a decrease in brown pigmentation without total absence of brown pigmentation, whereas I use the term depigmentation to refer to total absence of brown pigmentation.) Involvement can occur on any area of the skin surface.

A variation of the typical vitiligo lesion is the trichrome lesion of vitiligo in which there is a band of intermediate color between the depigmented area of a vitiligo lesion and the adjacent normally colored skin. Occasionally an entire lesion of vitiligo can be of the intermediate color. However, this intermediate color is not stable and over time evolves at an unpredictable rate to typical depigmentation.

When repigmentation of vitiligo occurs, it can occur around hair follicles, in which case there is perifollicular normal pigmentation within an area of depigmentation.

In some patients, lesions of vitiligo can develop at sites where cutaneous injury has occurred. This is a manifestation of the Koebner phenomenon, which is the development of a lesion of a particular cutaneous condition at sites where cutaneous injury has occurred.

Special considerations regarding vitiligo

The exact etiology/pathogenesis of vitiligo is unclear. Etiological/pathogenic factors include hereditary and autoimmune processes, among others.

Although most patients with vitiligo have no associated disorders, patients with vitiligo are at increased risk for ocular disorders (notably iritis), thyroid disease, diabetes mellitus, Addison's disease, pernicious anemia, multiple endocrinopathy syndrome, alopecia areata and halo melanocytic nevi. For discussions of alopecia areata and halo melanocytic nevi, see Chapter 12 and Chapter 24, respectively.

Also, a vitiligo-like condition can be associated with malignant melanoma. For discussion of malignant melanoma, see Chapter 26.

In my experience, virtually none of the patients I have seen with vitiligo have had associated disorders.

Management of vitiligo

Protection

In terms of the management of vitiligo, patients with the condition should be instructed to avoid sun exposure (even on cloudy days); keep the areas of involvement covered with clothing and, if appropriate, a hat when outdoors during the daytime; wear a broad-brimmed hat when outdoors during the daytime for involvement on the face; and use a sunscreen with an SPF of 15 or greater when outdoors during the daytime. Sun exposure can burn the skin, especially lesions of vitiligo, thereby causing a worsening of the vitiligo via the Koebner phenomenon, which was described above; sun exposure can also tan normal skin without tanning the vitiligo lesions, thereby making the patient's vitiligo more noticeable as a result of the development of increased contrast between the vitiligo lesions and the tanned, normal skin; and lesions of vitiligo, because of their lack of melanin protection, are particularly susceptible to the carcinogenic effects of sun exposure.

Camouflage

For cosmetic purposes, patients can use a specialized, corrective make-up such as Dermablend®, which can be matched to the patient's normal skin color. Alternatively, the patient can use an over-the-counter skin dye preparation such as Vita-Dye®. However, the more recent over-the-counter 'sunless, self-tanning' preparations seem to be superior in appearance to older skin dye preparations such as Vita-Dye.

Topical steroids

Topical steroids applied to the vitiligo involvement can promote repigmentation but should be used when the involvement being treated is not extensive.

Hydrocortisone (e.g. Hytone®) cream 1% can be used in adults daily for limited involvement on the face [excluding the eyelids and periorbital regions, for involvement on which I would use hydrocortisone (e.g. Delcort®) cream 0.5%], ears, area around the ears, genitals and skin folds. For limited involvement in these areas in pediatric patients, I would generally use hydrocortisone cream 0.5%.

Triamcinolone (e.g. Kenalog® or Aristocort®) cream 0.1% can be used in adults daily for limited involvement on the scalp, neck, trunk, arms and legs. For limited involvement in these areas in pediatric patients, I would generally use hydrocortisone cream 1%.

Fluocinonide (e.g. Lidex®) cream can be used in adults daily for limited involvement on the hands and feet. For limited involvement in these areas in pediatric patients, I would generally use hydrocortisone cream 1%.

One regimen for employing the topical steroid treatment involves having the patient use the topical steroid daily for periods of 3 weeks at a time with each 3-week period of topical steroid use being separated by a 1-week period during which time the patient does not use the topical steroid. This should minimize the risk of topical steroid-induced adverse effects. (See Chapter 1 for discussion of topical steroid-induced adverse effects.) If the vitiligo has not responded following 2 months of topical steroid treatment, this treatment modality should be abandoned. If there is a response to this treatment, the treatment should be continued, and the patient should be monitored every 2 months for signs of topical steroid-induced adverse effects (such as striae and atrophy – see Chapter 1 for a more detailed discussion of topical steroid-induced adverse effects).

PUVA

For vitiligo patients for whom no other approach is satisfactory, referral to a dermatologist for consideration of PUVA therapy should be considered. PUVA therapy consists of the use of psoralen in conjunction with exposure to ultraviolet A (UVA) light.

It should be noted that PUVA therapy has definite limitations, which include the fact that it is associated with an increased risk for the development of skin cancers.

When PUVA therapy is administered, the dermatologist can prescribe the psoralen in a form that is administered orally or topically. Whether the psoralen is used orally or topically generally depends on the extent of the involvement. Also, the dermatologist can administer the UVA light via an artificial light box or via sun exposure. I do not recommend the latter, because ultraviolet light dosage can be much more precisely controlled with the former.

Surgical-type treatment

Mention should be made of surgical techniques for treating vitiligo. Patients for whom these may be appropriate should ideally have stable vitiligo (e.g. stable for 2 years) without koebnerization. Also, preceding treatment with PUVA should ideally have been done in order to determine the areas that do not repigment with PUVA (these would be the areas ideally suited for surgical treatment.)

The surgical techniques for the treatment of vitiligo basically involve placing grafts (e.g. punch grafts) of pigmented skin in lesions of vitiligo.

If surgical intervention is being considered, the patient should be referred to a dermatologist.

Depigmentation treatment

Vitiligo can also be treated by permanently depigmenting the patient's normal skin so that all of the patient's skin matches. Patients who are candidates for this approach are patients whose vitiligo involvement is more extensive than is his or her normally pigmented skin and/or for whom other approaches have been unsatisfactory.

The depigmentation approach involves the use of monobenzylether of hydroquinone (MBEH) cream 20%, which generally produces depigmentation that is permanent and is not reversible. (Hydroquinone, which was discussed earlier in this chapter, produces hypopigmentation that is not permanent and is reversible, unlike MBEH 20%.)

Generally, when MBEH depigmentation is performed for the treatment of vitiligo, all of the patient's normally pigmented skin is treated in order to produce depigmentation of this, such that the color of the patient's entire skin surface matches. If only a portion of the patient's normally pigmented skin is treated with MBEH, depigmentation can occur unpredictably at distant sites.

If depigmentation therapy of vitiligo is being considered, the patient should be referred to a dermatologist.

DISTINGUISHING VARIOUS TYPES OF HYPOPIGMENTED/ DEPIGMENTED CONDITIONS

Features that aid in distinguishing various types of hypopigmented/ depigmented conditions are as follows.

Lesions of post-inflammatory hypopigmentation/post-inflammatory depigmentation are at sites where inflammation had been present previously.

Pityriasis alba has lesions that tend to be slightly, finely scaly and hypopigmented with non-sharp, poorly defined borders.

Idiopathic guttate hypomelanosis tends to have lesions that are small and porcelain-white with sharp, well-defined borders.

Vitiligo tends to have large lesions that are depigmented (although trichrome vitiligo lesions can be present, as described above), with sharp, well-defined scalloped borders.

Pityriasis versicolor (see Chapter 18) tends to have scaly lesions that are hypopigmented (hyperpigmented lesions may also be present), the lesions may fluoresce a yellowish color when exposed to the ultraviolet light of a Wood's lamp, and a KOH preparation (see Chapter 18) should be positive.

Chemically induced leukoderma is associated with a history of exposure to phenol-type disinfectants.

Leprosy occurs in endemic areas, and it has anesthetic lesions.

The depigmented patches that can occur with systemic or cutaneous lupus erythematosus can have associated erythema and cutaneous atrophy.

Serological testing for lupus erythematosus may be positive, and skin biopsy may show characteristic findings.

The hypopigmented macules or patches that can occur with cutaneous T-cell lymphoma and with sarcoidosis have characteristic findings on skin biopsy.

The hypopigmented macules of tuberous sclerosis are typically congenital, stable and off-white, and can vary in size from 0.4 cm to 12 cm (average size is 1–3 cm). Off-white confetti (tiny, 2–3-mm) macules are also seen.

Nevus depigmentosus consists of congenital, stable, somewhat dermatomal hypopigmentation that is of no medical significance.

Piebaldism is an autosomal dominant condition that is congenital and typically stable, and the pigmentary changes characteristically consist of a white forelock (an area of white hair typically involving the midline frontal scalp), depigmented cutaneous patches and hyperpigmented cutaneous patches, some of which may be present within the confines of depigmented patches, within which there may also be normally pigmented patches.

8

Hypertrophic scars and keloids

OVERVIEW

Hypertrophic scars and keloids are sometimes tender, sometimes itchy, firm, raised scars. Hypertrophic scars generally flatten over time, whereas keloids stay the same or enlarge, sometimes beyond their original confines, over time. Darker-skinned individuals (e.g. Blacks, Hispanics and Asians) seem to be more susceptible to the development of hypertrophic scars and keloids, but it should be emphasized that this type of scarring is not limited to such individuals.

TREATMENT OF HYPERTROPHIC SCARS AND KELOIDS

Intralesional steroids

A good treatment for hypertrophic scars and keloids consists of intralesional steroid injections (billed as 'intralesional injections'). These are given as discussed and described in Chapter 2 for intralesional injectible Kenalog® (triamcinolone) suspension injections of prurigo nodularis lesions, except that the Kenalog concentration that I recommend for intralesional injections of hypertrophic scars and keloids can range from 2.5 mg/ml to 10 mg/ml. I sometimes need to use a concentration of ≥ 20 mg/ml, but because such a high concentration has a much greater potential for adverse effects, I do not recommend its use unless the healthcare provider is especially skilled and confident in the use of intralesional steroid injections.

The appropriate concentration of injectable Kenalog suspension is made up as described for intralesional Kenalog injections of prurigo nodularis lesions in Chapter 2. One ml of Kenalog suspension 2.5 mg/ml is made by using 0.25 ml of 10 mg/ml injectable Kenalog suspension and 0.75 ml of injectible saline solution or injectable 1% plain lidocaine solution. Injectable plain lidocaine solution on injection causes a 'burning' sensation but provides an anesthetic effect after the injection, whereas injectable saline solution produces no such 'burning' sensation on injection but provides no anesthetic effect after injection. One milliliter of 5 mg/ml Kenalog suspension is made by using 0.5 ml of 10 mg/ml injectable Kenalog suspension and 0.5 ml of injectable saline solution or injectable 1% plain lidocaine solution. For a 10 mg/ml suspension of Kenalog, the suspension can be taken directly from the bottle of 10 mg/ml injectable Kenalog suspension, or 0.25 ml of 40 mg/ml injectable Kenalog suspension and 0.75 ml of injectable saline solution or injectable 1% plain lidocaine solution can be used to make 1 ml of 10 mg/ml suspension of Kenalog. One milliliter of 20 mg/ml suspension of Kenalog can be made by using 0.5 ml of 40 mg/ml injectable Kenalog suspension and 0.5 ml of injectable saline solution or injectable 1% plain lidocaine solution.

Obviously, the higher the concentration of Kenalog that is intralesionally injected, the greater is the efficacy of the injections, but also the greater is the potential for adverse effects (such as atrophy at the site of injection) resulting from the injections. I recommend starting out using a low concentration of injectable Kenalog suspension. The concentration of the injectable Kenalog suspension can be varied, depending on response, for subsequent intralesional Kenalog treatments, if such treatments are needed.

After the area to be injected is cleaned with an alcohol swab and then dried with sterile gauze, the hypertrophic scar or keloid is injected intradermally (using a 30-gauge needle) with an appropriate concentration of the injectable Kenalog suspension, ideally until the lesional area being injected blanches from the pressure of the intralesional intradermal injecting, but be aware that such blanching does not always occur, especially when the medication is being injected slowly. (Injecting slowly is less painful for the patient than is injecting more rapidly.) In order to prevent accidental intravascular injection of medication, aspiration (pulling back on the syringe's plunger) should be done immediately prior to the injection of the medication.

Since hypertrophic scars and particularly keloids can be quite firm, it can be difficult to achieve enough pressure in the intralesional injecting process to get the suspension into the lesion. To overcome this problem, it is sometimes useful to insert the needle intradermally into the hypertrophic scar or keloid and then inject the suspension as the needle is withdrawn from the lesion. (This technique can be thought of as creating a 'needle track' or 'channel' into which the triamcinolone suspension can be more easily injected.) Also, before injection, the hypertrophic scar or keloid to be injected can be 'softened' in order to facilitate the insertion of the Kenalog suspension into the lesion. The 'softening' is done by first treating the hypertrophic scar or keloid with liquid nitrogen. One must be very careful in the handling and use of liquid nitrogen because contact with it can cause severe frostbite at the site of contact – this is due to the extremely low temperature of liquid nitrogen. Also, liquid nitrogen should be placed only in containers made of appropriate material [e.g. Styrofoam® (polystyrene) cups] or in containers with linings made of appropriate material (e.g. special, Thermos®-like, lined vessels). Liquid nitrogen should never be kept in a closed container without appropriate venting (otherwise, pressure can build up in the container to the point where a pressure explosion occurs). The 'softening' of the hypertrophic scar or keloid with liquid nitrogen is done in the following way. Liquid nitrogen is placed in a Styrofoam cup. A cotton-tipped applicator is then dipped into the liquid nitrogen, after which the hypertrophic scar or keloid is touched with the liquid nitrogen-soaked cotton-tipped applicator so that a transient 'whitening' of the lesion at the site of the touching occurs as a result of the coldness of the liquid nitrogen-soaked cotton-tipped applicator. (The cotton-tipped applicator should have a solid wooden handle because liquid nitrogen spurts from the hollow channel in cotton-tipped applicators with hollow plastic handles and because the plastic of cotton-tipped applicators with plastic handles can crack when such applicators are placed in the liquid nitrogen in the Styrofoam cup.) This sequence of dipping the cotton-tipped applicator into the liquid nitrogen followed by touching the hypertrophic scar or keloid with the liquid nitrogen-soaked cotton-tipped applicator is done repeatedly until the whole lesion has been sequentially transiently white. It should be noted that, when the liquid nitrogen-soaked cotton-tipped applicator is touched to the lesion with greater pressure, the warm blood in the cutaneous blood vessels associated with the lesion is 'pushed away' so that less heat can be transferred from the warm blood to the site of the liquid nitrogen application. As result of this, this site of liquid nitrogen application gets colder, and therefore the 'freezing' effect (including 'freezing' destruction) is greater than when less pressure is applied to the lesion through contact with the liquid nitrogen-soaked cotton-tipped applicator. The liquid nitrogen treatment should soften the hypertrophic scar or keloid, which, after the whiteness disappears, is cleaned with an alcohol swab, then dried with sterile gauze, and then injected with the Kenalog suspension as described above. This injection should proceed more easily and require less pressure on the syringe plunger during the injection process as a result of the softening of the lesion by the above-described preceding liquid nitrogen treatment of the lesion. Be aware that, if the liquid nitrogen treatment is excessive, frostbite can result from the treatment; blistering, crusting and necrosis can develop within the next day or so; and this can result in further scar formation. Also be aware that liquid nitrogen treatment can cause post-inflammatory pigmentary alteration (hypopigmentation/depigmentation, hyperpigmentation), especially in dark-skinned individuals (see Chapter 7).

The intralesional injections of Kenalog are generally carried out every 4–6 weeks until the desired response is achieved. For the treatment of keloids in adults, I do not use more than a total of 20 mg of intralesionally injected Kenalog every 4–6 weeks. Excessive use of intralesionally injected corticosteroids can result in the clinical manifestations of Cushing's syndrome and hypothalamic–pituitary–adrenal axis suppression, as is the case with all forms of corticosteroid use.

I generally do not use intralesionally injected Kenalog, particularly large amounts, in pregnant or breast-feeding patients unless its use is approved by the patient's obstetrician or breast-fed baby's pediatrician, respectively. Likewise, I would use intralesionally injected Kenalog in pediatric patients with particular caution, if at all (pediatric patients can be considered to be especially susceptible to its adverse effects); in any case, pediatric patients are generally not compliant enough to undergo this treatment.

Cordran® tape

The use of the topical steroid preparation Cordran (flurandrenolide) tape is an alternative, but generally less effective, treatment for hypertrophic scars and keloids. It is used in the treatment of hypertrophic scars and keloids as discussed and described for the treatment of lichen simplex chronicus/prurigo nodularis in Chapter 2.

Silicone gel sheeting

Another modality for the treatment of hypertrophic scars and keloids is the prescription product Epi-Derm®, which is a brand of silicone gel sheeting. This product should not be used on open wounds and is contraindicated for patients who have dermatological conditions that disrupt the skin's integrity in the areas that would be covered by the silicone gel sheeting. When this product is used, proper hygiene as described below must be meticulously maintained.

When silicone gel sheeting is used for the treatment of a hypertrophic scar or keloid, a piece of the silicone gel sheeting is applied so that it fully covers the hypertrophic scar or keloid and extends one-quarter of an inch (0.5 cm) all of the way around the scar border. The exposed surface of the silicone gel sheeting should be covered with a plastic wrap or non-irritating paper tape or bandage to prevent sticking to clothing or other surfaces. The silicone gel sheet should be worn 24 h/day and should be removed every 12 h in order to wash both the scar and the silicone gel sheet in mild soapy water. For washing the silicone gel sheet, a basin should be filled with warm water and a small amount of lather should be worked up with a glycerin-based soap. The silicone gel sheet should be gently washed in the soapy water, rinsed and then patted dry. After washing, rinsing and drying of the scar site, the silicone gel sheet should be re-applied to the scar site. If it is not possible for the patient to wear the silicone gel sheet for the recommended 24-h period, the patient should wear it for a minimum of 12 h/day and should perform the washing as described above once during that period. Treatment with the silicone gel sheet should be carried out as described for 10–14 days. At about this time, the silicone gel sheet should begin to lose its adhesive quality and/or may become imbedded with surface dirt and should therefore be discarded and replaced by a new silicone gel sheet. This process of applying the silicone gel sheet, washing twice daily for 10–14 days, discarding the sheet at about 10–14 days of use, and applying a new sheet should be continued for 8–12 weeks.

If inflammation occurs as a result of the use of the silicone gel sheeting, the silicone gel sheeting should be applied for a 12-h period followed by 12 h during which the sheeting is not applied, and if the inflammation persists, treatment with the silicone gel sheeting should be discontinued.

The manufacture cites possible complications that can occur as a result of treatment with silicone gel sheeting. These possible complications include superficial maceration of the skin associated with the occlusive dressing, rash (inflammation) and pruritus.

More detailed instructions for the use of Epi-Derm silicone gel sheeting in the treatment of hypertrophic scars and keloids come with the product when it is purchased.

9

Seborrhea and acne

SEBORRHEA

Seborrhea is the condition in which the patient has excessive sebum production resulting in excessively oily skin. I have found that when a patient presents with this condition in conjunction with acne, the topical preparations used to treat the patient's acne (see below) generally also satisfactorily take care of the patient's seborrhea. When a patient presents solely with seborrhea, I have found that the use of Sebanil® or Seban Oil Inhibitor® (both of which are over-the-counter products intended solely for the treatment of seborrhea) works well for this problem. Another, newer product is Clinac O.C. Oil Control Gel®, which is available over the counter.

ACNE

Overview

Acne is a condition characterized by open comedones, closed comedones, erythematous papules, pustules, erythematous nodules and/or cysts typically involving the face, chest and/or back. Open comedones are also called 'blackheads', and closed comedones are also called 'whiteheads'. An open comedone is a hair follicle that contains a keratin plug and that has a wide orifice on the surface of the skin, whereas a closed comedone is a hair follicle that contains a keratin plug and that has a narrow orifice on the surface of the skin. Keratin is a protein that is produced by keratinocytes and is the substance of which hair, nails and the stratum corneum are composed. Keratinocytes are the cells that comprise the bulk of the epidermis, which is the superficial cutaneous layer that is located immediately above the dermis. The stratum corneum is the dead, horny, most superficial layer of the epidermis. Papules are small, solid bumps. Nodules are large, solid bumps. True cysts are rare in acne, and what we traditionally call acne cysts can actually be considered to be large, abscessed, fluctuant acne nodules.

It is not uncommon for women with acne to experience premenstrual flares of the inflammatory component of their acne. (One week before a woman's menstrual period starts, the woman will be in her menstrual cycle's luteal phase, during which time her physiological androgens normally increase, as discussed in the following section of this chapter.)

Although mild acne is often present at birth and may continue for a period of time during the neonatal period (probably as a result of adrenal androgens), onset of acne is usually during adolescence, with the condition spontaneously resolving in most patients a few years later.

Post-inflammatory pigmentary alteration (e.g. post-inflammatory hyper-pigmentation and/or post-inflammatory hypopigmentation/depigmenta-tion) and/or atrophic (depressed) and/or hypertrophic/keloidal (raised) scarring may be present following healing of inflammatory acne lesions. Post-inflammatory pigmentary alteration and scarring may spontaneously improve in appearance over time. Post-inflammatory pigmentary alter-ation is discussed in Chapter 7, and hypertrophic scars and keloids are discussed in Chapter 8.

I use the term 'physiological acne' to refer to acne that is not caused by any undeniably pathological process or medication. The above-described neonatal acne can be considered to be physiological in that it is probably a result of adrenal androgens that are non-pathologically present during the neonatal period, as mentioned above. The above-described acne that usu-ally begins during adolescence and spontaneously resolves in most patients a few years later can also be considered to be physiological in that it can be considered to result from an increased local skin (i.e. 'target tissue') response to a normal level of circulating androgen (e.g. testosterone), in which case the circulating androgen (e.g. testosterone) is converted locally in the skin to a more highly potent androgen (e.g. dihydrotestosterone) which leads to a more highly potent androgenic effect being exerted locally on the skin, thereby producing acne. This can be considered to occur, at least to some extent, in nearly all individuals during a certain, usually self-limited period of time during their lifetimes.

On the other hand, I use the term 'non-physiological acne' to refer to acne that is caused by undeniably pathological processes that result in hyperandrogenism (e.g. systemic androgenic excess, as discussed below) – a manifestion of which is increased levels of circulating androgenic com-pounds – thereby resulting in non-physiological acne. Non-physiological acne can also refer to acneiform eruptions that have been associated with certain medications [e.g. systemic steroids, lithium, medroxyprogesterone (Provera®), oral contraceptives].

RULING OUT THE PRESENCE OF NON-PHYSIOLOGICAL CAUSES OF ACNE

In patients with early onset of acne (e.g. in early childhood, such as 7–9 years of age or younger, excluding the neonatal period – see above) or late onset of acne (e.g. in the fourth decade of life or later), I check to see whether the patient is taking any medication that has been associated with acneiform eruptions (see above), and I consider doing an endocrinological work-up to rule out a pathological etiology if it is otherwise clinically indicated. It should be noted that menstrual dysfunction (e.g. irregular or infrequent periods, amenorrhea, infertility) in premenopausal women can result from hyperandrogenism (e.g. systemic androgenic excess), which can result in acne. Hyperandrogenism should be considered particularly in older female patients with treatment-resistant acne and particularly in female patients with severe acne, acne of sudden onset, or acne associated with irregular menstrual periods or hirsutism, which is discussed in Chapter 11. Hyperandrogenism, in addition to resulting in acne, menstrual dysfunction and hirsutism, can result in deepened voice, increased muscle mass, clitoral hypertrophy and androgenic alopecia, which is discussed in Chapter 13. Severe hyperandrogenism, which can result in frank virilization (the features of which can include a deepened voice, increased muscle mass and clitoral hypertrophy), is not common, and patients with this problem should be thoroughly evaluated for a serious condition such as an androgen-producing tumor.

The endocrinological work-up can include taking a history, performing a physical examination and carrying out laboratory tests.

The history should include checking for menstrual dysfunction (see above), which can result from hyperandrogenism, which can result in acne. The history should also include checking for symptoms and signs of Cushing's syndrome or disease, with which hyperandrogenism and acne can be associated. (Cushing's syndrome or disease symptoms and signs that can be elicited from the history include fatigue, loss of libido, easy bruising, amenorrhea in a premenopausal woman, history of spontaneous fractures of ribs and/or vertebrae, history of carbohydrate intolerance or diabetes mellitus, and history of emotional disturbances.) The health-care provider should also check for a history of inappropriate galactorrhea, which can result from hyperprolactinemia, with which hyperandrogenism can be associated.

The physical examination should include checking for signs of hyperandrogenism (see above), particularly in a child or woman. The physical examination should also include checking for signs of Cushing's syndrome or disease, with which hyperandrogenism and acne can be associated. Cushing's syndrome or disease signs that can be observed on physical examination include central (truncal) obesity, hirsutism, facial rounding and fullness (moon facies), facial plethora, buffalo hump (fat deposition in the region of the base of the posterior aspect of the neck), purple skin striae, thin skin, proximal muscle weakness and hypertension. The health-care provider should also check for the presence of inappropriate galactorrhea, which can result from hyperprolactinemia, with which hyperandrogenism can be associated.

The laboratory tests should include serum dehydroepiandrosterone sulfate (DHEAS), total testosterone and free testosterone, and 17-hydroxyprogesterone between 07.00 and 09.00 and, for premenopausal women, 1 week before the patient's menstrual period starts or right when the woman finishes her menstrual period. [DHEAS is an adrenal androgen. Testosterone is a gonadal androgen. 17-hydroxyprogesterone has been used as a screening test for late-onset congenital adrenal hyperplasia, with which hyperandrogenism can be associated. Between 07.00 and 09.00, peak serum DHEAS, 17-hydroxyprogesterone and testosterone levels occur. One week before a woman's menstrual period starts, the woman will be in her menstrual cycle's luteal phase, during which time androgens increase. Right when a woman finishes her menstrual period, she will be in her menstrual cycle's follicular phase, during which time follicle stimulating hormone (FSH), which is discussed below, peaks and drops.] If the patient is a premenopausal woman who also has menstrual dysfunction (see above), I also test serum prolactin level as well as luteinizing hormone (LH) and FSH levels. Menstrual dysfunction can result from hyperprolactinemia, with which hyperandrogenism can be associated. Patients with polycystic ovary syndrome have high LH and normal or low FSH levels (i.e. increased LH/FSH ratio) as well as such findings that can include menstrual dysfunction, clinical hyperandrogenism, anovulation, obesity, insulin resistance and enlarged cystic ovaries. (The diagnosis of polycystic ovary syndrome is confirmed by the presence of enlarged cystic ovaries on ultrasound examination.) If the patient has amenorrhea, I also obtain an estradiol level. If the patient has any signs or symptoms of Cushing's syndrome or disease (see above), I in addition do a dexamethasone suppression test. When a dexamethasone suppression test is done, the patient takes dexamethasone 1 mg orally at 23.00 on any day that is after the day that the blood for the other above-described tests is drawn (so that the dexamethasone suppression test does not have an effect on the results of the other above-described tests), and this is followed by a serum cortisol level at 08.00 the following morning (normal for this test is a serum cortisol level that is less than 5). An alternative to the dexamethasone suppression test is the 24-h urine for free cortisol test, which is generally more expensive and less convenient for the patient than is the dexamethasone suppression test. Finally, if the patient has inappropriate galactorrhea, I obtain a serum prolactin level. (Inappropriate galactorrhea can result from hyperprolactinemia, with which hyperandrogenism can be associated.)

If there are any abnormal findings, the patient should be referred to an endocrinologist and, as appropriate, a gynecologist.

TREATMENT OF ACNE

Non-specific/indirect acne treatment

Obviously, the first step in the treatment of acne is to take care of any underlying non-physiological causes that are found (see above). Next, make certain that the patient uses only non-comedogenic (i.e. not acne-causing) products (e.g. make-up, moisturizers, sunscreens); if a product is non-comedogenic, this is usually stated on the product's label. There is no evidence that particular foods cause acne, so it is therefore not necessary for patients with acne to avoid particular foods.

Specific/direct acne treatment

Overview

More specific treatment is geared toward the treatment of comedones and inflammatory acne lesions, which develop from microcomedones and closed comedones, as described below. (Microcomedones are early microscopic closed comedones, whereas closed comedones, *per se,* are macroscopic.)

Treatment of comedones primarily and inflammatory acne lesions secondarily

The best and most specific treatment for comedones and microcomedones consists of the use of retinoids – one topical form of which is tretinoin and another, possibly superior, topical retinoid-like compound is adapalene – which reduce comedones and microcomedones, the reduction of which, as discussed below, secondarily ultimately results in a reduction of inflammatory acne lesions (sometimes preceded by a transient flare of inflammatory acne lesions). Retinoids are vitamin A derivatives, which can, in general, cause dryness and irritation of the skin and increased sensitivity of the skin to artificial and natural sunlight. Tretinoin is retinoic acid, one brand of which is Retin-A®. A formulation of Retin-A called Retin-A Micro Microsphere® is reported to be more effective than the mildest form of the regular Retin-A formulation, but is reported to be no more irritating and usually less irritating than the mildest form of the regular Retin-A formulation. However, in using it for my patients, I personally have not been particularly impressed with Retin-A Micro Microsphere in regard to these claims, and I therefore generally do not use this formulation of Retin-A. Another, possibly superior, brand of tretinoin is Avita®. The brand of adapalene is Differin®.

The only systemic retinoid approved for the treatment of acne is isotretinoin (the brand of which is Accutane®), which is taken orally and which is approved only for the treatment of severe recalcitrant nodular acne because of significant adverse effects associated with its use. In reference to the approved use of isotretinoin, nodular acne is defined as acne that is characterized by inflammatory acne lesions with a diameter of 5mm or greater; 'severe' is defined as 'many' as opposed to 'few or several' lesions of nodular acne; and recalcitrant refers to unresponsiveness to conventional therapy, including oral antibiotics (see below). Treatment with isotretinoin is discussed further below.

I do not use retinoids in pregnant or breast-feeding patients, and isotretinoin in particular is contraindicated in pregnant and breast-feeding patients.

Treatment of inflammatory acne lesions primarily

Overview   Treatment more specifically geared directly toward the reduction of inflammatory acne lesions consists of the use of antibacterial medications. Antibacterial medications reduce the number of *Propionibacterium acnes* bacteria (which are part of the normal skin flora), which metabolize sebum in hair follicles to produce free fatty acids, which traditionally in the past have been felt ultimately to lead to the rupture of the hair follicles associated with microcomedones and closed comedones, thereby resulting in the production of inflammatory acne lesions, although it is now felt that there are other probably more important mechanisms involving *P. acnes* regarding the development of inflammatory acne lesions.

It should be noted that if a patient responds to a topical or oral antibiotic with inflammatory acne improvement, this improved state can end after a period of time. This has been felt to be due to mutation of the bacteria so that they are no longer susceptible to the particular antibiotic that is being used. When this happens, the patient should be switched to a different antibiotic, after which the patient frequently improves again in terms of his or her inflammatory acne, and this has been felt to be due to the bacteria being susceptible to the new antibiotic. Sometimes after a period of time on the new antibiotic, the improved state ends again, and this has been felt to be due to the bacteria mutating so that they are now not susceptible to the new antibiotic. If the patient is again switched to another antibiotic (even sometimes back to the original antibiotic), improvement of the inflammatory acne may again be seen after a period of time, and this has been felt to be due to the bacteria being susceptible to the latest antibiotic (or, if the patient was at this point instead switched back to the original antibiotic, and improvement was seen with this, it has been felt that this improvement was due to the bacteria mutating back, so that they are now again susceptible to the original antibiotic). It is important to be aware that this changing susceptibility to antibiotics of the bacteria associated with inflammatory acne can occur so that changes in antibiotic therapy, when appropriate, can be made, thereby again resulting in improvement.

Topical antibacterial medications   Topical antibacterial medications include benzoyl peroxide (an effective brand of which with a low potential for irritation is Benzac AC® gel); erythromycin solution or gel (a brand of which is A/T/S® solution or gel); and clindamycin solution, gel, or lotion (a brand of which is Cleocin-T® solution, gel, or lotion), which, even in this topical form, has been reported to cause diarrhea, bloody diarrhea and colitis (including pseudomembranous colitis). Therefore, this medication, even though it is topical, is contraindicated in patients with a history of regional enteritis, ulcerative colitis, or antibiotic-associated colitis.

The topical preparation with probably the second greatest antibacterial effect is benzoyl peroxide, and the topical preparation that has probably one of the greatest antibacterial effects is Benzamycin gel (which is the brand of a topical preparation consisting of a combination of benzoyl peroxide and erythromycin). However, it should be noted that Benzamycin gel for some patients can be more irritating than Benzac AC gel and, unlike other benzoyl peroxide preparations, Benzamycin gel requires refrigeration after it has been dispensed to the patient.

I generally do not use topical erythromycin, topical benzoyl peroxide, or Benzamycin in pregnant or breast-feeding patients unless their use is approved by the patient's obstetrician or breast-fed baby's pediatrician, respectively. I generally do not use topical clindamycin in pregnant patients unless its use is approved by the patient's obstetrician, and topical clindamycin should not be used in breast-feeding patients.

Oral antibacterial medications   For additional antibacterial effect (along with a reported non-specific anti-inflammatory effect – unrelated to antibacterial activity – associated with some antibiotics), the most common oral anti-biotics used for the treatment of inflammatory acne are the tetracyclines and erythromycin. The tetracyclines include tetracycline (which can be abbre-viated TCN), doxycycline (brands of which include Doryx®, Monodox®, and Vibramycin®) and minocycline (a brand of which is Minocin®). For most patients, the tetracyclines tend to work better in treating acne than does erythromycin, but in some patients, erythromycin works better. In some patients with severe acne, when the oral tetracyclines and oral erythro-mycin do not seem to help, the oral combination drug trimethoprim/ sulfamethoxazole (brands of which include Septra DS® and Bactrim DS®) is sometimes effective.

Mention should be made of Gram-negative folliculitis, which is an uncommon complication of oral antibiotic therapy for the treatment of acne and is typically manifested by the development of pustules on the face. The diagnosis of Gram-negative folliculitis is confirmed by obtaining a bacterial culture and sensitivities (C&S) of pustule contents (which are accessed by piercing pustule roofs with a 20-gauge needle or a no. 11 scalpel). The condition is treated by switching from the oral antibiotic cur-rently being used to a course of an oral antibiotic chosen on the basis of the bacterial C&S results.

Of the tetracyclines, I have generally found minocycline to be the most effective in treating acne, but a disadvantage is that it can be more likely to cause pigmentation of the teeth, conjunctiva, and fingernail and toenail units. It can be more likely to cause bluish or blue-gray discoloration that is due to deposition of pigment in the dermal layer of the skin at sites where inflammatory acne lesions have healed (the dermal layer of the skin is the layer that is immediately below the epidermis, which is the superfi-cial layer of the skin). It can also be more likely to cause blue-gray discol-oration that is due to deposition of pigment in the dermal layer of previously normal skin, especially on the anterior lower legs, feet, fore-arms, gingiva, hard palate and the area around the eyes. It can be more likely to cause diffuse brown discoloration that is more prominent in sun-exposed areas and is due to an increased amount of melanin in the epidermal layer of the skin (melanin is a pigment that is normally found in the epidermis). Although it has been felt that minocycline-induced pigmentation may follow ingestion of 100–200 mg of minocycline daily for 1–3 years (there are cases in which pigmentation developed following shorter courses and lower doses of minocycline), in my experience minocycline-induced pigmentation has been quite rare. In 18 years of clinical practice, I have not noted any cases of discoloration due to minocycline ingestion other than one case of bluish discoloration (which resolved a few weeks following discontinuation of the minocycline) at sites of healed inflammatory acne lesions and one case of nail unit pigmentary changes (which slowly faded over time following discontinuation of the minocycline). In any case, it has been said that minocycline-induced pigmentary changes gradually resolve over a period of months to years following cessation of the minocycline, and it has been reported that one treatment with the Q-switched Nd : YAG laser at 532 nm provided excellent results. Other adverse effects of minocycline include lightheadedness, dizziness and vertigo (see below).

In my experience, doxycycline is probably in general the second most effective of the tetracyclines, but its disadvantage is that it is more likely to cause photosensitivity (as manifested by an exaggerated sunburn reaction) than are the other tetracyclines.

Probably, in general, the least effective of the tetracyclines, but still very effective in its own right, is tetracycline itself.

None of the tetracyclines should be used in pregnant or breast-feeding patients or in pediatric patients (I do not use tetracyclines for acne in patients younger than 12 years of age), and all of the tetracyclines can make the skin more sensitive to sunlight (as manifested by an exaggerated sunburn reaction).

I generally do not use oral erythromycin for acne in pregnant or breast-feeding patients. Hepatic dysfunction and hepatocellular and/or cholestatic hepatitis, with or without jaundice, have been reported to occur in patients receiving oral erythromycin products. Trimethoprim/sulfamethoxazole is contraindicated in pregnant and breast-feeding patients. Trimethoprim/sulfamethoxazole should not be used for the treatment of acne in patients with folate deficiency, and it should be noted that, with the use of trimethoprim/sulfamethoxazole in patients with glucose-6-phosphate dehydrogenase deficiency, hemolysis may occur (this reaction is frequently dose related). Trimethoprim/sulfamethoxazole is contraindicated in patients with severe renal insufficiency when renal function status cannot be monitored and in patients with marked hepatic damage. It should be noted that there have been rare fatalities due to severe reactions (including

Stevens-Johnson syndrome, toxic epidermal necrolysis, fulminant hepatic necrosis, agranulocytosis, aplastic anemia and other blood dyscrasias) associated with administration of sulfonamides. Trimethoprim/sulfamethoxazole should be discontinued at the first appearance of skin rash or any sign of adverse reaction. Trimethoprim/sulfamethoxazole is contraindicated in pediatric patients less than 2 months of age.

Before prescribing one of the tetracyclines, erythromycin, or trimethoprim/sulfamethoxazole, a check, as with all drugs, should be made regarding drug interactions, which include, but are not limited to, oral contraceptives being rendered less effective.

Miscellaneous agents

Azelaic acid   As a separate type of topical anti-acne medication, mention should be made of azelaic acid cream (the brand of which is Azelex Cream®), the active ingredient in which, azelaic acid, is a dietary constituent (found in whole-grain cereals and animal products) and can be formed endogenously. Its mechanism of action in the treatment of acne is unknown, but there is evidence that it causes normalization of keratinization leading to an anti-comedonal effect suggesting an ability to decrease microcomedone formation. There is also evidence that it has antimicrobial activity against *P. acnes*.

It has been reported that, in isolated cases, hypopigmentation has occurred following use of azelaic acid cream, so patients, particularly dark-skinned patients, being treated with this medication should be monitored for this potential complication.

I generally do not use azelaic acid cream in pregnant or breast-feeding patients unless its use is approved by the patient's obstetrician or breast-fed baby's pediatrician, respectively.

Ortho Tri-Cyclen® and Estrostep®   For physicians who are knowledgeable in terms of prescribing oral contraceptives, mention should be made of the oral contraceptives Ortho Tri-Cyclen (norgestimate/ethinyl estradiol) and Estrostep (norethindrone acetate/ethinyl estradiol), which are indicated for the treatment of moderate acne in females who are 15 years of age or older, have no known contraindications to oral contraceptive therapy, desire oral contraception, have achieved menarche and are unresponsive to topical anti-acne medications. In addition, Estrostep should be used for the treatment of acne only if the patient desires an oral contraceptive for birth control and plans to stay on it for at least 6 months. When prescribing Ortho

Tri-Cyclen and Estrostep, as with all medications, one should bear in mind potential drug interactions, which for oral contraceptives include decrease in their efficacy when used in conjunction with certain medications, which include certain antimicrobials, including the tetracyclines. Oral contraceptives are contraindicated in pregnant patients and should not be used in breast-feeding patients.

General principles regarding acne treatment

It should be noted that, when treating acne, it can generally take as long as 6–12 weeks of continuous treatment with a given regimen before improvement of the acne involvement is seen, and this should be discussed with the patient so that the patient understands and will therefore be appropriately patient and not become disappointed in this regard.

When topical anti-acne preparations are used as described below, the patient should be advised to apply them to the general areas of acne involvement and not just to individual acne lesions, because acne treatment is in general more effective in preventing the development of new lesions than it is in getting rid of existing lesions.

It should be explained to the patient that if the topical medications are too drying and/or irritating, the patient should use them less often, and then, if possible and as tolerated, should try to increase the frequency of application in step-wise fashion up to the prescribed frequency described below. The patient should also be told that he or she can use a non-comedogenic moisturizer (such as Nutraderm Lotion®) as frequently as necessary to try to counteract dryness and/or irritation. Also, it should be explained to the patient that if a topical medication causes burning or stinging on application – if the medication is applied too soon after the patient has dried his or her skin after it has been wet with water – he or she should wait about 15–20 min after the skin has been dried before applying the medication.

For normal hygiene, the patient should bathe using a gentle, non-irritating cleanser such as white, unscented Dove Bar® or Purpose Bar®. (Ivory® soap, which can be very drying and irritating, should not be used.)

If a retinoid or a tetracycline is used, the patient should be told that the retinoid or tetracycline can cause increased sensitivity of the skin to artificial or natural sunlight, and he or she should therefore accordingly avoid sunlamp and sun exposure, keep covered, wear a broad-brimmed hat (which provides supplemental sun protection for the face), and use a SPF 15 or greater, non-comedogenic sunscreen (such as Presun 29®) when outdoors during the daytime.

If a retinoid is used, it has been recommended that the patient should not undergo wax epilation on skin treated with the retinoid because of the potential for the development of skin erosions, and retinoids should not be used on sunburned, irritated or eczematous skin.

Also, if a retinoid is used, the patient should be told that his or her inflammatory acne component (i.e. the non-comedonal component) may get worse at first and flare, but he or she should also be told that the flare will be only temporary and will generally get better with continued use of the retinoid.

Other than carrying out what is described in the non-specific treatment section (see above) and performing acne surgery (see below), I generally do not treat pregnant or breast-feeding patients for acne.

A treatment regimen for the treatment of minimal to moderate acne

In general, I tell the patient to use only non-comedogenic products in terms of make-up, moisturizers and sunscreens (as discussed above). For normal hygiene (as discussed above), I have the patient use a gentle, non-irritating cleanser such as white, unscented Dove Bar or Purpose Bar. (Ivory soap, which can be very drying and irritating, should not be used.)

I prescribe Retin-A cream 0.025% to be applied to the general areas of acne involvement and not just to individual acne lesions (as discussed above) nightly at bedtime; Benzamycin gel to be applied to the general areas of acne involvement and not just to individual acne lesions (as discussed above) one to two times daily, not near the time of application of the Retin-A (which can be inactivated by benzoyl peroxide); Nutraderm Lotion to be applied as frequently as necessary to try to counteract any dryness and/or irritation and Presun 29 sunscreen (as discussed above). I explain to the patient that the Retin-A can make his or her skin more sensitive to artifical and natural sunlight; I tell the patient that that is why Presun 29 sunscreen is being prescribed; and I tell the patient that he or she should accordingly avoid sun or sunlamp exposure, keep covered and wear a broad-brimmed hat (which provides additional sun protection for the face) when outdoors during the daytime (as discussed above). Wax epilation should not be performed on skin treated with the Retin-A (as discussed above), so the patient is told this accordingly. In addition, I tell the patient that the Retin-A should not be used on sunburned or irritated (which would include eczematous) skin (as discussed above). I also tell the patient that if the medications are too drying and/or irritating, he or she should use them every other day or every third day at first and then try to increase the frequency of application in step-wise fashion up to every day, if possible (as discussed above). In addition, I explain to the patient that if the medications cause burning or stinging on application, he or she should wait about 15–20 min after the skin has been dried before applying the medications (as discussed above). I also explain to the patient that it can take as long as 6–12 weeks before improvement of the acne is seen, and the inflammatory acne component may flare at first as a result of use of the Retin-A, but I also tell the patient that the flare will be only temporary and will generally get better with continued use of the Retin-A (as discussed above). (I tell patients that the flare that can be associated with the use of Retin-A is as though the Retin-A were drawing out the pimples that are hidden underneath the skin. This seems to help patients feel better regarding the flare that may occur with the use of Retin-A.)

If the Retin-A is tolerated well, but improvement of the acne is not satisfactory, stronger Retin-A cream (i.e. 0.05% and then 0.1%) can be successively tried instead. Bear in mind that, at equal concentrations, Retin-A solution is generally more effective but also more irritating than is Retin-A gel, which is generally more effective but also more irritating than is Retin-A cream. I generally never use Retin-A solution at all; I only very occasionally use Retin-A gel 0.01% and 0.025%; I occasionally use Retin-A cream 0.1%; I sometimes use Retin-A cream 0.05% and if I am going to use Retin-A, I usually start out using Retin-A cream 0.025% (which is generally the best tolerated of all of the Retin-A formulations) and sometimes switch to one of the other Retin-A preparations if needed.

In general, I have found generic tretinoin preparations to be clinically equivalent to Retin-A, and I use them interchangeably with Retin-A.

As a rule, I have found that Avita (tretinoin) cream 0.025%, which is a newer preparation, is better tolerated and possibly more effective than are Retin-A (tretinoin) cream 0.025% and generic tretinoin cream 0.025% because Avita has a better cream vehicle. Because of this, I am increasingly inclined to start a patient on Avita cream 0.025% instead of Retin-A cream 0.025% or generic tretinoin cream 0.025%, when formulary restrictions are not involved. Also, in my experience the topical retinoid-like medication Differin (adapalene) gel 0.1%, which is a newer medication, seems to be more effective and less irritating than are Retin-A cream 0.025%, generic tretinoin cream 0.025% and even Avita cream 0.025%, so I am even more inclined to start a patient on Differin gel 0.1% instead of Retin-A cream 0.025%, Avita cream 0.025% or generic tretinoin cream 0.025%, when formulary restrictions are not involved. Another advantage of Differin gel over Retin-A, Avita and generic tretinoin is that Differin gel is not made less effective by benzoyl peroxide, so benzoyl peroxide preparations can be applied right after Differin gel has been applied and has dried, and the patient does not need to have an interval of time between applications of the two preparations. (When using benzoyl peroxide preparations with Retin-A, Avita, or generic tretinoin, the benzoyl peroxide preparation should not be applied near the time of application of the Retin-A, Avita, or generic tretinoin, because these preparations are made less effective by benzoyl peroxide.) It should be noted that Differin also comes in a solution preparation, which may be more irritating but more effective than is Differin gel, and a cream preparation, which may be less irritating than is Differin gel.

I generally have the patient return to see me in 6–8 weeks, or sooner if needed. At each visit, I monitor the patient's status, and after cleaning with an alcohol swab the lesions to be injected, I then dry the lesions with sterile gauze, after which I intralesionally inject (billed as 'intralesional injections') large inflammatory acne lesions with injectible Kenalog® (triamcinolone) suspension 2.5 mg/ml as discussed and described for intralesional steroid injections of prurigo nodularis lesions in Chapter 2. However, for inflammatory acne cysts, I insert the syringe needle into the cavity of the cyst and inject the Kenalog into the cavity until the cavity is filled, and for inflammatory acne nodules (which are solid), I insert the syringe needle into the dermis of the nodule, and I inject the Kenalog intradermally into the lesion, ideally until the lesional area being injected blanches from the pressure of the intralesional intradermal injecting. Be aware that such blanching does not always occur, however, especially when the medication is being injected slowly. (Injecting slowly is less painful for the patient than is injecting more rapidly.) In order to prevent accidental intravascular injection of medication, aspiration (pulling back on the syringe's plunger) should be done immediately prior to injection of the medication.

In addition, after the lesions to be injected are cleaned with an alcohol swab and then dried with sterile gauze, I intralesionally inject with injectible Kenalog suspension any hypertrophic scars or keloids that resulted from healed inflammatory acne lesions. These intralesional Kenalog injections of hypertrophic scars and keloids are carried out as discussed and described in Chapter 8, in which treatment of hypertrophic scars and keloids with Cordran® (flurandrenolide) tape and with Epi-Derm® silicon gel sheeting is also discussed.

Also, after the lesions to be incised are cleaned with an alcohol swab and then dried with sterile gauze, I incise comedones and pustules with a no. 11 scalpel or a 20-gauge needle. A Schamberg comedo expressor, which is a metal instrument consisting of a handle with a loop of metal at each end of the handle, is then used to express the contents of the comedones and pustules. This is done by placing the Schamberg comedo expressor so that the previously described incision is in the center of one of the loops at the end of the comedo expressor and then applying pressure to the comedo expressor, sometimes while sliding the loop of the comedo expressor on the skin surface. This expresses the contents of the lesion that was incised (this is called 'acne surgery' and is billed as such). It should be noted that the incision and expression of comedones proceeds more easily after the patient has been on retinoid therapy for a few weeks.

Benzac AC (benzoyl peroxide) gel 5% can be substituted for Benzamycin gel if Benzamycin gel is not tolerated well or is not otherwise acceptable to the patient, although it should be remembered that, in my experience, Benzac AC is not as effective as Benzamycin. Benzac AC gel 2.5% can instead be used if Benzac AC gel 5% is too drying and/or irritating, and Benzac AC gel 10% can instead be used if Benzac AC gel 5% is well tolerated but not satisfactorily effective. I have generally found that benzoyl peroxide washes are not particularly effective, so I usually do not prescribe them.

For additional antibacterial effect or for substitution for other preparations that are being used but are not being tolerated or are not helping, a topical antibiotic such as topical erythromycin (A/T/S) or topical clindamycin (Cleocin-T) can be used (see above). Likewise, topical azelaic acid (Azelex Cream) can be used (see above).

Other than carrying out what is described in the non-specific treatment section (see above) and performing acne surgery (see above), I generally do not treat pregnant or breast-feeding patients for acne.

A treatment regimen for moderate to severe acne

For moderate to severe acne, I start out using an oral antibiotic along with the topical regimen using a topical retinoid and a benzoyl peroxide preparation as described above. I commonly start out with tetracycline 500 mg one pill twice a day if not otherwise unadvisable and have the patient accordingly avoid sun and sunlamp exposure, keep covered, wear a broad-brimmed hat and use Presun 29 sunscreen when outdoors during the daytime (see above). For maximum absorption, the tetracycline should be taken on an empty stomach (i.e. 1 h before meals or 2 h after meals). I tell the patient that it can take 6–12 weeks of treatment before we start to see improvement. I also tell the patient that if he or she reaches a point where for a long period of time (weeks) he or she is doing very well and has no inflammatory acne lesions, he or she can decrease the tetracycline to 500 mg one pill daily; if he or she continues to do very well and has no inflammatory acne lesions for a continued long period of time (weeks), he or she can decrease the tetracycline to 500 mg one pill every other day; and if he or she continues to do very well for a continued long period of time as described previously, he or she can discontinue the tetracycline. I tell the patient that if at any point after decreasing the tetracycline dosage the inflammatory acne component worsens, he or she can go back to the last dose that was controlling the acne and, if necessary, he or she can increase the dose up to a maximum of 500 mg one pill twice a day. I also tell the patient that if at any point he or she is not tolerating the tetracycline well, he or she should discontinue it and call me. I generally have the patient return to see me in 6 weeks, or sooner if needed, and at every visit I monitor the patient's status and perform intralesional Kenalog injections and incise and express lesions as described above.

In place of tetracycline, doxycycline 100 mg one pill daily, with the same sunlight precautions as described above for tetracycline, can be prescribed. Unlike tetracycline, doxycycline can be taken with or without food. Again, I tell the patient that it can take 6–12 weeks of treatment before improvement of the acne is seen. I explain to the patient that if he or she reaches a point where for a long period of time (weeks) he or she is doing very well and has no inflammatory acne lesions, he or she can decrease the doxycycline to 100 mg one pill every other day, and if he or she continues to do very well and continues to have no inflammatory acne lesions for a continued long period of time (weeks), he or she can discontinue the doxycycline. I tell the patient that if at any point after decreasing the doxycycline dosage the inflammatory acne component worsens, he or she can go back to the last dose that was controlling the acne and, if necessary, he or she can increase the dose up to a maximum of 100 mg one pill daily. I also tell the patient that if at any point he or she is not tolerating the doxycycline well, he or she should discontinue it and call me.

Instead of tetracycline or doxycycline, minocycline 100 mg one pill every 12 h, with the same sunlight precautions as described above for the other tetracyclines, can be prescribed. Unlike tetracycline, minocycline can be taken with or without food. It should be noted that lightheadedness, dizziness and vertigo can occur with minocycline therapy, but these symptoms may disappear during minocycline therapy and usually disappear rapidly when minocycline is discontinued, and I discuss this with the patient. The patient can adjust the minocycline dosage according to the patient's response as described above for tetracycline, and I tell the patient that if at any point he or she is not tolerating the minocycline well, he or she should discontinue it and call me.

Instead of the tetracyclines, erythromycin 500 mg one pill twice a day can be used, if not otherwise unadvisable. It should be noted that for some formulations of oral erythromycin, optimal absorption occurs when the erythromycin is taken on an empty stomach (i.e. 1 h before meals or 2 h after meals), but other formulations of oral erythromycin can be taken without regard to meals (consult the package insert of the particular formulation of erythromycin being prescribed). The patient can adjust the erythromycin dosage according to the patient's response as described above for tetracycline, and I tell the patient that if at any point he or she is not tolerating the erythromycin well, he or she should discontinue it and call me.

Although many dermatologists do not do this, I monitor organ function as follows while patients are on oral tetracycline, doxycycline, minocycline, or erythromycin therapy for acne (package inserts recommend such monitoring during long-term treatment as is the case with acne therapy): I generally obtain a complete blood count (CBC) with white blood cell (WBC) differential and platelet count – liver function panel, creatinine level and urinalysis every 4–6 months.

If the tetracyclines and erythromycin are not successful or cannot be used, I consider using instead Bactrim DS or Septra DS (trimethoprim/ sulfamethoxazole) one pill daily for severe acne, if not otherwise unadvisable. The patient can adjust the Bactrim DS or Septra DS dosage according to the patient's response as described above for doxycycline, and I tell the patient that if at any point he or she is not tolerating the medication well, he or she should discontinue it and call me. Since hemolysis that is frequently dose related may occur when trimethoprim/sulfamethoxazole is used in patients with glucose-6-phosphate dehydrogenase deficiency, I consider testing the glucose-6-phosphate dehydrogenase level in patients who may be at risk for having deficiency of this enzyme. (Glucose-6-phosphate dehydrogenase deficiency is more common among Black Americans, Asians and persons of Mediterranean descent.) Also, when I use trimethoprim/sulfamethoxazole for the treatment of acne, I generally obtain a CBC (with WBC differential and platelet count), urinalysis with microscopic examination, blood urea nitrogen, creatinine and liver function panel at 2 weeks of therapy, at 4 weeks of therapy and at 8 weeks of therapy, and I then obtain CBCs approximately every month and the other tests approximately every 2–4 months thereafter.

Other than carrying out what is described in the *non-specific treatment* section (see above) and performing acne surgery (see above), I generally do not treat pregnant or breast-feeding patients for acne.

A treatment regimen for severe, recalcitrant, nodular acne that is unresponsive to conventional therapy

If a patient has severe, recalcitrant nodular acne that is unresponsive to conventional therapy, including oral antibiotics, I consider treating the patient with isotretinoin (Accutane), if not otherwise unadvisable as determined by the drug's approved indication and as discussed below. Severe, recalcitrant nodular acne that is unresponsive to conventional therapy, including oral antibiotics, is the only approved indication for isotretinoin (Accutane) treatment. In reference to the approved use of isotretinoin, nodular acne is defined as acne that is characterized by inflammatory acne lesions with a diameter of 5 mm or greater, and 'severe' is defined as 'many' as opposed to 'few or several' lesions of nodular acne.

It should be emphasized that Accutane is highly teratogenic and is contraindicated in female patients of childbearing potential unless the patient meets all of the following contitions: the patient must not be pregnant or breast feeding; the patient must be capable of complying with the mandatory contraceptive measures that are required for Accutane therapy for females of childbearing potential (see below); the patient must understand behaviors associated with an increased risk of pregnancy; and the patient must be reliable in understanding and carrying out instructions. Patients must not be pregnant while on Accutane therapy and for 1 month following discontinuation of Accutane therapy.

Accutane must be prescribed under the manufacturer's (Roche) System to Manage Accutane Related Teratogenicity (SMART). In order to prescribe Accutane, the prescriber must obtain a supply of yellow self-adhesive Accutane qualification stickers. To obtain these stickers, the prescriber must read the booklet entitled '*System to Manage Accutane Related Teratogenicity (SMART) Guide to Best Practices*' and must sign and return the completed SMART Letter of Understanding (the prescriber can obtain this booklet and letter by phoning 1-800-93-ROCHE and selecting Option 1 and then selecting Option 1 again). When Accutane is prescribed to any patient (male or female), a yellow self-adhesive Accutane qualification sticker must be affixed to the prescription.

For female patients, the yellow self-adhesive Accutane qualification sticker confirms that the patient has had two negative urine or serum pregnancy tests with a sensitivity of at least 25 mIU/ml before receiving the initial Accutane prescription. The first pregnancy test is a screening test that is obtained by the prescriber when it is decided to pursue qualification of the patient for Accutane. The second pregnancy test is a confirmation test that is done during the first 5 days of the menstrual period immediately preceding the beginning of Accutane therapy. For patients with amenorrhea, the second test should be done at least 11 days after the last act of unprotected intercourse, where unprotected intercourse refers to intercourse during which two effective forms of contraception were not used. The patient must have a negative serum or urine pregnancy test monthly during Accutane therapy, and the pregnancy test must be obtained monthly prior to the patient receiving her monthly prescription for Accutane. (Roche will provide urine pregnancy test kits and instructions on how to use them, and the prescriber can obtain these by calling 1-800-93-ROCHE and selecting Option 1 and then selecting Option 3.)

The yellow self-adhesive Accutane qualification sticker also confirms for female patients that the patient is using two forms of effective contraception simultaneously. At least one of these forms of contraception must be a primary form, unless absolute abstinence is the chosen method of contraception or unless the patient has undergone a hysterectomy. Primary forms of contraception include tubal ligation, partner's vasectomy, intrauterine devices, birth control pills, and injectible/implantable/insertable hormonal birth control products, while secondary forms of contraception include diaphragms, latex condoms, and cervical caps (each of these secondary forms of contraception must be used with a spermicide). Any birth control method can fail. Therefore, patients must receive written warnings about the rates of possible contraception failure [these written warnings are included in the patient booklets (see below) that the prescriber can obtain by calling 1-800-93-ROCHE and selecting Option 1 and then selecting Option 3]. It should be noted that micro-dosed progesterone preparations (so-called 'minipills' that do not contain an estrogen) may be an inadequate method of contraception during Accutane therapy. Also, prescribers should consult the package insert of any medication administered concomitantly with hormonal contraceptives to determine if that medication has the potential for decreasing the efficacy of hormonal contraceptives. In addition, patients using hormonal contraceptives should be warned not to use the herbal supplement St. John's Wort (depression has been associated with the use of Accutane in some patients) because of the potential for decreasing the efficacy of hormonal contraceptives. Female patients must use the two forms of contraception for at least 1 month prior to initiation of Accutane therapy, during Accutane therapy, and for 1 month after discontinuing Accutane therapy.

Counseling about contraception and behaviors associated with an increased risk of pregnancy must be repeated monthly.

In addition, the yellow self-adhesive Accutane qualification sticker confirms that female patients have signed the patient information/consent form that contains warnings about the risk of potential birth defects if a fetus is exposed to isotretinoin, and that the patient has been informed of the purpose and importance of participating in the Accutane survey and has been given the opportunity to enroll in this survey. (The prescriber can obtain a supply of the booklets (see below) that contain the patient information/consent forms and material regarding the Accutane survey by calling 1-800-93-ROCHE and selecting Option 1 and then selecting Option 3.)

If pregnancy occurs during treatment with Accutane or within 1 month of discontinuing Accutane, the desirability of continuing the pregnancy must be discussed with the patient. Prescribers should report all cases of pregnancy to Roche at 1-800-526-6367, where a Roche Pregnancy Prevention Program Specialist will be available, or to the Food and Drug Administration Med/Watch Program at 1-800-FDA-1088.

Accutane also has the potential for severe adverse reactions that can involve virtually any organ system. Most adverse reactions associated with Accutane therapy are reversible when Accutane is discontinued, however some adverse reactions have persisted following discontinuation of Accutane therapy. More specifically, some of the adverse reactions (in addition to teratogenicity in pregnant patients) include pseudotumor cerebri (benign intracranial hypertension); psychiatric disorders; acute pancreatitis; hypertriglyceridemia, hypercholesterolemia, and decrease in high-density lipoproteins (HDL); hearing impairment and tinnitus; hepatotoxicity; inflammatory bowel disease; hyperostosis; premature epiphyseal closure; and visual impairment, including decreased night vision, all of which are discussed in more detail below.

The use of Accutane has been associated with cases of pseudotumor cerebri. Some of these cases involved the concomitant use of tetracyclines, so tetracyclines should not be used when Accutane is being used. Symptoms and signs of pseudotumor cerebri include headache, nausea, vomiting, visual disturbances, and papilledema. Patients having these symptoms and/or signs should be checked for the presence of papilledema, and if papilledema is present, the Accutane should be discontinued immediately, and the patient should be referred to a neurologist for further evaluation and care.

Accutane may cause depression, psychosis, and, rarely, suicidal ideation, suicide attempts, and suicide. It may be insufficient merely to discontinue Accutane, and further evaluation and follow-up may be necessary following discontinuation of Accutane.

Accutane therapy has been associated with the development of acute pancreatitis in patients with either elevated or normal serum triglyceride levels, and in rare instances fatal hemorrhagic pancreatitis has occurred. If hypertriglyeridemia cannot be controlled at an acceptable level or if symptoms and/or signs of pancreatitis develop, Accutane should be discontinued.

Accutane therapy can be associated with hypertriglyceridemia, which is usually dose-related. In clinical trials, approximately 25% of patients on Accutane developed marked hypertriglyceridemia in excess of 800 mg/dl. Also, about 15% of patients developed decreased levels of HDL, and about 7% of patients developed hypercholesterolemia. These lipid effects were reversible on cessation of Accutane therapy in clinical trials. In some patients it is possible to reverse hypertriglyceridemia by weight reduction, dietary fat and alcohol restriction, and Accutane dose reduction while continuing Accutane. Blood lipid determinations should be performed before Accutane therapy is initiated and then weekly or biweekly until the lipid response to Accutane is established (which usually occurs within 4 weeks). Whether or not Accutane should be used in patients at high risk for lipid abnormalities should be carefully considered. (Patients at high risk for lipid abnormalities include those with diabetes mellitus, obesity, increased alcohol consumption, personal history of lipid metabolism disorder, and/or familial history of lipid metabolism disorder.) If Accutane therapy is instituted in such patients, more frequent checks of serum lipid and/or blood sugar levels should be done.

Hearing impairment and tinnitus have been associated with Accutane therapy, and in some patients impaired hearing has persisted following discontinuation of Accutane therapy. If a patient develops hearing impairment or tinnitus while he or she is on Accutane, the Accutane should be discontinued, and the patient should be referred for appropriate specialized evaluation and care.

Clinical hepatitis occurring in patients taking Accutane has been reported. In addition, about 15% of patients treated with Accutane in clinical trials had mild to moderate elevations of liver enzymes. Some of the patients with elevated liver enzymes showed normalization of these values with dosage reduction or continued administration of Accutane. Liver function tests should be performed before Accutane therapy is initiated and then weekly or biweekly until the response to Accutane has been established. Accutane should be discontinued and further evaluation initiated if normalization of abnormal liver function tests does not readily occur or if hepatitis is suspected during Accutane therapy.

In patients without a prior history of intestinal disorders, Accutane therapy has been associated with inflammatory bowel disease, including regional ileitis. In some patients, the problem has persisted following discontinuation of Accutane therapy. Accutane should be discontinued immediately in patients who have such symptoms and signs as abdominal pain, severe diarrhea, or rectal bleeding.

Accutane therapy has been associated with skeletal hyperostosis and calcification of ligaments and tendons. The skeletal effects are not known for multiple courses of Accutane treatment.

Although it is not known whether there is a causal relationship with Accutane, premature epiphyseal closure has been reported in patients on Accutane. As noted in the previous paragraph, the skeletal effects are not known for multiple courses of Accutane treatment.

Accutane should be discontinued, and opthalmological examination should be done for any Accutane patient who is having a visual problem. It should be noted that Accutane therapy has been associated with decreased night vision, and in some patients the problem has persisted following discontinuation of Accutane. Patients should be warned of the possibility of the development of this problem and should be told to be cautious when operating any vehicle at night.

Accutane therapy has been associated with problems in the control of blood sugar in some patients. Although no causal relationship has been determined, there have been cases in which the diagnosis of diabetes mellitus has been made during therapy with Accutane.

There have been patients who have had elevated CPK levels while underdoing vigorous physical activity while taking Accutane, but the clinical significance of this is not known.

Accutane therapy has been associated with anemia, leukopenia, thrombocytopenia, neutropenia, and, more rarely, agranulocytosis. Accutane therapy has been associated with hyperuricemia. Accutane therapy has been associated with glomerulonephritis, proteinuria, white cells in the urine, microscopic hematuria, and gross hematuria. Accutane therapy has been associated with alopecia, which in some cases has persisted following cessation of Accutane therapy; abnormal wound healing (e.g. delayed wound healing and development of exuberant granulation tissue with crusting); dry lips; dry mouth; dry skin; dry eyes; dry nasal passages; epistaxis, and increased susceptibility to sunburn.

Patients on Accutane should be warned not to donate blood while they are on Accutane therapy and for 1 month following discontinuation of Accutane therapy (because such donated blood could be given to a pregnant patient).

Patients should be advised that there may be a transient worsening of their inflammatory acne, most commonly during the early stages of

Accutane therapy. Patients should be warned that wax epilation and skin resurfacing procedures (such as laser resurfacing, dermabrasion) should not be performed while the patient is on Accutane and for at least 6 months following discontinuation of Accutane therapy (because of the possibility of scarring).

Patients should be warned not to have prolonged exposure to ultraviolet (UV) rays or sunlight.

Patients taking Accutane should be warned not to take vitamin supplements containing vitamin A (this is to avoid additive toxic effects that could occur as a result of Accutane's relationship to vitamin A) and should not take tetracyclines (Accutane has been associated with a number of cases of pseudotumor cerebri, some of which involved the concomitant use of tetracyclines), and patients using hormonal contraceptives should be warned not to use the herbal supplement St John's Wort because of the potential for decreasing the efficacy of hormonal contraceptives. In addition, microdosed progesterone preparations may be an inadequate method of contraception during Accutane therapy.

Before prescribing Accutane, the prescriber must be thoroughly familiar with the contents of its package insert. This is the case with all medications but is especially important with Accutane. Also, it should be noted that the Accutane package insert states: "Accutane should be prescribed only by prescribers who have demonstrated special competence in the diagnosis and treatment of severe recalcitrant nodular acne, are experienced in the use of systemic retinoids, have read the *SMART Guide to Best Practices*, signed and returned the completed SMART Letter of Understanding, and obtained yellow self-adhesive Accutane qualification stickers." (As noted previously, all these are available by phoning 1-800-93-ROCHE and selecting Option 1 and then selecting Option 1 again.)

The necessary laboratory test monitoring for patients on Accutane is as follows. At baseline, obtain fasting triglycerides, cholesterol, HDL, SGOT, SGPT, GGT, alkaline phosphatase, LDH, total bilirubin, albumin, appropriate pregnancy test for females of childbearing potential, CBC, platelet count, urinalysis with microscopic exam, blood sugar, CPK, and uric acid. At 2 weeks, obtain fasting triglycerides, SGOT, SGPT, GGT, alkaline phosphatase, LDH, total bilirubin, albumin, CBC, platelet count, and blood sugar. At 4 weeks, obtain fasting triglycerides, cholesterol, HDL, SGOT, SGPT, GGT, alkaline phosphatase, LDH, total bilirubin, albumin, appropriate pregnancy test for females of childbearing potential, CBC, platelet count, urinalysis with microscopic exam, blood sugar, CPK, and uric acid. Every 4 weeks thereafter while the patient is undergoing Accutane therapy, obtain fasting triglycerides, SGOT, SGPT, GGT, alkaline phosphatase,

LDH, total bilirubin, albumin, appropriate pregnancy test for females of childbearing potential, CBC, platelet count, urinalysis with microscopic exam, blood sugar, CPK, and uric acid.

Before starting a patient on Accutane and before obtaining the pre-treatment baseline laboratory tests, it is essential to discuss the risks, adverse effects, benefits, and precautions of Accutane (see above) with the patient. Also, male patients need to read the material in the booklet '*Be Smart, Be Safe, Be Sure, Accutane Risk Management Program for Men*, and female patients need to read the material in the booklet *Be Smart, Be Safe, Be Sure, Accutane Pregancy Prevention and Risk Management Program for Women* (the prescriber can obtain a supply of these booklets by calling 1-800-93-ROCHE and selecting Option 1 and then selecting Option 3). Female patients of childbearing potential should also be given the opportunity to view the videotape that deals with contraception and teratogenic drugs (the prescriber can obtain copies of this videotape for loan to patients by phoning 1-800-93-ROCHE and selecting Option 1 and then selecting Option 3). If the patient still wishes to proceed with Accutane therapy, male patients need to sign the appropriate form that is contained in the booklet *Be Smart, Be Safe, Be Sure, Accutane Risk Management Program for Men*, and female patients need to sign the appropriate forms that are contained in the booklet *Be Smart, Be Safe, Be Sure, Accutane Pregancy Prevention and Risk Management Program for Women*. Copies of the signed forms are then placed in the patients' charts, and for all patients the above-described pretreatment baseline lab tests are obtained. Also, with the use of the referral form that is contained in *Be Smart, Be Safe, Be Sure, Accutane Pregnancy Prevention and Risk Management Program for Women* woman may have free contraception counseling (reimbursed by Roche) by a reproductive specialist, the two reliable forms of birth control, and the appropriate second pregnancy test as described above. A copy of the referral form is placed in the patient's chart.

Before starting the patient on Accutane, I tell him or her not to take vitamin A or supplements containing vitamin A whilst on Accutane; I tell the patient not to use any other acne treatment, especially tetracyclines, during Accutane therapy (Accutane has been associated with a number of cases of pseudotumor cerebri, some of which involved the concomitant use of tetracyclines; Accutane by itself is very drying, and using other topical acne preparations can add to this drying); patients using hormonal con-traceptives should be warned not to use the herbal supplement St John's Wort (depression has been associated with the use of Accutane in some patients) because of the potential for decreasing the efficacy of hormonal contraceptives; I warn the patient that they may have decreased night vision both whilst on Accutane treatment and after it has been discontinued, and they should therefore take appropriate precautions; I also warn the patient that other visual disturbances can occur, and that they must discontinue the Accutane and notify me immediately if any visual disturbances occur (at which time I refer the patient to an ophthalmologist); I warn the patient not to donate blood during Accutane therapy and for 1 month after stopping Accutane therapy; I arrange for diabetic patients to have their blood sugars followed closely while they are on Accutane therapy; I explain to the patient that they may develop a flare of the acne (such a flare can be controlled with intralesional triamcinolone injections as described above and, if severe, with a 4 week tapering course of prednisone as described for generalized non-specific dermatitis in Chapter 2); I warn the patient that they should not undergo wax epilation or elective surgery (including laser resurfacing or dermabrasion) during Accutane therapy and for at least 6 months following cessation of Accutane therapy because there may be abnormal wound healing associated with Accutane therapy; I explain to the patient that during Accutane therapy, he or she may develop significant dryness of the skin and mucous membranes (including the lips, mouth, and nasal passages, dryness of the latter of which may result in epistaxis), and he or she should use a non-comedogenic moisturizer (e.g. Nutraderm Lotion) frequently for dry skin, Vaseline Petroleum Jelly frequently for dry lips, and a thin film of Vaseline Petroleum Jelly applied with a cotton-tipped applicator for dry nasal passages near the nostril openings; I explain to the patient that Accutane can make the skin more sensitive to sunlight (and sunlamps), so he or she should accordingly avoid sun (and sunlamp) exposure, keep covered, wear a broad brimmed hat, and use an SPF 15 or greater non-comedogenic sunscreen (e.g. Presun 29 sunscreen) when outdoors during the daytime; I have the patient discontinue the Accutane and notify me immediately if they develop any signs or symptoms of pseudotumor cerebri, psychological/emotional problems (including depression), acute pancreatitis, clinical hepatitis, or inflammatory bowel disease, as discussed previously in this chapter; I have the patient discontinue the Accutane and notify me if they begin developing any hearing impairment or tinnitus (at which time I refer the patient for appropriate specialized evaluaton and care); and I have the patient notify me if they begin developing alopecia.

If the pretreatment baseline lab tests are okay, men, and women who are not of childbearing potential, are started on the Accutane treatment regimen that is discussed below. For female patients of childbearing potential with okay pretreatment baseline lab tests, one must also obtain from the gynecologist the completed copy of the referral form confirming that contraception counseling and the required contraception have been provided and that the appropriate negative second pregnancy test has been obtained, if the patient has been on the required contraception for at least 1 month, the completed copy of the referral form is put in the patient's chart, and the patient is also started on Accutane as discussed below. In addition, female patients of childbearing potential should be encouraged to enroll in the Accutane Survey (a survey enrollment form is enclosed in each Prescription Pack of Accutane and is also enclosed in each *Be Smart, Be Safe, Be Sure, Accutane Pregnancy Prevention and Risk Management Program for Women* booklet).

When I start patients on Accutane, I generally start them on 1 mg/kg/day with this total daily dose being given in two divided doses. The recommended dosage range is 0.5–2 mg/kg/day with the total daily dose being given in two divided doses for 15–20 weeks (Accutane should be taken with food). Patients with very severe disease or with disease that is mainly on the body may require up to the maximum dose of 2 mg/kg/day. During treatment, the dose may be adjusted according to response and/or adverse effects, some of which may be dose-related. Female patients of childbearing potential should not be given their initial prescription for Accutane until they have been on the required contraception for at least 1 month as discussed above and until they have had negative results from the two pregnancy tests described previously. For all Accutane patients, no more than a 1-month supply of Accutane can be prescribed, and there can be no automatic refills. A yellow self-adhesive Accutane qualification sticker must be affixed to all prescriptions for Accutane.

While on Accutane, the patient must be monitored for the above-described adverse effects and for general monitoring when the monitoring lab tests are obtained (i.e. at 2 weeks of therapy, at 4 weeks of therapy, and then every 4 weeks thereafter while the patient is on Accutane) if the patient is doing well and having no problems. At each visit, intralesional Kenalog injections of appropriate inflammatory acne nodules, inflammatory acne cysts, hypertrophic scars, and keloids are done as described previously in this chapter. I generally do not intralesionally inject a given lesion with Kenalog more often than every 4 weeks, and I do not use more than 20 mg total of intralesionally injected Kenalog per 4–6 weeks. (In any case, an inflammatory acne nodule or cyst generally resolves within a few days after it has been intralesionally injected with Kenalog.) In addition, for female patients, counseling about contraception and behaviors associated with an increased risk of pregnancy needs to be repeated at each visit.

If there are no problems, the Accutane is continued for 15–20 weeks. After a period of 2 months or more after finishing Accutane therapy (during which time continued acne improvement can occur) and if warranted by persistent or recurring severe nodular acne, a second course of Accutane therapy can be prescribed in the same fashion as was done for the first course of Accutane as described above. It should be noted that for patients who have not completed skeletal growth, the optimal interval before retreatment is instituted has not been defined. It should also be noted that it has been observed that following completion of a course of Accutane therapy, many patients respond better to conventional acne treatment (as described earlier in this chapter) than they did prior to undergoing the course of Accutane therapy.

Treatment of hypertrophic scars, keloids, and post-inflammatory hyperpigmentation resulting from healed inflammatory acne lesions

Hypertrophic scars and keloids resulting form healed inflammatory acne lesions can be treated with intralesional Kenalog injections, Cordran (flurandrenolide) tape, or Epi-Derm silicone gel sheeting as mentioned previously in this chapter and as described and discussed in Chapter 8. Post-inflammatory hyperpigmentation resulting from healed inflammatory acne lesions can be treated as described in Chapter 7.

Other treatment for acne scarring, the appearance of which usually improves somewhat with time, is reserved for when the patient's acne is no longer active or is under excellent control. Also, a period of time needs to be observed following completion of Accutane therapy before surgical procedures are carried out to correct acne scarring. As discussed previously, Accutane causes abnormal wound healing, and therefore such surgical procedures should not be performed during Accutane therapy and for at least 6 months following cessation of Accutane therapy. When appropriate, as just described, patients with facial atrophic (depressed) acne scars can be referred to a dermatologist, who can arrange for treatment of these scars with intralesional collagen injections of the scars to 'fill them in'. The results of this are not permanent, and the effect resolves after a period of time, at which time the collagen injections are repeated, if desired. Alternatively, standard excisions of the scars followed by primary closure of the wounds and/or punch excisions of the scars followed by primary closure of the wounds or by punch grafting of the wounds can be done. In addition, when appropriate, as described above, patients with more extensive facial acne scarring can be referred to a dermatologist, who can arrange for treatment of this scarring with laser resurfacing, chemical peels, or dermabrasion, all of which are intended to 'even out' the scarred skin surface.

10

Acne-like skin conditions

Acne-like skin conditions include rosacea, perioral dermatitis, steroid-dependent facial dermatosis, acne keloidalis nuchae and hidradenitis suppurativa.

ROSACEA

Overview

Rosacea is a skin condition that develops during adulthood and consists of three cutaneous components, which in my experience may occur individually or in combination. The first cutaneous component is persistent erythema involving primarily the central face. After erythema has been present for a prolonged period of time, telangiectases can develop within the area of erythema. (Telangiectases are fine, red, superficial, cutaneous blood vessels.) Also, there can be episodes of flushing associated with the erythema. If a patient has flushing that is clearly not associated with the presence of rosacea, if the flushing episodes are spontaneous (in that they are not triggered by anger, embarrassment, or other such emotions), and if it is otherwise clinically indicated, I consider carrying out the following work-up to rule out causes of flushing other than rosacea: 24-h urine for total free catecholamines, vanillylmandelic acid (VMA) and metanephrines to rule out pheochromocytoma; 24-h urine for 5-hydroxyindoleacetic acid (5-HIAA) to rule out carcinoid; and 24-h urine for histamine to rule out mastocytosis.

The second cutaneous component of rosacea consists of recurrent acneiform erythematous papules involving primarily the central face; in addition, there may be recurrent acneiform pustules in association with the papules. This component of rosacea, unlike acne, does not exhibit comedones and premenstrual flares (see Chapter 9).

The third cutaneous component of rosacea consists of connective tissue hyperplasia manifested diffusely by coarse thickening of the skin involving the central face (particularly the nose) and also consists of discrete sebaceous gland hyperplasia manifested by persistent yellowish papules also involving the central face (particularly the nose). A severe form of connective tissue and sebaceous gland hyperplasia is called rhinophyma, which is a disfiguring condition of the nose.

Some patients with cutaneous rosacea also have ophthalmic rosacea, the onset of which can precede the onset of cutaneous rosacea. The components of ophthalmic rosacea are blepharitis, conjunctivitis, iritis, iridocyclitis, hypopyoniritis and/or keratitis. I refer all patients with ophthalmic rosacea to an ophthalmologist.

Treatment of cutaneous rosacea

Topical treatment

I feel that a good topical medication for cutaneous rosacea is MetroGel® (metronidazole gel 0.75%) or MetroCream® (metronidazole cream 0.75%). These medications are for the treatment of the acneiform papules and pustules, have little effect on the erythema and have no effect on the telangiectases and connective tissue and sebaceous gland hyperplasia. MetroGel is preferably used in patients with oily skin, whereas MetroCream can be used in all patients but particularly patients with dry and/or sensitive skin (MetroGel can be drying and irritating).

As is the case with acne (see Chapter 9), preventing the development of new acneiform papules and pustules of rosacea is more easily accomplished than is getting rid of acneiform papules and pustules that are already present. Therefore, when MetroGel or MetroCream is applied, it should be applied to the general areas of papulopustular rosacea involvement and not just to individual lesions. The medication should be applied one to two times daily, and it can take 6–12 weeks of treatment before improvement of the papulopustular involvement is seen.

A newer medication is Noritate (metronidazole cream 1%), which is indicated for treatment of the the erythema as well as the papulopustular lesions of rosacea, is applied once daily, and potentially may be less irritating than are MetroGel and MetroCream. (Noritate's vehicle contains fewer known irritants than do the vehicles of Metrogel or Metrocream).

I use topical metronidazole in pregnant patients only if its use is approved by the patient's obstetrician. Topical metronidazole should not be used in breast-feeding patients.

Another topical medication that can be used in place of topical metronidazole is sodium sulfacetamide 10%/sulfur 5% lotion (Sulfacet-R Lotion® or Novacet Lotion®), which is used the way topical metronidazole is used but is contraindicated in patients with kidney disease. I use sodium sulfacetamide/sulfur lotion in pregnant or breast-feeding patients only if its use is approved by the patient's obstetrician or breast-fed baby's pediatrician, respectively. Other topical products that can be used in place of topical metronidazole include benzoyl peroxide, topical erythromycin, Benzamycin® (benzoyl peroxide in combination with erythromycin) and topical clindamycin, which can be used as described for acne in Chapter 9.

Systemic treatment

For more severe papulopustular rosacea involvement, oral tetracycline, minocycline, doxycycline, or erythromycin (in conjunction with topical treatment as described above) can be used as described for acne in Chapter 9. It should be noted that, as described for acne in Chapter 9, the tetracyclines tend to work better than erythromycin in the treatment of the papulopustular involvement of rosacea in most patients, but in some patients, erythromycin may work better. Again, it should be noted that it can take 6–12 weeks of treatment before improvement of the papulopustular rosacea involvement is seen.

Physical/surgical treatment of telangiectases, diffuse facial erythema and rhinophyma   For telangiectases due to rosacea, patients can be referred to a dermatologist who can arrange for electrodesiccation (which is an electrosurgical procedure) or laser treatment of the telangiectases for cosmetic purposes. Patients with diffuse facial erythema due to rosacea can also be referred for cosmetic purposes to a dermatologist who can arrange for this problem to be treated with intense pulsed light (IPL) therapy, which differs from laser therapy and has provided beneficial results in the treatment of this problem. A dermatologist can also arrange for electrosurgical or laser treatment of rhinophyma for cosmetic purposes.

PERIORAL DERMATITIS

Overview

Perioral dermatitis is not a 'true' dermatitis, as described in Chapter 2, but clinically consists of an erythematous, sometimes scaly eruption of small papules, with small papulopustular or papulovesicular lesions sometimes being present, involving the skin of the perioral region.

Treatment of perioral dermatitis

The etiology of perioral dermatitis is unclear. Many dermatologists, with whom I am in agreement, feel that this condition in some cases can be caused or exacerbated by topical steroids. Therefore, in treating perioral dermatitis, topical steroids should not be used and should be discontinued in patients who are using them. Also, it is felt that, if a patient with perioral dermatitis is using a potent topical steroid that is abruptly withdrawn, the perioral dermatitis will undergo a rebound flare. To avoid this potential problem, patients with perioral dermatitis being treated with potent topical steroids should be tapered off the potent topical steroid by the use of successively lower-potency topical steroids over a few weeks until the patient is no longer on topical steroid therapy.

The best medication for the treatment of most patients with perioral dermatitis is oral tetracycline, which is used as described for the treatment of acne in Chapter 9. It may take 6–12 weeks of treatment before improvement is seen. The use of oral doxycycline or minocycline as described for the treatment of acne in Chapter 9 is also effective in treating perioral dermatitis. Oral erythromycin as described for the treatment of acne in Chapter 9 can also be effective in treating perioral dermatitis, but it is generally not as effective as are the tetracyclines.

If oral antibiotics cannot be used, perioral dermatitis can be treated with topical erythromycin or topical clindamycin as described for the treatment of acne in Chapter 9.

It is unclear why antibiotic therapy is successful in treating perioral dermatitis.

STEROID-DEPENDENT FACIAL DERMATOSIS

Overview

I have not uncommonly seen patients with what can be called steroid-dependent facial dermatosis, in which patients who have been using topical steroids on the face for any reason for a period of time can develop burning erythema, sometimes associated with erythematous papules and/or scaling, on the face as a result of the prolonged use of topical steroids on the face. Some patients with this condition may have underlying rosacea, and others may have underlying perioral dermatitis, but most patients whom I have seen with this condition seem to have had neither rosacea nor perioral dermatitis underlying the condition. When the topical steroids are abruptly withdrawn from these patients, a rebound flare of this condition frequently occurs.

Treatment of steroid-dependent facial dermatosis

For treatment of this condition, the topical steroid use needs to be discontinued. If the topical steroid being used is potent, the patient should be tapered off it by the use of successively lower-potency topical steroids over a few weeks until the patient is no longer on topical steroid therapy. In addition, if not otherwise unadvisable, I start the patient on oral tetra-cycline 500 mg one pill twice daily as described for oral tetracycline treat-ment of acne in Chapter 9. If the patient cannot take oral tetracycline but can take oral erythromycin, I would prescribe oral erythromycin 500 mg one pill twice daily as described for oral erythromycin treatment of acne in Chapter 9.

Because the patient's facial skin is very sensitive at this point, I have the patient apply nothing to the face other than cool plain water open wet compresses (which are soothing) as described for non-specific dermatitis in Chapter 2 and, if tolerated and if needed for dryness, a soothing, bland, non-irritating emollient such as Lubriderm Seriously Sensitive Lotion®.

In my experience, the problem completely resolves with this treatment within a few weeks, at which time all treatment can be discontinued. If the underlying problem (e.g. rosacea, perioral dermatitis, or other problem) subsequently becomes apparent, it can be treated accordingly (for example, rosacea or perioral dermatitis should be treated as described above) with-out use of topical steroids.

It is very important to give patients with what can be called steroid-dependent facial dermatosis insight regarding this condition (this insight helps them deal with the condition until it resolves) by explaining to them that, although topical steroid use keeps the condition from worsening, it is also somewhat paradoxically promoting the condition, so it is necessary to withdraw the topical steroid use as described above. Along these lines, the patients should also be advised that the condition may flare at first when the topical steroid is withdrawn, but with continued treatment as described above, it will get better and eventually resolve completely – I have had no patients for whom this was not the case.

ACNE KELOIDALIS NUCHAE

Overview

Acne keloidalis nuchae is manifested by recurrent, acneiform, erythema-tous papules, typically involving the occipital region of the scalp and the upper portion of the posterior aspect of the neck; in addition, there may be recurrent acneiform pustules in association with the papules. Some of the papules and pustules heal without sequelae while others heal with the formation of firm keloidal papules that may coalesce to form keloidal plaques.

I have seen this condition only in post-adolescent individuals, and I have rarely seen it in women.

Treatment of acne keloidalis nuchae

Treatment consists of the use of oral antibiotics (such as tetracycline, doxycycline, minocycline, or erythromycin as described for acne in Chapter 9) for the acneiform papules and pustules and the use of intralesional injectible Kenalog® (triamcinolone) suspension injections of acneiform papules and firm keloidal lesions as described for prurigo nodularis lesions in Chapter 2 and hypertrophic scars/keloids in Chapter 8, respectively. It can take 6–12 weeks of treatment before overall improvement of the acneiform component is seen. Improvement of the firm keloidal component can be seen after one or more intralesional Kenalog injections.

HIDRADENITIS SUPPURATIVA

Overview

Hidradenitis suppurativa in my experience is a not uncommon member of the group of what have been considered to be related skin conditions comprising the so-called 'follicular occlusion triad', which consists of acne conglobata and dissecting folliculitis of the scalp (also called perifolliculitis capitis abscedens et suffodiens of Hoffman) in addition to hidradenitis suppurativa. I consider acne conglobata to be a severe form of acne (acne was discussed in Chapter 9), although many consider it to be a condition that is separate from acne, partially because coagulase-positive staphylococci are frequently isolated and β-hemolytic streptococci are sometimes isolated from lesions of acne conglobata. Dissecting folliculitis of the scalp (also called perifolliculitis capitis abscedens et suffodiens of Hoffman) is quite rare in my experience, so it will not be discussed further here.

Hidradenitis suppurativa involves the apocrine gland-bearing areas of the skin, which include the axillae, groins and perineum. The clinical manifestations consist of recurrent cutaneous abscesses with subsequent resultant associated scarring, fistulas and sinus tracts. Hidradenitis suppurativa generally occurs in persons of adolescent age and older.

In my experience and in my opinion, the inflammatory lesions of hidradenitis suppurativa can be sterile (in which case normal skin flora contaminants are isolated on bacterial culture and sensitivities (C&S) of pus from inflamed lesions), somewhat analogous to the typical inflammatory lesions of acne (see Chapter 9), or they can contain pathogenic bacteria, somewhat analogous to furuncles and carbuncles (see Chapter 17).

Treatment of hidradenitis suppurativa

For treatment of hidradenitis suppurativa, local skin care consists of gentle washing with antiseptic soaps, the avoidance of tight-fitting clothing and the avoidance of deodorants. If not otherwise unadvisable, long-term use of oral antibiotics such as tetracycline, doxycycline, minocycline, or erythromycin (as described for acne treatment in Chapter 9) as well as cephalexin 500 mg every 12 h (with dosage adjustment and laboratory monitoring as described for tetracycline treatment of acne in Chapter 9) may be beneficial. As described for acne in Chapter 9, it may be necessary to switch from one antibiotic to another as the bacteria become resistant to the preceding antibiotic. (Also as described for acne in Chapter 9, the bacteria, after being treated in the interim with other antibiotics to which they are susceptible, can eventually become susceptible again to the anti-biotic to which they had become resistant.) If there is severe inflammation, a course of prednisone, as described for non-specific dermatitis in Chapter 2, may be useful if not otherwise unadvisable and if there is no pathogenic bacterial component to the involvement (see above). The use of Accutane® (isotretinoin) as described for nodular acne in Chapter 9, if not otherwise unadvisable, has been used with some success in patients with severe inflam-matory hidradenititis suppurativa, although this is not a package insert indication for Accutane.

I feel that hidradenitis suppurativa abscesses should not be incised and drained unless they are fluctuant and on the verge of spontaneously drain-ing, because I feel that incision and drainage can otherwise lead to sinus tract formation. If a hidradenitis suppurativa abscess is fluctuant and on the verge of spontaneously draining, it can be incised and drained (billed as 'incision and drainage of cutaneous abscess') as follows. (Before incision and drainage are performed in any patient with a heart murmur and/or artifical implant, the American Heart Association guidelines regarding incision and drainage of infected tissue in such patients should be consulted and followed accordingly to prevent bacterial seeding of the heart or artificial implant.) The local anesthetic 1% lidocaine with or without epinephrine is drawn into a 3-ml syringe with a large-bore needle such as a 20-gauge needle, which is then replaced with a small-bore needle such as a 30-gauge needle. Epinephrine decreases bleeding and prolongs the local anesthetic effect via vasoconstriction. However, I do not use epinephrine on such sites as the fingers, toes, and penis – some dermatologists recommend not using epinephrine on the nose and ear lobes also – because epinephrine can excessively decrease arterial blood flow at such sites, and this can result in tissue necrosis. The area to be incised is cleaned with an alcohol swab and then dried with sterile gauze. The 1% lidocaine is then injected intradermally into the site to be incised (a wheal will develop). In order to prevent accidental intravascular injection of anesthetic, aspiration (pulling back on the syringe's plunger) should be done immediately prior to the injection of the anesthetic. A no. 11 scalpel is then used to make a small puncture incision through the skin into the abscess cavity. Bacterial C&S of the draining pus are then obtained. The remaining pus is then gently expressed from the abscess cavity, and this can be facilitated by the gentle and careful insertion and withdrawal of a closed hemostat through the incision. The abscess cavity is not packed. If there is oozing of blood, pressure is applied to the oozing area with sterile gauze in order to stop the oozing. The area is then cleaned again with an alcohol swab and dried with sterile gauze, after which Polysporin Ointment® (polymyxin B sulfate/bacitracin zinc) is applied to the incision with a sterile cotton-tipped applicator, and a fresh piece of sterile gauze, held in place by paper tape, is then placed to cover the incision. If the patient is allergic to Polysporin Ointment but is not allergic to iodine, brown Betadine Ointment® (povidone-iodine) can be used in place of Polysporin Ointment. (Allergy to Polysporin Ointment, or to any other topical preparation, can be manifested by the development of increased inflammation or by non-healing of a wound without associated increased inflammation.) Clear Betadine Ointment should not be used in this situation, because it contains the same active ingredients that Polysporin Ointment contains. Beginning the next day, the patient removes the dressing, cleans the incision with hydrogen peroxide and a sterile cotton-tipped applicator, dries the area with sterile gauze, applies the antibiotic ointment with a fresh sterile cotton-tipped applicator and then covers the incision with a fresh piece of sterile gauze held in place with paper tape. (I tell the patient that if the dressing sticks to the wound and is therefore hard to remove, soaking the dressing with hydrogen peroxide prior to removal of the dressing will facilitate its removal.) The patient carries out this wound care twice daily until any drainage stops. An oral antibiotic is selected on the basis of the bacterial C&S results.

Abscesses can also be injected intralesionally with injectible Kenalog (triamcinolone) suspension, as described for inflammatory acne cysts in Chapter 9, if there is no pathogenic bacterial component to the involvement (see above).

If the patient is not doing well or not responding to treatment, consultation with a dermatologist should be obtained.

If involvement is severe with scarring, sinus tracts and fistulas, the patient can be referred to a dermatologist, who can arrange surgical intervention such as exteriorization of the sinus tracts and fistulas or complete excision of the involved area.

Complications of hidradenitis suppurativa

Hidradenitis suppurativa can uncommonly lead to rectal or urethral fistulas and strictures, and aggressive squamous cell carcinoma (see Chapter 26) can rarely develop in the sinus tracts or scarring of long-standing hidradenitis suppurativa.

11

Hirsutism and hypertrichosis

DEFINITIONS

I use the term hirsutism when referring to excessive hair in an adult male pattern occurring in females or boys, whereas I use the term hypertrichosis when referring to excessive hair that is not in an adult male pattern.

HIRSUTISM

Overview

When hirsutism is familial or idiopathic, it can be considered to be physiological (i.e. normal) in that the hirsutism is not caused by any undeniably pathological process or medication. Physiological (i.e. familial or idiopathic) hirsutism can be considered to result from an increased local skin ('target tissue') response to a normal level of circulating androgen (e.g. testosterone), in which case the circulating androgen (e.g. testosterone) is converted locally in the skin to a more highly potent androgen (e.g. dihydrotestosterone), which leads to a more highly potent androgenic effect being exerted locally on the skin, thereby producing hirsutism.

On the other hand, non-physiological hirsutism can refer to hirsutism that is caused by undeniably pathological processes that result in hyperandrogenism (e.g. systemic androgenic excess, as discussed below) – a manifestion of which is increased levels of circulating androgenic compounds – thereby resulting in non-physiological hirsutism. Non-physiological hirsutism can also refer to hirsutism that has been associated with certain medications (e.g. phenytoin (Dilantin®), danazol (Danocrine®), medroxyprogesterone (Provera®), oral contraceptives).

Ruling out the presence of non-physiological causes of hirsutism

In patients for whom hirsutism is not clearly familial, I check to see whether the patient is taking any medication that has been associated with hirsutism, and I consider performing an endocrinological work-up to rule out a pathological etiology if it is otherwise clinically indicated. It should be noted that menstrual dysfunction (e.g. irregular or infrequent periods, amenorrhea, infertility) in premenopausal women can result from hyperandrogenism (e.g. systemic androgenic excess), which can result in hirsutism. In addition to resulting in menstrual dysfunction and hirsutism, hyperandrogenism can result in acne, which is discussed in Chapter 9, deepened voice, increased muscle mass, clitoral hypertrophy and androgenic alopecia, which is discussed in Chapter 13. Severe hyperandrogenism, which can result in frank virilization (the features of which can include a deepened voice, increased muscle mass and clitoral hypertrophy), is not common, and patients with this problem should be thoroughly evaluated for a serious condition such as an androgen-producing tumor.

The endocrinological work-up can include taking a history, performing a physical examination, and carrying out laboratory tests.

The history should include checking for menstrual dysfunction (see above), which can result from hyperandrogenism, which can result in hirsutism. The history should also include checking for symptoms and signs of Cushing's syndrome or disease, with which hyperandrogenism and hirsutism can be associated. (Cushing's syndrome or disease symptoms and signs that can be elicited from the history include fatigue, loss of libido, easy bruising, amenorrhea in a premenopausal woman, history of spontaneous fractures of ribs and/or vertebrae, history of carbohydrate intolerance or diabetes mellitus and history of emotional disturbances.) The health-care provider should also check for a history of inappropriate galactorrhea, which can result from hyperprolactinemia, with which hyperandrogenism can be associated.

The physical examination should include checking for signs (see above) of hyperandrogenism. The physical examination should also include checking for signs of Cushing's syndrome or disease, with which hyperandrogenism and hirsutism can be associated. (Cushing's syndrome or disease signs that can be observed on physical examination include central (truncal) obesity, acne, facial rounding and fullness (moon facies), facial plethora, buffalo hump (fat deposition in the region of the base of the posterior aspect of the neck), purple skin striae, thin skin, proximal muscle weakness and hypertension.) The health-care provider should also check for the presence of inappropriate galactorrhea, which can result from hyperprolactinemia, with which hyperandrogenism can be associated.

The laboratory tests should include serum dehydroepiandrosterone sulfate (DHEAS), total testosterone and free testosterone, and 17-hydroxy-progesterone between 07.00 and 09.00 and, for premenopausal women, 1 week before the patient's menstrual period starts or right when the woman finishes her period. DHEAS is an adrenal androgen. Testosterone is a gonadal androgen. 17-Hydroxyprogesterone has been used as a screening test for late-onset congenital adrenal hyperplasia, with which hyperandrogenism can be associated. Between 07.00 and 09.00, peak serum DHEAS, 17-hydroxyprogesterone and testosterone levels occur. One week before a woman's menstrual period starts, the woman will be in her menstrual cycle's luteal phase, during which time androgens increase. Right when a woman finishes her menstrual period, she will be in her menstrual cycle's follicular phase, during which time follicle stimulating hormone (FSH), which is discussed below, peaks and drops. If the patient is a premenopausal woman who also has menstrual dysfunction (see above), I also test the prolactin level as well as levels of luteinizing hormone (LH) and FSH. Menstrual dysfunction can result from hyperprolactinemia, with which hyperandrogenism can be associated. Patients with polycystic ovary syndrome have high LH and normal or low FSH levels (i.e. increased LH/FSH ratio) as well as such findings that can include menstrual dysfunction, clinical hyperandrogenism, anovulation, obesity, insulin resistance and enlarged cystic ovaries. (The diagnosis of polycystic ovary syndrome is confirmed by the presence of enlarged cystic ovaries on ultrasound examination). If the patient has amenorrhea, I also obtain an estradiol level. If the patient has any signs or symptoms of Cushing's syndrome or disease (see above), I in addition include a dexamethasone suppression test. When a dexamethasone suppression test is carried out, the patient takes dexamethasone 1 mg orally at 23.00 on any day that is after the day that the blood for the other above-described tests was drawn (so that the dexamethasone suppression test does not have an effect on the results of the other above-described tests), and this is followed by a serum cortisol level at 08.00 the following morning (normal for this test is a serum cortisol level that is less than 5). An alternative to the dexamethasone suppression test is the 24-h urine for free cortisol test, which is generally more expensive and less convenient for the patient than is the dexamethasone suppression test. Finally, if the patient has inappropriate galactorrhea, I obtain a prolactin level. (Inappropriate galactorrhea can result from hyperprolactinemia, with which hyperandrogenism can be associated.)

If there are any abnormal findings, the patient should be referred to an endocrinologist and, as appropriate, a gynecologist.

Excessive hair and acromegaly

It should be mentioned that excessive hair can be seen in patients with acromegaly. However, the excessive hair in these patients differs from that seen in patients with virilizing conditions in that the excessive hair seen in patients with acromegaly spares the beard area.

Treatment of hirsutism

Obviously, the first step in the treatment of hirsutism is to take care of any underlying non-physiological causes that are found (see above). The following can also be performed for cosmetic purposes: bleaching of the hair in appropriate patients, use of over-the-counter depilatory creams that are intended for use on the face, plucking of hairs, waxing, referral to an electrologist for removal of hairs via electrolysis and/or referral to a dermatologist, who can arrange for removal of hairs via laser. Shaving can also be done, but be aware that there are women who are uncomfortable with this approach.

Vaniqa® (eflornithine) cream, which is an ornithine decarboxylase inhibitor, is available for the cosmetic slowing of growth of unwanted hair on the face and adjacent involved areas under the chin in women. Patients using Vaniqua should be informed that they will probably need to continue to use a hair removal technique (as described above) in conjunction with the use of Vaniqa, which is not a depilatory but retards the growth of hair, and within about 8 weeks following discontinuation of treatment with Vaniqa, hair growth may return to pretreatment levels. I would not recommend using Vaniqa, which is a medication used for cosmetic purposes, in pregnant or breast-feeding patients. The safety and efficacy of Vaniqa in patients under 12 years of age have not been established.

HYPERTRICHOSIS

Evaluation of hypertrichosis

For patients with hypertrichosis, evaluation for an underlying etiology should be pursued. Such etiology includes underlying malignancy or soon-to-develop underlying malignancy, acquired porphyria cutanea tarda (a test for which is a 24-h urine for porphyrins), association with certain hereditary conditions (including erythropoietic protoporphyria, variegate prophyria, porphyria cutanea tarda), use of certain drugs (including cyclosporin, minoxidil, phenytoin (Dilantin)), multiple sclerosis, hypothyroidism, anorexia nervosa and starvation.

Treatment of hypertrichosis

As with hirsutism, if an underlying problem is found, this obviously should be taken care of first. Also, the same cosmetic approaches as those described above for hirsutism can also be used for hypertrichosis.

12

Alopecia areata

Alopecia areata is a somewhat common hair-loss condition that can affect any part of the body, and it can be associated with nail changes, particularly fine pitting of the nails. Typically, alopecia areata involves the scalp with one or more characteristic well-demarcated patches of complete alopecia within which the scalp usually looks clinically uninflamed and normal.

Since secondary syphilis (see Chapter 27) can present with patchy, 'moth-eaten' alopecia of the scalp, it should be considered in the differential diagnosis of alopecia areata if the clinical circumstances are appropriate. Secondary syphilis can be ruled out by obtaining a negative rapid plasma reagin (RPR) or Venereal Disease Research Laboratories (VDRL) test.

Tinea capitis (discussed further in Chapter 18) also presents with patchy scalp hair loss, but it is usually associated with some inflammation of the scalp. To test for tinea capitis, a potassium hydroxide (KOH) preparation and/or fungal culture of scrapings and plucked hairs (which can be plucked using a small hemostat with or without rubber tubing placed on its clamping arms), as described in more detail in Chapter 18, from affected areas involving the scalp can be done. If the health-care provider is not qualified to run the laboratory portion of these tests in his or her office, the specimens can be sent to a clinical laboratory, which can run these tests, as described in more detail in Chapter 18.

Alopecia areata can also be manifested by diffuse (non-patchy) scalp hair loss (characterized by decreased hair density over the entire scalp without well-demarcated patches of complete hair loss) that can resemble anagen effluvium. See Chapter 13 for discussion of anagen effluvium and other conditions that should also be considered when considering diffuse alopecia areata.

The total loss of all scalp hair due to alopecia areata is called alopecia totalis. The total loss of all body and scalp hair due to alopecia areata is called alopecia universalis. The loss of scalp hair in a band at the periphery of the scalp due to alopecia areata is called ophiasis. In comparison, diffuse alopecia areata, as described above, is characterized by the loss of scalp hair diffusely, so that there is a decrease in hair density over the entire scalp without well-demarcated patches of complete hair loss.

In my experience, alopecia totalis, alopecia universalis, ophiasis and diffuse alopecia areata are much less common than is the above-described, more limited, patchy type of alopecia areata involving the scalp.

PROBLEMS ASSOCIATED WITH ALOPECIA AREATA

It is felt that alopecia areata is due to an autoimmune process directed against hair follicles. Alopecia areata has other autoimmune associations in that it has been associated with autoimmune thryoid disease, vitiligo (which has been felt to be an autoimmune disease), other autoimmune diseases and multiple autoantibodies (although patients with alopecia areata who have these autoantibodies generally do not develop an associated autoimmune disease). For a discussion of vitiligo, see Chapter 7. Alopecia areata has also been associated with atopy. For a discussion of atopy, see the section on atopic dermatitis in Chapter 2. In my experience, I have seen very few patients with alopecia areata who have had the above-described associated conditions.

PROGNOSTIC FACTORS PERTAINING TO ALOPECIA AREATA

Patchy alopecia areata not uncommonly spontaneously resolves, but spontaneous resolution is uncommon for alopecia totalis and alopecia universalis. Factors that have been reported to be prognostic of low likelihood of spontaneous resolution or poor response to treatment of alopecia areata include the ophiasis pattern of involvement, associated atopy, long duration of hair loss in a given area, onychodystrophy (abnormal nails) and onset in childhood (although nearly all of the patients I have seen with childhood alopecia areata with limited patchy scalp involvement have had spontaneous resolution or good response to treatment of their alopecia areata). I have frequently noted alopecia areata to be chronic or to relapse and remit spontaneously or with treatment over time.

TREATMENT OF ALOPECIA AREATA

Overview

Treatment of alopecia areata (i.e. inducing hair regrowth) is geared toward directly reducing inflammation (which is felt to be the result of the putative autoimmune etiology of the condition); stimulating inflammation (such as causing contact dermatitis; see Chapter 2) either by producing a non-hypersensitivity, non-allergic, irritant reaction or by producing a hypersensitivity, allergic reaction; or non-specifically stimulating hair growth by other means. It is not known why stimulating inflammation is beneficial – one thought is that the inflammation produced gets rid of the putative hair follicle antigen that triggers the putative autoimmune etiology of alopecia areata.

It should be noted that there are some patients who decide not to undergo treatment and prefer to wear hairpieces. (This tends to occur only in patients with extensive involvement.)

Treatment of alopecia areata by reducing inflammation

Topical steroids

Inflammation can be reduced by the application of a topical steroid such as non-augmented betamethasone dipropionate (Diprosone®) cream, which is a high mid-potency class III topical steroid (see Chapter 1), to the affected areas on the scalp twice daily in adults. (Other topical steroids in classes I to V have also been used to treat this condition.) In pediatric patients, I would generally use hydrocortisone cream 1% in place of the non-augmented betamethasone dipropionate (Diprosone) cream. If this form of therapy is successful for a given patient, it can take many months for adequate regrowth of hair to occur. When this therapy is used, the patient should be watched for the development of the adverse effects associated with topical steroid use (see Chapter 1), and this therapy should be used with particular caution in pediatric patients (as discussed in Chapter 1). I generally do not use this therapy in pregnant or breast-feeding patients unless its use is approved by the patient's obstetrician or breast-fed baby's pediatrician, respectively.

Intralesional steroids

Therapy using intralesional steroids (billed as 'intralesional injections') is more effective and more rapidly effective (early hair regrowth can sometimes be seen as soon as 4–6 weeks after an intralesional steroid injection) than is therapy using topical steroids, but the risk of developing adverse effects (steroid-induced adverse effects are discussed in Chapter 1) is greater with intralesional steroid therapy than it is with topical steroid therapy, and intralesional steroid therapy carries with it a particular risk for producing steroid atrophy at the site of treatment (i.e. at the site of injection).

Intralesional steroid therapy using injectible Kenalog® (triamcinolone) suspension 2.5 mg/ml for alopecia areata lesions on the scalp is performed as described for intralesional steroid therapy using injectible Kenalog suspension 2.5 mg/ml for prurigo nodularis lesions in Chapter 2, except that, for the intralesional steroid therapy for alopecia areata scalp lesions, the needle is placed in the deep dermis (i.e. deeply intradermally) or immediately subdermally (so that the Kenalog suspension will be injected at the level of the bases of the hair follicles) after the area to be injected is cleaned with an alcohol swab and then dried with sterile gauze. Immediately prior to injection, aspiration (pulling back on the syringe's plunger) should be done in order to prevent accidental intravascular injection. The Kenalog suspension is then injected just to the point where the injected area becomes palpable or, in addition, slightly raised. (If the injection is done in this fashion, no wheal should form as it does with standard intradermal injections.) This injection process is repeated until all involvement that is to be treated during the visit has been injected as just described. This treatment is repeated every 4–6 weeks until hair regrowth is satisfactory (assuming that the treatment is successful).

In the treatment of alopecia areata in adults, I intralesionally inject no more than a total of 20 mg of Kenalog every 4–6 weeks. The patient should be watched for intralesional steroid-induced adverse effects (as noted above, steroid-induced adverse effects are discussed in Chapter 1). In terms of intralesional steroid-induced local adverse effects, local steroid atrophy of the skin and/or subcutis can occur, especially, but not only, when the amount of steroid injected is excessive. (Local steroid atrophy of the skin and/or subcutis can be manifested by thinning of the skin itself as well as by depression of the skin at the sites of intralesional steroid injection.) In terms of systemic adverse effects, hypothalamic–pituitary–adrenal axis suppression as well as the clinical manifestations of Cushing's syndrome can occur as the result of excessive use of intralesionally injected steroids, as is the case with all forms of steroid use.

I generally do not use intralesionally injected Kenalog, particularly large amounts, in pregnant or breast-feeding patients unless its use is approved by the patient's obstetrician or breast-fed baby's pediatrician, respectively. Likewise, I would use intralesionally injected Kenalog in pediatric patients with particular caution, if at all (pediatric patients can be considered to be especially susceptible to its adverse effects); in any case, pediatric patients are generally not compliant enough to undergo this treatment.

Treatment of alopecia areata by stimulating inflammation

Inducing irritant contact dermatitis

Alopecia areata therapy involving stimulation of inflammation is probably most commonly done by using anthralin (Drithocreme®), which is used to create irritant contact dermatitis. Anthralin can be used for the treatment of alopecia areata in the same way that it is used for the treatment of psoriasis (described in Chapter 4), except that, when treating alopecia areata, Drithocreme (anthralin) 1% is applied to the scalp involvement and thoroughly washed off 10–20 min later, and this treatment is repeated daily.

Alternatively, Drithocreme (anthralin) in increasing concentrations and/or with increasing duration of application can be used for the treatment of alopecia areata, in which case it is used in the same way as it is used for the treatment of psoriasis (as described in Chapter 4), except that, in treating alopecia areata, the concentration and/or duration of application of Drithocreme is progressively increased until mild erythema is attained, and this is maintained until satisfactory hair regrowth occurs or until it is decided that this form of therapy is not working.

Inducing allergic contact dermatitis

Alopecia areata therapy involving stimulation of inflammation by causing allergic contact dermatitis can be performed using immunogens such as dinitrochlorobenzene (DNCB), which has not uncommonly been used by dermatologists in the past for the treatment of extensive or unresponsive alopecia areata (however, DNCB has been shown by the Ames bacterial test of mutagenicity to be mutagenic, so its use is controversial); diphencyprone; and squaric acid dibutyl ester. For this type of treatment, the patient would need to be referred to a dermatologist who performs such treatment or who can arrange for such treatment to be undertaken.

Treatment of alopecia areata by non-specifically stimulating hair growth

Non-specific stimulation of hair growth can sometimes be achieved by the application of the over-the-counter product topical minoxidal solution (Rogaine®). This medication is generally well tolerated, but it does have the potential for systemic adverse effects such as edema, cardiac irregularities and widespread hypertrichosis, especially when used in children or with the application of more than 2 ml/day over large areas. I would not use this medication in pregnant patients, breast-feeding patients, or pediatric patients unless its use is approved by the patient's obstetrician, breast-fed baby's pediatrician, or pediatrician, respectively.

Treatment of alopecia areata by using PUVA

If the patient has large areas of involvement, he or she can be referred to a dermatologist, who can arrange for therapy using the compound psoralen in conjunction with ultraviolet A (UVA) light (PUVA), which I feel probably works by reducing inflammation (by causing an immuno-suppressant effect) and/or by stimulating inflammation (by causing irritation). It should be noted that this therapy increases the risk for the delayed development of skin cancers and photoaging/photodamage on a generally dose-related basis.

13

Diffuse non-lesional alopecia of the scalp

In my experience, women (much more commonly than men) present with a complaint that I call diffuse, non-lesional alopecia of the scalp. This consists of diffuse (non-patchy) decreased density of scalp hair, frequently over the entire scalp (which is otherwise normal), with or without a complaint of increased shedding of scalp hair. In my experience, the problem most commonly ends up being androgenetic alopecia (this is discussed below). However, when there is significant associated increased shedding of scalp hair over the entire scalp, the problem most commonly is transient telogen effluvium (this is discussed below), but persistent pathological etiologies should be ruled out (this is discussed below) if clinically indicated.

TELOGEN EFFLUVIUM

Overview

Telogen effluvium is the increased, diffuse shedding of telogen (the 'resting' phase in the hair growth cycle) hairs from the scalp, sometimes with a perceptible decrease in scalp hair density, but telogen effluvium does not lead to total scalp hair loss. The scalp hair shedding of telogen effluvium generally occurs about 3–4 months following the occurrence of certain inciting conditions. If the inciting condition does not continue and is no longer present, the shedding will resolve over the next few months, and the hair density will return to its normal state over the next 6–12 months. On the other hand, if the inciting condition persists, the increased hair shedding and decreased hair density can persist and become chronic.

To confirm the presence of increased shedding of scalp hair, I generally have the patient collect and count all hairs shed during a 24-h period (normal is 50–100 hairs) because some patients feel that they are experiencing increased scalp hair shedding when in reality they are having no increase in scalp hair shedding.

Inciting conditions for telogen effluvium

Inciting conditions for telogen effluvium include parturition, hypothyroidism, hyperthyroidism, iron deficiency, zinc deficiency, protein deficiency, caloric deficiency, anemia, surgery, systemic illness, psychological stress and medication use. Medications that can cause telogen effluvium include β-blockers, anticoagulants, antimitotic agents, lithium, angiotensin-converting enzyme inhibitors and oral contraceptives (some patients can develop telogen effluvium as as result of starting oral contraceptives, and some can develop it as a result of discontinuing oral contraceptives).

ANDROGENETIC ALOPECIA

Overview

Androgenetic alopecia is a type of hair loss that is genetic (it has been said to be autosomal dominant with variable penetrance) and dependent on the presence of androgens. It occurs both in men and in women.

Androgenetic alopecia can be considered to be physiological (e.g. normal) in that it can be considered that androgenetic alopecia is not caused by any undeniably pathological process or medication. Androgenetic alopecia can be considered to result from a genetically determined increased local skin (i.e. 'target tissue') response to a normal level of circulating androgen (e.g. testosterone), in which case the circulating androgen (e.g. testosterone) is converted locally in the skin to a more highly potent androgen (e.g. dihydrotestosterone) which leads to a more highly potent androgenic effect being exerted locally on the skin, thereby producing androgenetic alopecia.

Androgenetic alopecia in men

Androgenetic alopecia in men usually begins in the third to fourth decade of life (although severe cases can begin immediately after puberty), may continue to worsen for years, and involves the development of decreased hair density (which may progress to total hair loss in the affected scalp areas) usually involving the bitemporal areas (bitemporal recession), the frontal area (frontal recession), the vertex and the top of the scalp. (This pattern of hair loss can be called 'male-pattern baldness'.) Rarely, androgenetic alopecia in men may manifest itself as a diffuse decrease in hair density over the entire scalp.

Androgenetic alopecia in men can be considered to be of cosmetic significance only, and it is treated only if the patient requests such treatment.

Androgenetic alopecia in women

Androgenetic alopecia in women should refer to women in whom there is no hyperandrogenism (e.g. systemic androgenic excess) present. If hyperandrogenism is present, the problem should more precisely be called androgenic alopecia (this is discussed below).

Androgenetic alopecia in women usually begins in the third to fourth decade of life (although severe cases can begin immediately after puberty), may continue to worsen for years, involves the development of decreased hair density (which generally does not progress to total hair loss) usually involving the top of the scalp diffusely, usually begins with a progressively widening 'part' running longitudinally anterior–posterior on the top of the scalp, and usually lacks frontal hairline recession or hair loss. (This pattern of hair loss can be called 'female-pattern hair thinning'.) Androgenetic alopecia in women may also manifest itself as a diffuse decrease in hair density over the entire scalp. Also, androgenetic alopecia in women may less commonly manifest itself in the usual male pattern ('male-pattern baldness') described above for androgenetic alopecia in men, although in women the condition generally does not progress to total hair loss in the affected scalp areas.

As is the case in men, androgenetic alopecia in women can be considered to be of cosmetic significance only, and it is treated only if the patient requests such treatment.

ANDROGENIC ALOPECIA

As noted above, androgenetic alopecia in women should refer to women who have no hyperandrogenism (e.g. systemic androgenic excess) present. If hyperandrogenism – a manifestion of which is increased levels of circulating androgenic compounds – is present, the problem should more precisely be called androgenic alopecia, which is less common than is androgenetic alopecia and indicates the presence of a non-physiological process, which should be treated. In addition to resulting in androgenic alopecia, hyperandrogenism can result in menstrual dysfunction (e.g. irregular or infrequent periods, amenorrhea, infertility) in premenopausal women; hirsutism, which is discussed in Chapter 11; acne, which is discussed in Chapter 9; deepened voice; increased muscle mass; and clitoral hypertrophy. Severe hyperandrogenism, which can result in frank virilization (the features of which can include a deepened voice, increased muscle mass and clitoral hypertrophy), is not common, and patients with this problem should be thoroughly evaluated for a serious condition such as an androgen-producing tumor.

ANAGEN EFFLUVIUM AND DIFFUSE ALOPECIA AREATA

Mention should be made of anagen effluvium, which is a type of diffuse hair loss resulting from shedding of anagen (the 'active growth' phase in the hair growth cycle) hairs from the scalp. It is typically caused by radiation therapy to the head or by systemic chemotherapy. Normal regrowth of hair occurs rapidly in most cases after the systemic chemotherapy is discontinued, although alopecia following high-dose busulfan may be permanent. Regrowth of hair following radiation therapy to the head depends on various radiation therapy parameters.

Anagen effluvium can also be caused by such toxic agents as mercury, boric acid, thallium and colchicine, and by ingestion of certain toxic plants. Severe protein malnutrition can also cause anagen effluvium.

Mention should also be made of diffuse alopecia areata (see Chapter 12), which can be manifested by diffuse scalp hair loss that can resemble anagen effluvium.

EVALUATION OF A WOMAN PRESENTING WITH DIFFUSE, NON-LESIONAL SCALP ALOPECIA OF UNCLEAR ETIOLOGY

When a woman presents with diffuse non-lesional scalp alopecia of unclear etiology, I ask her if she has been having increased shedding of scalp hair. If she says that she has been having increased shedding of scalp hair, I have her collect and count all hairs shed during a 24-h period (normal is 50–100 hairs) to confirm the presence of increased shedding of scalp hair. If indeed the patient has increased shedding of scalp hair, I find out whether or not she has had any serious illness, febrile illness, surgery, parturition, initiation of a new drug, trauma, or initiation of stress occurring about 3–4 months prior to the onset of the increased scalp hair shedding (to rule out some of the inciting causes of telogen effluvium as discussed above).

If the patient is premenopausal, I also inquire as to whether or not she has menstrual dysfunction (e.g. irregular or infrequent periods, amenorrhea, infertility).

In addition, the patient should have a general assessment of her health status. I also order the following tests as indicated: complete blood count (CBC), rapid plasma reagin (RPR) or Venereal Disease Research Laboratories (VDRL) tests, comprehensive chemistry panel, thyroid stimulating hormone (TSH), antinuclear antibodies (ANA), ferritin, zinc, dehydro-epiandrosterone sulfate (DHEAS), total testosterone and free testosterone, and 17-hydroxyprogesterone between 07.00 and 09.00 and, for premenopausal women, 1 week before the patient's menstrual period starts or right when the woman finishes her period. A negative RPR or VDRL test will rule out secondary syphilis (see Chapter 27), which can be cutaneously manifested solely by diffuse non-lesional alopecia of the scalp as well as by patchy 'moth-eaten' alopecia of the scalp. A negative ANA test will help rule out systemic lupus erythematosus, a manifestation of which can be diffuse non-lesional alopecia of the scalp. DHEAS is an adrenal androgen. Testosterone is a gonadal androgen. 17-Hydroxyprogesterone has been used as a screening test for late-onset congenital adrenal hyperplasia, with which hyperandrogenism, which was discussed above, can be associated. Between 07.00 and 09.00 peak serum DHEAS, 17-hydroxyprogesterone and testosterone levels occur. One week before a woman's menstrual period starts, she will be in her menstrual cycle's luteal phase, during which time androgens increase. Right when a woman finishes her menstrual period, she will be in her menstrual cycle's follicular phase, during which time follicle stimulating hormone (FSH), which is discussed below, peaks and drops. If the patient is a premenopausal woman who also has menstrual dysfunction (e.g. irregular or infrequent periods, amenorrhea, infertility), I also obtain a serum prolactin level as well as serum luteinizing hormone (LH) and FSH levels. Menstrual dysfunction can result from hyperprolactinemia, with which hyperandrogenism can be associated. Patients with polycystic ovary syndrome have high serum LH and normal or low serum FSH levels (i.e. increased LH/FSH ratio) as well as such findings that can include menstrual dysfunction, clinical hyperandrogenism, anovulation, obesity, insulin resistance and enlarged cystic ovaries. (The diagnosis of polycystic ovary syndrome is confirmed by the presence of enlarged cystic ovaries on ultrasound examination.) If the patient has amenorrhea, I also obtain an estradiol level. If the patient has any signs and/or symptoms of Cushing's syndrome or disease, with which hyperandrogenism can be associated, I in addition perform a dexamethasone suppression test. Signs and symptoms of Cushing's syndrome or disease include central (truncal) obesity, facial rounding and fullness (moon facies), facial plethora, acne, hirsutism, buffalo hump (deposition of fat in the region of the base of the posterior aspect of the neck), purple skin striae, thin skin, easy bruising, proximal muscle weakening, amenorrhea in premenopausal women, hypertension, carbohydrate intolerance or diabetes mellitus, fatigue, loss of libido, spontaneous fractures of ribs and/or vertebrae, and emotional disturbances. When a dexamethasone suppression test is done, the patient takes dexamethasone 1 mg orally at 23.00 on any day that is after the day that the blood for the other above-described tests was drawn (so that the dexamethasone suppression test does not have an effect on the results of any of the other above-described tests), and this is followed by a serum cortisol level at 08.00 the following morning (normal for this test is a serum cortisol level that is less than 5). An alternative to the dexamethasone suppression test is the 24-h urine for free cortisol test, which is generally more expensive and less convenient for the patient than is the dexamethasone suppression test. Finally, if the patient has inappropriate galactorrhea, I obtain a serum prolactin level. (Inappropriate galactorrhea can result from hyperprolactinemia, with which hyperandrogenism can be associated.)

If there are any abnormal findings, appropriate action should be taken, and this might include referral to an endocrinologist and/or a gynecologist, as appropriate.

EVALUATION OF A MAN PRESENTING WITH DIFFUSE, NON-LESIONAL SCALP ALOPECIA OF UNCLEAR ETIOLOGY

When a man presents with diffuse non-lesional scalp alopecia that is clearly not androgenetic alopecia and is of unclear etiology, I inquire as to whether or not he has been having increased shedding of scalp hair. If he says that he has been having increased shedding of scalp hair, I have him collect and count all hairs shed during a 24-h period (normal is 50–100 hairs) to confirm the presence of increased shedding of scalp hair. If indeed the patient has increased shedding of scalp hair, I find out whether or not he has had any serious illness, febrile illness, surgery, initiation of a new drug, trauma, or initiation of stress occurring about 3–4 months prior to the onset of the increased scalp hair shedding (to rule out some of the inciting causes of telogen effluvium). In addition, he should have a general assessment of his health status. I also order the following tests as indicated: CBC, RPR or VDRL, comprehensive chemistry panel, TSH, ANA, ferritin, and zinc. A negative RPR or VDRL will rule out secondary syphilis (see Chapter 27), which can be cutaneously manifested solely by diffuse non-lesional alopecia of the scalp as well as by patchy, 'moth-eaten' alopecia of the scalp. A negative ANA will help rule out systemic lupus erythematosus, a manifestation of which can be diffuse non-lesional alopecia of the scalp.

If there are any abnormal findings, appropriate action should be taken.

TREATMENT OF DIFFUSE, NON-LESIONAL ALOPECIA OF THE SCALP

In treatment of diffuse, non-lesional alopecia of the scalp in a man or a woman, any abnormalities that are discovered, as described above, should obviously be taken care of first.

As described above, androgenetic alopecia in men can be considered to be of cosmetic significance only, and it is treated only if the patient requests such treatment. Such treatment includes topical minoxidal solution, which is available over the counter as Rogaine®. Also, there is the oral prescription drug Propecia® (finasteride), which in my patients has been more effective than Rogaine has been. (Both Rogaine and Propecia generally require months of treatment with the medication before benefit is seen in those who receive benefit, and when treatment with either medication is stopped, any hair regrowth that resulted from the use of the medication will subsequently disappear.) In addition, patients can be referred to a dermatologist who performs surgical intervention regarding androgenetic alopecia, and probably the most common procedure for this problem is hair transplantation. Finally, hairpieces can be worn.

Androgenetic alopecia in women can also be considered to be of cosmetic significance only, and it also is treated only when such treatment is requested by the patient. As with men, treatment options include Rogaine (topical minoxidal solution), which I do not use in pregnant or breast-feeding patients unless its use is approved by the patient's obstetrician or breast-fed baby's pediatrician, respectively; surgical intervention such as hair transplants; and hairpieces. However, oral finasteride (Propecia) is not FDA approved for use in women because the use of this medication in a pregnant woman can cause her baby, if a male, to have genital deformity.

Since women with androgenic alopecia have the presence of systemic androgen excess, such patients should be evaluated and treated in conjunction with an endocrinologist and, if indicated, a gynecologist.

14

Hyperhidrosis and xerosis

HYPERHIDROSIS

Overview

Hyperhidrosis is excessive sweating. It most commonly involves and is limited to the palms, soles and/or axillae and, as such, is triggered by states of mental stress such as anxiety.

In patients with generalized hyperhidrosis, the presence of an underlying internal medical problem should be considered. Such internal medical problems include thyrotoxicosis, menopause, diabetes mellitus, hypoglycemia, congestive heart failure, hyperpituitarism, anxiety, dumping syndrome, carcinoid, pheochromocytoma, drug reaction (e.g. fluoxetine (Prozac®) and cyclobenzapine (Flexeril®)), brain lesions, or fever.

In patients with generalized hyperhidrosis occurring at night (i.e. night sweats), an underlying infectious disease or malignancy as well as hyperthyroidism, diabetes mellitus, hypoglycemia due to insulinoma, systemic vasculitis, pheochromocytoma, carcinoid syndrome, dysautonomic states, acromegaly and Prinzmetal's angina pectoris should be considered.

Treatment of hyperhidrosis of the axillae

Xerac AC Solution®

Regarding hyperhidrosis of the axillae, I first confirm that the patient has tried unsuccessfully a product such as Mitchum Antiperspirant®. If he or she has, I recommend the product Xerac AC Solution® (aluminum chloride (hexahydrate) 6.25% in anhydrous ethyl alcohol). Xerac AC Solution is applied to the axillae at bedtime, and the area should be completely dry prior to application in order to prevent irritation. (Xerac AC Solution should not be applied to broken or irritated skin.) It should be noted that transient stinging or itching may occur after application of Xerac AC Solution, and this may be prevented or reduced by applying the medication only to completely dry skin. If necessary, the medication can be removed by washing the area with soap and water. If actual skin irritation occurs, the medication should be discontinued.

Drysol Solution®

For hyperhidrosis of the axillae that is not responsive to treatment with Xerac AC Solution, I recommend the product Drysol Solution® (aluminum chloride (hexahydrate) 20% in anhydrous ethyl alcohol), which is applied to the axillae once daily only at bedtime, and, as with Xerac AC Solution, the area of application should be completely dry prior to application in order to prevent irritation. (Drysol Solution should not be applied to broken, irritated, or recently shaved skin.) It should be noted that Drysol Solution may produce a burning or prickling sensation. If actual skin irritation occurs, Drysol Solution should be discontinued.

Drysol Solution under occlusion   If the use of Drysol Solution as described above is not working satisfactorily, the effect of Drysol Solution can be enhanced by covering the treated area with Saran Wrap® (plastic clingfilm) held in place by a snugly fitting T-shirt or body shirt (the Saran Wrap should never be held in place with tape), with the treated area being washed the following morning. The hyperhidrosis may cease after two or more treatments, after which the Drysol Solution is then applied once or twice weekly or as needed.

Treatment of hyperhidrosis of the palms and/or soles

Drysol Solution and Drysol Solution under occlusion

Hyperhidrosis of the palms and/or soles is treated with Drysol Solution as described above for the treatment of hyperhidrosis of the axillae, except that, if Saran Wrap is used, it is held in place by a snugly fitting mitten and/or sock, accordingly.

Iontophoresis

Tap water iontophoresis, which requires an iontophoresis device, is an alternative modality for the treatment of hyperhidrosis of the palms and/or soles, but I have not found the need to prescribe this.

Hyperhidrosis treatment using local cutaneous injections of Botox®

It should be noted that some dermatologists are using local cutaneous injections of Botox® (botulinum toxin type A) to treat patients who have refractory hyperhidrosis that is unresponsive to other treatment modalities. (This is not a package insert indication for Botox.) Referral to a dermatologist should be considered for patients who have refractory hyperhidrosis.

XEROSIS

Overview

Xerosis (also called asteatosis), which is commonly pruritic, is dry skin (which is typically rough and scaling). Traditional thinking is that what is seen as dry skin is a manifestation of decreased water in the stratum corneum. (The stratum corneum is the dead, horny, most superficial layer of the epidermis and is composed of the protein keratin. The epidermis is the superficial skin layer that is located immediately above the dermis.) It has been thought that xerosis can result from dry air that is present in heated rooms during the winter. Xerosis is commonly associated with aging and is a common problem in elderly individuals.

Xerosis can also be associated with myxedema (hypothyroidism), hypoparathyroidism, chronic nephritis, chronic renal failure, HIV infection, hypervitaminosis A, atopic dermatitis (see Chapter 2), internal malignancy and drugs. Such drugs include niacin, other cholesterol-lowering drugs, atropine-like drugs and retinoids. Retinoids are vitamin A derivatives that include isotretinoin (Accutane®), which is used in the treatment of severe, recalcitrant nodular acne, and acitretin (Soriatane®), which is used in the treatment of severe psoriasis. For discussions of acne and psoriasis, see Chapters 9 and 4, respectively.

Treatment of xerosis

Overview

Standard symptomatic treatment of xerosis involves judicious bathing along with the use of moisturizer lotions, creams, or ointments.

Bathing

Frequent bathing in hot water and bathing with drying soaps can exacerbate xerosis. I recommend that patients with xerosis bathe less often, and when they bathe, they should take brief showers every other day and should use tepid water and a mild, non-irritating cleanser such as white, unscented Dove Bar® or Purpose Bar®. ('Dirty' areas such as the anogenital region and axillae can be bathed more frequently.) Another cleanser that can be used is Olay Daily Renewal Body Wash® (which is soap-free and contains petrolatum). Ivory soap, which is very drying, should not be used.

Moisturizers

Traditionally, some moisturizers have been thought of as acting as 'sealants' by 'sealing' the surface of the skin in order to facilitate retention of water in the skin. Such moisturizers include Aquaphor® ointment and Eucerin® cream, which should ideally be applied after bathing (with the goal of 'sealing in' water that is absorbed by the skin during bathing) as well as frequently throughout the day as needed.

Other moisturizers have been thought of as acting as hygroscopic agents that bind water in the skin. Such moisturizers contain hygroscopic agents such as α-hydroxy acids (e.g. lactic acid) and urea. Lac-Hydrin® (ammonium lactate) 12% lotion and cream are very effective lactic acid-based moisturizers for very dry skin. Very effective urea-based moisturizers include Carmol 10® (10% urea) lotion for 'total body' very dry skin and Carmol 20® (20% urea) cream for rough, very dry skin.

There are also many other elegant moisturizers that include Nutraderm 30® lotion, Cetaphil Moisturizer® lotion and cream, Moisturel® lotion and cream, and Lubriderm Seriously Sensitive Lotion® (which, in my experience, has been the least likely to cause irritation in the very few patients who could not tolerate other moisturizers).

15

Stasis ulcer

OVERVIEW

Clinical features

A stasis ulcer results from venous insufficiency occurring in the legs and consists of a somewhat nondescript ulcer typically involving the skin of the medial distal lower extremity (most commonly, in my experience, involving the ankle or the region immediately proximal to the ankle).

Associated with the stasis ulcer, there may be other signs of venous insufficiency in the area of the stasis ulcer, and these can include edema involving the distal lower extremity; varicose veins involving the lower extremity; stasis dermatitis involving the distal lower extremity; and brown skin pigmentation, usually resulting from deposition of hemosiderin in the dermis of the skin and/or resulting from increased amounts of cutaneous melanin developing as post-inflammatory hyperpigmentation following involution of stasis dermatitis. For discussion of stasis dermatitis, see Chapter 2. The dermis is the skin layer that is located immediately below the epidermis, which is the superficial layer of the skin. Melanin is a pigment that is normally present in the epidermis. For discussion of post-inflammatory hyperpigmentation, see Chapter 7. There may also be the presence of skin fibrosis, resulting in induration clinically, involving the area where the stasis ulcer is located.

The stasis ulcer itself may be crusted or non-crusted and dry or oozing.

Special considerations

The pedal pulses (i.e. the dorsalis pedis and posterior tibial pulses) should be checked in patients who present with stasis ulcers in order to rule out the coexistence of arterial insufficiency.

I generally perform periodic bacterial cultures and sensitivities (C&S) of the ulcer to rule out the presence of secondary bacterial infection, which, if present, should be treated with an at least 10-day course of an appropriate oral antibiotic, which is selected on the basis of the sensitivity results of the bacterial culture.

TREATMENT OF STASIS ULCERS

A good treatment regimen

The stasis ulcer care regimen that I prescribe is as follows. If the patient has no arterial insufficiency or diabetes mellitus, I have him or her elevate the leg while lying supine (with the ankle at about the level of the heart) as often as possible and for as long as possible. The patient should clean the ulcer (and not the surrounding skin) with hydrogen peroxide-soaked cotton-tipped applicators. (There are physicians who do not recommend the use of hydrogen peroxide because they consider it to be excessively tissue destructive. However, I have never encountered a problem in this regard in the many years during which I have prescribed hydrogen peroxide.) The patient should then dry the ulcer with gauze. Using a fresh cotton-tipped applicator, the patient should apply Polysporin Ointment® (polymyxin B sulfate/bacitracin zinc ointment) to the ulcer (and not to the surrounding skin). I do not recommend the use of Neosporin Ointment® (polymyxin B sulfate/bacitracin zinc/neomycin ointment) because many patients develop or already have an allergy to the neomycin in the preparation. The patient performs this ulcer care regimen using hydrogen peroxide and Polysporin Ointment twice daily until the ulcer heals completely. In addition to the antibacterial effects of hydrogen peroxide and Polysporin Ointment, the ointment base of Polysporin Ointment softens any crusting that may be present, and this softening facilitates the removal of the crusting by the hydrogen peroxide-soaked cotton-tipped applicators, thereby resulting in a good débridement-like effect.

If the patient's peripheral circulation is not otherwise impaired (for example, there is no arterial insufficiency) and the patient does not have diabetes mellitus, the patient covers the ulcer during the day with a gauze pad after the application of the Polysporin Ointment, after which the patient wraps an Ace Bandage® around the affected lower extremity from the foot to the knee (being careful not to wrap it so tightly as to impair arterial circulation). Overnight, the patient leaves the ulcer open to air (i.e. not covered with a gauze pad or Ace Bandage). I tell the patient that if the gauze pad is sticking to the ulcer wound when he or she is trying to remove the gauze pad prior to performing the ulcer care described above, he or she should soak the gauze pad with hydrogen peroxide prior to removing it, and this will loosen the gauze pad from the wound, thereby facilitating its removal.

Special considerations

If the patient develops inflammation of the skin surrounding the ulcer, the inflammation may be due to bacterial infection of the ulcer, and therefore a bacterial C&S of the ulcer should be obtained to rule out the presence of bacterial infection, which, if present, should be treated with an at least 10-day course of an appropriate oral antibiotic, which is selected on the basis of the sensitivity results of the bacterial culture. It should be remembered that bacterial culture results can be falsely negative.

Also, the development of such inflammation may be due to the patient applying the hydrogen peroxide to the surrounding skin and not just to the ulcer itself, thereby resulting in an irritant contact dermatitis (see Chapter 2). If this is the case, the patient should be reminded not to apply the hydrogen peroxide to the surrounding skin. If necessary, saline solution can be substituted for hydrogen peroxide (bearing in mind that I have generally found saline solution to be less effective than hydrogen peroxide in the treatment of stasis ulcers). If necessary, the irritant contact dermatitis can in addition be treated with a topical steroid (such as triamcinolone 0.025% cream or triamcinolone 0.1% cream) as described for contact dermatitis and non-specific dermatitis in Chapter 2.

The development of such inflammation can also be due to an allergic reaction to the Polysporin Ointment, thereby resulting in allergic contact dermatitis (see Chapter 2). This problem is dealt with by discontinuing the Polysporin Ointment and using in its place (if the patient is not allergic to iodine) brown Betadine Ointment® (povidone-iodine ointment). Clear Betadine Ointment should not be used in this situation, because it contains the same active ingredients that Polysporin Ointment contains. If necessary, the allergic contact dermatitis can also be treated with a topical steroid, as described above for irritant contact dermatitis due to hydrogen peroxide.

Lastly, inflammation of the skin in the area of the ulcer can also be due to stasis dermatitis (see Chapter 2), which is treated as described for stasis dermatitis in Chapter 2.

It should be noted that I have seen allergy to Polysporin Ointment and allergy to other topical preparations cause non-healing of skin ulcers, such as stasis ulcers, without any other indication of allergic reaction, in which case the ulcers healed following discontinuation of the offending topical agent. Otherwise, I have virtually never had a patient whose stasis ulcer did not heal as expected with the stasis ulcer treatment regimen described above. I have never found it necessary to use any of the currently available 'high tech' skin ulcer products and dressings, which are generally quite expensive.

If the ulcer does not heal as expected, the patient should be referred to a dermatologist to rule out other etiologies, including malignant neoplasm, which I have seen manifested as a non-descript skin ulcer (which in some cases was also secondarily infected with *Staphylococcus aureus*). Also, it should be noted that aggressive squamous cell carcinoma (see Chapter 26) can develop in long-standing, chronic skin ulcers.

16

Scabies and pediculosis

SCABIES

Overview

Scabies is a cutaneous parasitic infestation by the mite *Sarcoptes scabiei* var. *hominis*, which burrows into the stratum corneum. (The stratum corneum is the dead, horny, outermost layer of the epidermis and is composed of the protein keratin. The epidermis is the superficial skin layer that is located immediately above the dermis.) It is felt that a hypersensitivity reaction plays a role in the clinical manifestations of scabies.

It is common for persons (e.g. family members or sexual partners) who have had close contact with a patient with scabies to have scabies also, although I have seen more than one case in which persons who had had close contact with a patient with scabies never developed scabies. Non-sexual close contact can occur, for example, when a bed is used by a person without the bed linen being washed or changed after the patient with scabies used it; when a sleeping bag is used by a person without it's being washed after the patient with scabies used it; when clothes are worn by a person without their being washed after the patient with scabies wore them; or when a caretaker provides close care for a patient with scabies.

When a patient gets scabies for the first time, the patient typically develops tiny, itchy, erythematous papules involving the finger webs, anterior wrists, axillary folds (folds of skin that are anterior and posterior to each axilla), umbilicus region, waist, genitals, buttocks and thighs as well as elsewhere on the neck, trunk and extremities some weeks after infestation (it generally takes the host that long to become sensitized to the mite's excreta and saliva, and it also takes the mites a period of time to become numerous enough to be noticeable). Although in infants involvement can be on all parts of the body, involvement is usually limited to the neck and below in patients older than 3 or 4 years of age.

The characteristic lesion of scabies is the burrow, which is a small, narrow, raised linear lesion that is about 5 mm long and frequently has a tiny papule at its end. The scabies mite is in this burrow, and no mites are generally found in most of the other tiny papules that are not associated with burrows. It is felt that in the majority of patients, burrows are not found, but this has been considered to be due to inadequate searching for burrows in many cases.

I have found that itchy, erythematous nodules on the genitals (accompanied by more typical involvement elsewhere) tend to be confirmative in making the diagnosis of scabies on a clinical basis.

Mention should be made of the variant of scabies called Norwegian scabies, which typically is seen in immunologically compromised patients and is manifested by crusted lesions that can be similar in appearance to lesions of dermatitis (see Chapter 2) or psoriasis (see Chapter 4). The lesions of Norwegian scabies contain numerous mites.

Absolute confirmation of the diagnosis of scabies

The diagnosis of scabies can be confirmed absolutely by a positive scraping of burrows. When this is done, burrows are moistened with mineral oil, after which the burrows are vigorously scraped with a no. 15 scalpel (I generally have the scalpel blade oriented perpendicularly to the skin surface when I do the scraping) so as to unroof the burrow (bleeding may be produced by this scraping, but bleeding is not necessary for an adequate scraping). The scrapings are placed on a glass slide, after which they can be covered with mineral oil and a coverslip. It should be noted that scraping for potassium hydroxide (KOH) preparation and fungal culture to rule out superficial fungal infection (see Chapter 18) should virtually never produce bleeding, because this scraping is performed much more superficially than the scraping for mites. The scrapings are then examined with a microscope under low power, and the diagnosis of scabies is confirmed if evidence of mites (e.g. mite body parts, eggs, or golden brown fecal pellets) is seen. If the health-care provider is not adequately skilled in terms of this examination for evidence of mites, the scrapings on the glass slide can be covered with another glass slide instead of a coverslip, the two glass slides can be held together by wrapping paper tape around one or both ends of the slides, and labeling information can then be written on the paper tape, after which the glass slides can be sent to a clinical laboratory for examination for evidence of mites. If no burrows are found, unexcoriated papules can be scraped as described above.

If the scrapings are negative for evidence of mites, the patient should still be treated for scabies if the clinical evidence indicates scabies. (False-negative scraping tests for scabies are not uncommon.)

Possible problems associated with scabies

For patients who acquired scabies sexually, evaluation for the presence of other sexually transmitted diseases should be done, and this evaluation should include, but is not limited to, obtaining a rapid plasma reagin (RPR) or Venereal Disease Research Laboratories (VDRL) and HIV test. Obviously, the patient's sexual partner should be evaluated and treated accordingly.

Treatment of scabies

Elimite cream®

Patients with scabies and, if not otherwise unadvisable (see below), their close contacts (as described above) are treated simultaneously with Elimite Cream® (permethrin), which is applied to the skin from the head to the soles of the feet. (Be sure that infants are treated on the scalp, temple and forehead.) Twelve hours after application, the medication is thoroughly washed off, but before the medication is washed off, the bed linen, clothes and underwear should be washed with hot water in a washing machine or dry-cleaned. This treatment with Elimite should be done once only.

Elimite should be used during pregnancy only if clearly needed. If Elimite is used in breast-feeding patients, breast feeding should be discontinued temporarily. Elimite has been shown to be safe and effective in pediatric patients of 2 months of age and older, but safety and effectiveness in infants younger than 2 months of age have not been established.

It should be noted that itching can persist for a period of weeks (occasionally months) after treatment of scabies, and this rarely indicates persistence of active scabies and need for retreatment. However, the presence of demonstrable living mites 2 weeks after treatment indicates treatment failure or reinfestation, in which case the patient should be retreated once only. If the problem persists, the patient should be refered to a dermatologist.

Eurax® lotion and cream

Eurax® is applied to the whole body from the chin down to the soles. Eurax is applied again 24 h later. Bed linen, clothes and underwear are changed the next morning. The contaminated bed linen, clothes and underwear should be washed in hot water in a washing machine or dry-cleaned. A cleansing shower is taken 48 h after the last application.

Eurax should not be applied to acutely inflamed, raw, or weeping skin until such acute inflammation has subsided.

Eurax should be used during pregnancy only if clearly needed. The safety and effectiveness of the use of Eurax in children have not been established.

If the problem does not resolve the patient must be referred to a dermatologist

Lindane lotion

Lindane has been banned in some places. In California, for example, its use in treating scabies and lice has been banned because of toxic environmental pollution considerations. However, before the ban, if it was decided that treatment failure with other therapy (see above) had occurred, I treated the patient with lindane lotion 1%, if not otherwise unadvisable or contraindicated. In places where it is not banned, lindane lotion is indicated for the treatment of scabies only in patients who have failed to respond to adequate doses of, or are intolerant of, other approved therapies. Lindane lotion is contraindicated for premature neonates, for patients with Norwegian scabies (see above) and for patients with known seizure disorders (lindane penetrates the skin, has the potential for central nervous system toxicity, and has the potential for causing seizures); lindane lotion should be used during pregnancy only if clearly needed, and pregnant patients should be treated no more than twice during a pregnancy; breast-feeding patients should discontinue breast feeding for 4 days after application of lindane lotion; and during lindane treatment, infants' hands and feet should be covered in order to prevent sucking, and licking of the applied lotion; if open wounds, cuts, or sores are present, lindane lotion should be used with caution, if at all.

Lindane treatment for scabies is as follows. Lindane lotion is applied to the entire body from the neck down, including the soles of the feet. Eight hours after application of the lindane, the patient takes a shower and thoroughly washes off the medication, but before the medication is washed off, the bed linen, clothes and underwear should be washed with hot water in a washing machine or dry-cleaned. This treatment with lindane should be done once only.

It should be made certain that the pharmacist gives the patient the lindane lotion manufacturer's instruction sheet that describes how scabies is treated with lindane lotion.

If the problem does not resolve, the patient should be referred to a dermatologist.

Adjunctive therapy

Topical steroids can be used for itchy scabetic papules and nodules (see above) as described for non-specific dermatitis in Chapter 2, and sedating or non-sedating oral antihistamines can be used for itching as described for non-specific dermatitis in Chapter 2. Persistent itchy erythematous nodules can be cautiously injected intralesionally with injectible Kenalog® (triamcinolone) suspension as described for prurigo nodularis in Chapter 2.

Secondary bacterial infection of scabies involvement

Possible secondary bacterial infection – which can result from frequent scratching – associated with scabies can be approached as described for possible secondarily infected non-specific dermatitis in Chapter 2.

PEDICULOSIS

Overview

Pediculosis is human lice infestation, of which there are three types: pediculosis capitis (head lice), pediculosis corporis (body lice) and pediculosis pubis (pubic lice).

Pediculosis capitis

Overview

Pediculosis capitis is caused by infestation of the scalp with the louse *Pediculus humanus capitis*. It is spread from one person to another through contact with fomites (such as combs, brushes, or hats) or through direct physical contact, and children are more commonly affected than are adults.

Patients with pediculosis capitis present with scalp itching. On clinical examination, adult lice are commonly not seen, but nits, which are louse egg sacs attached to hair shafts, are present. When the eggs are unhatched, the nits are tannish in color, and when the eggs are hatched, the nits are grayish in color. These egg sacs are attached to the side of the proximal portion of the hair shaft and grow out with the hair shaft as the hair shaft grows out. Typically, when nits are more than a few centimeters from the surface of the scalp, the eggs have most likely hatched, and when there are no nits less than a few centimeters from the scalp, the louse infestation is generally over. Nits can be distinguished from other artifacts (e.g. scale) attached to hair shafts in that nits are not easily moved on the hair shaft, unlike other artifacts that may be attached to the hair shaft.

Treatment of pediculosis capitis

Pediculosis capitis can be treated with Rid Shampoo® or Nix Creme Rinse® as described in the product's accompanying written information, which also tells the patient how to take care of nits and fomites. Rid Shampoo is an over-the-counter product that contains the active ingredients pyrethrum extract and piperonyl butoxide. Nix Creme Rinse is an over-the-counter product that contains the active ingredient permethrin, which should not be used on children less than 2 months of age, and I do not recommend using this product in pregnant or breast-feeding patients unless its use is approved by the patient's obstetrician or breast-fed baby's pediatrician, respectively.

As mentioned earlier, lindane has been banned in some places because of toxic environmental pollution considerations. In places where it is not banned, lindane shampoo 1% is indicated for the treatment of pediculosis capitis only in patients who have failed to respond to adequate doses of, or are intolerant of, other approved therapies; it is contraindicated for premature neonates and for patients with known seizure disorders (lindane penetrates the skin, has the potential for central nervous system toxicity, and has the potential for causing seizures). It should be used in pregnancy only if clearly needed, and pregnant patients should be treated no more than twice during a pregnancy; breast-feeding patients should discontinue breast feeding for 4 days after use of lindane shampoo; and if open wounds, cuts, or sores are present in the area to be treated, lindane shampoo should be used with caution, if at all.

If lindane shampoo 1% is used for the treatment of pediculosis capitis, it should be made certain that the pharmacist gives the patient the lindane shampoo manufacturer's instruction sheet that describes how pediculosis capitis is treated with lindane shampoo and how nits are taken care of, and the patient should be directed to follow these instructions closely.

In terms of taking care of fomites, I recommend that all personal headwear, scarves and bed linen be machine washed in hot water and then dried in a dryer using the hot cycle for at least 20 min. Items that cannot be washed and dried as just described should instead be dry-cleaned. Combs and brushes should be soaked in hot water for about 10 min.

Secondary bacterial infection of pediculosis capitis involvement

Possible secondary bacterial infection – which can result from frequent scratching – associated with pediculosis capitis can be approached as described for possible secondarily infected non-specific dermatitis in Chapter 2.

Treatment of head lice infestation of eyelashes

It should be noted that head lice can infest eyelashes. The best treatment for this is to apply petrolatum to the eyelashes three times daily for 3 days.

Pediculosis corporis

Overview

Pediculosis corporis is caused by infestation of the body by the louse *Pediculus humanus corporis*, which feeds on the skin of the body but lives on clothes, particularly in the seams of clothes. Infestation spreads from person to person via direct physical contact or via fomites such as clothes and bedding.

Typically, patients with pediculosis corporis present with itching and excoriations, and examination of frequently worn clothing, particularly the seams, reveals the presence of lice.

Possible problems associated with pediculosis corporis

For patients for whom it is felt that pediculosis corporis was acquired sexually, evaluation for the presence of other sexually transmitted diseases should be done, and this evaluation should include, but is not limited to, obtaining an RPR or VDRL and HIV test. Obviously, the patient's sexual partner should be evaluated and treated accordingly.

Treatment of pediculosis corporis

Treatment consists of use of an over-the-counter product such as Rid Shampoo (which contains the active ingredients pyrethrum extract and piperonyl butoxide) as described in the product's accompanying written information, which also tells the patient how to take care of fomites.

Secondary bacterial infection of pediculosis corporis involvement

Possible secondary bacterial infection – which can result from frequent scratching – associated with pediculosis corporis can be approached as described for possible secondarily infected non-specific dermatitis in Chapter 2.

Pediculosis pubis

Overview

Pediculosis pubis is caused by infestation of the pubic area by the louse *Phthirus pubis*. This infestation is primarily sexually acquired, but it can be spread via fomites such as bed linen and clothing.

Typically, patients with pediculosis pubis present with itching of the pubic area, where lice can be seen on the skin and nits (see pediculosis capitis above) are seen on the hairs. In hairy men, the infestation may also involve areas beyond the pubic region.

Possible problems associated with pediculosis pubis

Pediculosis pubis is primarily sexually acquired. Therefore, evaluation for the presence of other sexually transmitted diseases should be done accordingly, and this evaluation should include, but is not limited to, obtaining an RPR or VDRL and HIV test. Obviously, the patient's sexual partner should be evaluated and treated accordingly.

Treatment of pediculosis pubis

Treatment consists of use of an over-the-counter product such as Rid Shampoo (which contains the active ingredients pyrethrum extract and piperonyl butoxide) as described in the product's accompanying written information, which also tells the patient how to take care of nits and fomites.

In places where lindane is not banned, lindane shampoo 1% is indicated for the treatment of pediculosis pubis only in patients who have failed to respond to adequate doses of, or are intolerant of, other approved therapies; it is contraindicated for premature neonates and for patients with known seizure disorders (lindane penetrates the skin, has the potential for central nervous system toxicity, and has the potential for causing seizures). It should be used in pregnancy only if clearly needed, and pregnant patients should be treated no more than twice during a pregnancy; breast-feeding patients should discontinue breast feeding for 4 days after use of lindane shampoo; and if open wounds, cuts, or sores are present in the areas to be treated, lindane shampoo should be used with caution, if at all.

If lindane shampoo 1% is used for the treatment of pediculosis pubis, it should be made certain that the pharmacist gives the patient the lindane shampoo manufacturer's instruction sheet that describes how pediculosis pubis is treated with lindane shampoo and how nits are taken care of, and the patient should be directed to follow these instructions closely.

In terms of taking care of fomites, I recommend that bed linen and clothing, particularly underwear, be machine washed in hot water and then dried in a dryer for at least 20 min using the hot cycle.

Pediculosis pubis is primarily sexually acquired. Therefore, sexual partners should be simultaneously treated accordingly.

Secondary bacterial infection of pediculosis pubis involvement

Possible secondary bacterial infection – which can result from frequent scratching – associated with pediculosis pubis can be approached as described for possible secondarily infected non-specific dermatitis in Chapter 2.

Treatment of pubic lice infestation of eyelashes

It should be noted that pubic lice can infest eyelashes. The best treatment for this is to apply petrolatum to the eyelashes three times daily for 3 days as described above for the treatment of head lice infestation of eyelashes.

17

Impetigo/bullous impetigo, ecthyma, bacterial folliculitis, furuncles/carbuncles/cutaneous abscesses, and bacterial paronychia

IMPETIGO/BULLOUS IMPETIGO

Overview

Impetigo, which occurs more commonly in children than in adults, is a superficial cutaneous bacterial infection that typically presents to the health-care provider as 'honey-colored' crusting on an erythematous base at the site of the infection. It is due to *Staphylococcus aureus*, *Streptococcus pyogenes*, or a combination of the two organisms.

When due to certain uncommon strains of *S. pyogenes*, impetigo can lead to post-streptococcal glomerulonephritis. However, post-streptococcal glomerulonephritis can already be present when the patient is seen for impetigo. Impetigo does not lead to acute rheumatic fever.

Certain strains of *S. aureus* cause bullous impetigo, which presents as vesicles or bullae on an erythematous base. (Vesicles are small blisters. Bullae are large blisters.) When the vesicles or bullae rupture, erosions are present. The blister formation is caused by a toxin produced by the particular strains of *S. aureus* that cause bullous impetigo. When this toxin spreads systemically through the bloodstream, the staphylococcal scalded skin syndrome, which is characterized by extensive sloughing of the superficial layers of the skin, results.

Confirmative testing regarding impetigo/bullous impetigo

The diagnosis of impetigo or bullous impetigo and the antimicrobial sensitivities of the causative bacteria can be confirmed by obtaining a bacterial culture and sensitivities (C&S) of the crusting, erosions, or blister fluid that is present. The blister fluid is accessed by piercing the blister roof with a no. 11 scalpel or a 20-gauge needle.

Treatment of impetigo/bullous impetigo

Treatment consists of an at least 10-day course of an appropriate oral antibiotic based on bacterial C&S results and patient response.

For an otherwise healthy adult, I usually start out with cephalexin (Keflex®) 250–500 mg every 6 h, if not otherwise unadvisable, and modify the antibiotic therapy according to bacterial C&S results and patient response, with systemic antibiotic therapy being continued for at least 10 days. If the patient is allergic to cephalosporins or penicillins (there is evidence of partial cross-allergenicity of the penicillins and the cephalosporins) or if the patient is otherwise unable to take cephalexin, I instead start out with erythromycin 250–500 mg every 6 h, if not otherwise unadvisable. The dosages for children are based on the package insert recommendations for the patient's age and weight.

ECTHYMA

Overview

Ecthyma is a cutaneous bacterial infection, which, like impetigo, is caused by *S. aureus*, *S. pyogenes*, or a combination of the two organisms, but with ecthyma, the level of infection is deeper in the skin than it is with impetigo.

Patients with ecthyma typically present with a cutaneous ulcer covered by a crust and surrounded by erythema.

Confirmative testing regarding ecthyma and treatment of ecthyma

Confirmative testing regarding the diagnosis of ecthyma, confirmative testing regarding the antimicrobial sensitivities of the causative bacteria and treatment of ecthyma are as described above for impetigo.

Special considerations regarding ecthyma

It should be mentioned that I have seen cases of ecthymatous involvement of skin cancer (e.g. basal cell carcinoma – see Chapter 26) in which patients presented clinically with an ecthymatous-appearing, crusted ulcer with *S. aureus* infection of the ulcer confirmed by bacterial C&S. However, in these cases, the lesions did not resolve with appropriate ecthyma treatment, and subsequent skin biopsy revealed skin cancer.

BACTERIAL FOLLICULITIS

Overview

Bacterial folliculitis consists of a bacterial infection of hair follicles and is manifested by erythematous follicular papules and/or pustules that may be pierced by hairs and that can occur anywhere on the hairy skin. Remember that, even though hairs may not be visible with the naked eye, hair follicles are present throughout the skin surface, excluding such areas as the palms and soles.

Bacterial folliculitis is commonly caused by *S. aureus* but can be caused by other bacteria. When Gram-negative bacteria are the infecting agents, the term 'Gram-negative folliculitis' is used.

Confirmative testing regarding bacterial folliculitis

A bacterial C&S of pustule contents may confirm the diagnosis, determine the causative bacteria and confirm the antimicrobial sensitivities of the causative bacteria. Pustule contents can be accessed by piercing the pustule roof with a no. 11 scalpel or a 20-gauge needle. It is important to remember that false-negative bacterial culture results can occur.

Special considerations regarding bacterial folliculitis

If bacterial folliculitis involvement is extensive or frequently recurrent following adequate therapy (treatment of bacterial folliculitis is discussed below), an immunocompromised state and diabetes mellitus should be considered.

In terms of common differential diagnosis, if involvement is limited to shaved hairy areas, such as the bearded region in men, pseudofolliculitis barbae or pili incarnati (see Chapter 19), which is not due to infection but is an inflammatory reaction to ingrown hairs resulting from shaving, should be considered in the differential diagnosis. If the involvement is limited to hairy areas such as the bearded region in men or the scalp, superficial fungal infection (tinea barbae or tinea capitis – see Chapter 18) should be considered in the differential diagnosis. If a diagnosis of generalized bacterial folliculitis is being considered, the 'great mimickers' secondary syphilis (see Chapter 27) and drug eruption (see Chapter 3) should be considered in the differential diagnosis, if the clinical situation is appropriate. Papular pityriasis rosea (see Chapter 6) and viral eruption might also be considered in the differential diagnosis.

In my experience, there are viruses that can produce non-specific eruptions (see Chapter 6).

The differential diagnosis might also include acne (see Chapter 9); rosacea, perioral dermatitis, acne keloidalis nuchae, and possibly steroid dependent facial dermatosis (see Chapter 10); eruptive/guttate and pustular psoriasis (see Chapter 4); and scabies (see Chapter 16). In addition, the differential diagnosis might include papular cutaneous manifestations of HIV disease; papular acrodermatitis of childhood (Gianotti-Crosti syndrome); the papular type of chronic cutaneous graft-versus-host reaction; vasculitis; and erythema multiforme (for brief discussions of the preceding entities, see the *Common differential diagnosis of extensive/generalized non-specific dermatitis* section in Chapter 2).

A negative Venereal Disease Research Laboratories (VDRL) or rapid plasma reagin (RPR) test will rule out secondary syphilis; a complete blood count (CBC) showing lymphocytosis would be suggestive of a viral eruption, which may have associated constitutional symptoms and/or signs and typically presents as erythematous macules that may coalesce, erythematous papules, vesicles and/or pustules; and a CBC showing eosinophilia might be suggestive of a drug eruption. Severe, serious drug eruptions may show lymphocytosis with atypical lymphocytes and may have associated constitutional symptoms and/or signs along with other findings. Current evidence is that eosinophilia on CBC is an uncommon finding for common drug reactions and is a parameter that is of little value in diagnosing common drug reactions, but an eosinophil count higher than 1000/μl may be seen with severe, serious drug eruptions. A viral culture of pustule contents can be performed, and the diagnosis of viral eruption would be confirmed if a virus is cultured out, but be aware that false-negative viral culture results can occur.

The untreated rash of secondary syphilis would resolve spontaneously (at which time the patient would be said to have latent syphilis). If the diagnosis of secondary syphilis is made, this obviously should be evaluated, treated and followed accordingly, and if the patient is pregnant, her obstetrician should be notified because of the potential effect of syphilis on the fetus. It should be noted that viral eruption generally needs only symptomatic treatment since it is generally self-limited, but if the patient is pregnant, and viral eruption is considered, the patient's obstetrician should be notified regarding the possibility of associated harm to the fetus. If the diagnosis of a viral eruption is made, appropriate precautions need to be taken to prevent transmission of the condition to other individuals.

Treatment of bacterial folliculitis

The treatment of bacterial folliculitis consists of bathing with an antibacterial soap (such as Dial® soap) and taking a course of an appropriate oral antibiotic based on bacterial C&S results of pustule contents and patient response.

For an otherwise healthy adult, I usually start out with cephalexin (Keflex) 250–500 mg every 6 h, if not otherwise unadvisable, and modify the antibiotic therapy according to bacterial C&S results and patient response, with systemic antibiotic therapy being continued for at least 10 days. If the patient is allergic to cephalosporins or penicillins (there is evidence of partial cross-allergenicity of the penicillins and the cephalosporins) or if the patient is otherwise unable to take cephalexin, I instead start out with erythromycin 250–500 mg every 6 h if not otherwise unadvisable. The dosages for children are based on the package insert recommendations for the patient's age and weight. If there are no pustules from which a bacterial C&S can be obtained, I would start oral antibiotic therapy with cephalexin as described above, and if the patient cannot take cephalexin, I would instead start with erythromycin as described above, if not otherwise unadvisable, with the oral antibiotic therapy being modified according to patient response and with oral antibiotic therapy being continued for at least 10 days.

FURUNCLES/CARBUNCLES/CUTANEOUS ABSCESSES

Overview

A furuncle ('boil') is a follicular bacterial infection (generally due to *S. aureus*) that is present more deeply in the skin than is the case with bacterial folliculitis. Clinically, a furuncle is a tender, painful, erythematous nodule (large cutaneous bump) that can occur anywhere on the hairy skin.

When the lesion is larger and involves multiple adjacent hair follicles, it is called a carbuncle.

When the lesion becomes a fluctuant, pus-filled cavity, it has become an abscess.

Special considerations regarding furuncles/carbuncles/cutaneous abscesses

Carbuncles occur more frequently in patients with diabetes mellitus than in non-diabetics.

In patients who develop recurrent furuncles or carbuncles, I consider the possibilities of immunological impairment and diabetes mellitus.

When the involvement is limited to the bearded region of men or to the scalp, kerion (which occurs with the superficial fungal infections tinea barbae and tinea capitis) should be considered in the differential diagnosis. A KOH preparation and fungal culture of scrapings and plucked hairs from the surface of the lesion may confirm the diagnosis of tinea barbae or tinea capitis, but be aware that there can be false-negative KOH preparation and fungal culture results. (See Chapter 18 regarding tinea barbae, tinea capitis, kerions, KOH preparations, and fungal cultures.)

Treatment of furuncles/carbuncles/cutaneous abscesses

When a furuncle or carbuncle is not fluctuant, the degree of abscess formation within the lesion is not great enough to warrant incision and drainage. In this case, I have the patient treat the lesion with warm, plain water open wet compresses as described for non-specific dermatitis in Chapter 2, and I also place the patient on a course of an oral antibiotic such as cephalexin (Keflex) 500 mg every 6 h for otherwise healthy adults, if not otherwise unadvisable. If the patient is allergic to cephalosporins or penicillins (there is evidence of partial cross-allergenicity of the penicillins and the cephalosporins) or if the patient is otherwise unable to take cephalexin, I would instead prescribe a course of erythromycin 500 mg every 6 h, if not otherwise unadvisable. Dosages for children are as described in the package inserts and are based on age and weight.

If a furuncle or carbuncle evolves to the point where significant abscess formation has occurred within the lesion, the lesion becomes fluctuant – the presence of fluctuance is indicative of the presence of a cutaneous abscess. Treatment of a cutaneous abscess involves incision and drainage of the lesion (billed as 'incision and drainage of cutaneous abscess'). (Before incision and drainage are performed in any patient with a heart murmur and/or artificial implant, the American Heart Association guidelines regarding incision and drainage of infected tissue in such patients should be consulted and followed accordingly to prevent bacterial seeding of the heart or artificial implant.) I perform the incision and drainage as follows. I draw up 1% lidocaine with or without epinephrine into a 3-ml syringe with a large-bore needle, such as a 21-gauge needle. Epinephrine decreases bleeding and prolongs the local anesthetic effect via vasocon-striction. However, I do not use epinephrine on such sites as the fingers, toes, and penis – some dermatologists recommend not using epinephrine on the nose and ear lobes also – because epinephrine can cause excessively decreased arterial blood flow at such sites, and this can result in tissue necrosis. I then replace the large-bore needle with a small-bore needle, such as a 30-gauge needle. I clean the skin over and around the abscess with an alcohol swab and then dry it with sterile gauze, after which I provide local anesthesia by injecting the lidocaine intradermally so that it infiltrates the skin around the abscess and the skin overlying the abscess, with each injection beginning in the previously injected site and then extending beyond, because injecting local anesthetic in this way is less painful. (Injecting the local anesthetic slowly into the skin also lessens the pain of the injecting.) In order to prevent accidental intravascular injection of anesthetic, aspiration (pulling back on the syringe's plunger) should be done immediately prior to each time the anesthetic is injected. I use a no. 11 scalpel to incise through the skin into the pus-filled cavity of the abscess. Sometimes I place a second incision perpendicularly to the first incision so that a cruciate incision is formed. (A cruciate incision is less likely to close prematurely.) Alternatively, the incision can be made using a 3-mm or 4-mm punch, which is an instrument with a circular, sharp, metal ring at the end of a handle. (Disposable, sterile punches of various sizes can be purchased from medical instrument suppliers.) Pus is then expressed through the incision, and this can be facilitated by carefully and gently inserting and then withdrawing a closed hemostat through the incision. I also obtain a bacterial C&S of the pus as it comes out of the incision. I do not pack the abscess cavity. (I have found that packing the cavity has been unnecessary, and when the cavity is not packed and the treatment and follow-up care are performed as described here, the wound heals with a scar that is better in appearance than is the scar that occurs when the cavity is packed.) If there is brisk oozing of blood (which can result from hyperemia of the incised and drained skin), it can be stopped by the application of steady pressure to the briskly oozing area with sterile gauze for at least 15–20 min without peeking. I then clean the area again with an alcohol swab, dry the area with sterile gauze, and apply Polysporin Ointment® (polymyxin B sulfate/bacitracin zinc) to the incision with a sterile cotton-tipped applicator. I cover the incision with a fresh piece of sterile gauze held in place with paper tape. If the patient is allergic to Polysporin Ointment and not allergic to iodine, I use brown Betadine Ointment® (povidone-iodine) instead of Polysporin Ointment. (Allergy to Polysporin Oinment, or to any other topical preparation, can be manifested by the development of increased inflammation or by non-healing of a wound without associated increased inflammation.) Clear Betadine Ointment should not be used in this situation because it contains the same active ingredients that Polysporin Ointment contains. I start otherwise healthy adult patients on a course of cephalexin 500 mg every 6 h or, if cephalexin cannot be used, erythromycin 500 mg every 6 h, if not otherwise unadvisable, and I modify the antibiotic therapy according to the C&S results and patient response, with antibiotic therapy being continued for at least 10 days. Pediatric dosages are as described in the package inserts and are based on age and weight.

Beginning the next day, I have the patient remove the dressing, clean the incision with hydrogen peroxide-soaked cotton-tipped applicators, dry the site with sterile gauze, apply the antibiotic ointment to the incision with a fresh sterile cotton-tipped applicator and cover the incision with a fresh piece of sterile gauze held in place with paper tape. (I tell the patient that, if the gauze sticks to the wound and is therefore difficult to remove from the wound, soaking the gauze with hydrogen peroxide will loosen it from the wound and facilitate its removal.) I have the patient continue this wound care twice daily until the drainage has stopped. In my experience, this wound care in conjunction with an appropriate oral antibiotic seems to keep the incision open until there is no more pus to be drained such that I have found that packing the abscess cavity is unnecessary and, as described above, the wound seems to heal with less scarring in comparison to when the cavity is packed.

If the abscess is large or is in a critical area or if the health-care provider does not feel comfortable or has reservations about performing an incision and drainage, the patient should be referred to a dermatologist or a general surgeon for the procedure to be performed, in which case the referring health-care provider should ideally not start the patient on an oral antibiotic, so that when the dermatologist or the general surgeon performs the incision and drainage, he or she can obtain a bacterial C&S that is not altered by the patient being on an oral antibiotic before the C&S are obtained. At the time that he or she performs the incision and drainage, the dermatologist or general surgeon can start the patient on an appropriate oral antibiotic.

BACTERIAL PARONYCHIA

Overview

Bacterial paronychia is a proximal and/or lateral nail-fold bacterial infection. It is the usual cause of acute paronychia, typically follows injury to the cuticle or proximal or lateral nail fold, and is manifested by the acute development of typically tender, painful erythema and swelling of the proximal and/or lateral nail fold(s) of a finger or toe. (The proximal nail fold is the skin fold that is located at the proximal edge of the nail, and the lateral nail folds are the skin folds that are adjacent to the sides of the nail. The term paronychia is used to refer to proximal and/or lateral nail fold inflammation.) Sometimes pus can be expressed from the area between the skin of the proximal and/or lateral nail fold(s) and the underlying nail plate. If such pus is present, bacterial C&S of the pus should be obtained, and oral antibiotic therapy (see below) can be modified accordingly.

In my experience, bacterial paronychia is usually due to infection by *S. aureus*.

Special considerations regarding bacterial paronychia

Bacterial paronychia, which is the usual cause of acute paronychia, needs to be distinguished from candidal paronychia (see Chapter 18), which is a proximal and/or lateral nail fold candidal infection and is the usual cause of chronic paronychia.

Like bacterial paronychia, candidal paronychia is typically manifested by erythema and swelling of the proximal and/or lateral nail fold(s), and sometimes pus can be expressed from the area between the skin of the proximal and/or lateral nail fold(s) and the underlying nail plate. However, candidal paronychia usually develops slowly and typically follows excessive exposure of the proximal and lateral nail folds to water, whereas bacterial paronychia usually develops acutely and typically follows injury to the cuticle or proximal or lateral nail fold. Also, in my experience candidal paronychia tends to be less acutely tender and painful than is bacterial paronychia, and pus tends to be less commonly present with candidal paronychia than it is with bacterial paronychia. The evaluation and treatment of candidal paronychia are as described in Chapter 18.

Treatment of bacterial paronychia

If the lesion is non-fluctuant (which indicates lack of evolution to abscess formation), treatment of the lesion involves the use of warm, plain water open wet compresses and oral antibiotics as described above for the treatment of non-fluctuant furuncles or carbuncles.

If the lesion is fluctuant (which indicates evolution to abscess formation), the lesion is incised, drained, cultured and treated with oral antibiotics as described above for cutaneous abscesses, except 1% lidocaine without epinephrine (and *not* with epinephrine) is used because of the location being

18

Common superficial fungal infections, intertrigo and perleche

COMMON SUPERFICIAL FUNGAL INFECTIONS

Overview

Superficial fungal infections are fungal infections that generally involve the stratum corneum, hair and/or nails. The stratum corneum is the dead, horny, outer (i.e. most superficial) layer of the skin. The stratum corneum, hair and nails are composed of the protein keratin.

The fungi that commonly cause superficial fungal infections can generally be divided into two groups: molds, which are filamentous; and yeasts, which are single-celled.

The most common superficial fungal infections are those due to dermatophytes (which are molds), that called pityriasis versicolor (which is due to a fungus that exhibits yeast and filamentous forms) and those due to the genus *Candida*, most commonly *Candida albicans* (which is a yeast).

Dermatophytes

Overview

The dermatophytes comprise the group of filamentous fungi that produce ringworm, or what I will call 'true' tinea infections. (Ringworm has nothing to do with worms – it is a fungal infection caused by dermatophytes.) 'True' tinea infections, which are caused by dermatophytic fungi, should not be confused with the cutaneous fungal infection that has been called 'tinea versicolor', which is caused by the non-dermatophytic fungus called *Malassezia furfur*, and should instead be called 'pityriasis versicolor', which is discussed below, to avoid confusing it with 'true' tinea infections, which, as already stated, are caused by dermatophytic fungi.

There are three genera to which dermatophytic fungi belong: *Trichophyton, Microsporum* and *Epidermophyton*. Patients can acquire dermatophytic infections from other people, from animals and from soil.

Dermatophytic infection that involves the scalp can be called tinea capitis. Dermatophytic infection that involves the bearded region in men can be called tinea barbae. Dermatophytic infection that involves the face other than the bearded region can be called tinea facei (or tinea faciale). Dermatophytic infection that involves the trunk, buttocks, arms, legs, or non-bearded region of the neck can be called tinea corporis. Dermatophytic infection that involves the groins, pubic area, genitals, perineum, or perianal skin/intergluteal cleft can be called tinea cruris. (The intergluteal cleft is the area between the buttocks.) Dermatophytic infection that involves the feet can be called tinea pedis. Dermatophytic infection that involves the hands can be called tinea manuum. Dermatophytic infection that involves the nails can be called tinea unguium. The term onychomycosis refers to any fungal infection of the nails (onychomycosis can be due to a dermatophyte or to a non-dermatophyte), whereas tinea unguium refers specifically to a fungal nail infection that is due to a dermatophyte and not due to any other type of fungus. Non-dermatophytic onychomycosis is discussed later in this chapter.

Tinea capitis

Tinea capitis occurs mostly in children and generally presents as patches with varying degrees of inflammation (erythema and/or flaking) associated with broken hairs on the scalp. In some cases, one sees 'black dots', which result when the hair shaft breakage occurs at the level of the scalp, and in other cases, one sees short hairs (1–2 mm long), which result when the hair shaft breakage occurs more distally.

The degree of associated inflammation can range from minimal to severe. When the inflammatory reaction to the fungus is severe, it can produce a boggy, purulent mass resembling a furuncle (see Chapter 17), and this is called a 'kerion'. Follicular pustules may also be present, resembling bacterial folliculitis (see Chapter 17).

Tinea barbae

Tinea barbae occurs in men, involves the bearded region and is characterized by patches with annular vesiculopustular borders and central scaling, by areas of erythema associated with erythematous papules and pustules resembling bacterial folliculitis (see Chapter 17), or by a boggy, purulent mass representing a kerion, which resembles a furuncle (see Chapter 17). The differential diagnosis of tinea barbae also includes pseodofolliculitis barbae (pili incarnati), which is not due to infection but is an inflammatory response to ingrown hairs resulting from shaving (see Chapter 19); acne (see Chapter 9); and rosacea, perioral dermatitis, and steroid dependent facial dermatosis (see Chapter 10).

Tinea facei (tinea faciale), tinea corporis and tinea cruris

Tinea facei (tinea faciale) occurs on non-bearded areas of the face. Tinea corporis occurs on the trunk, buttocks, arms, legs, or non-bearded areas of the neck. Tinea cruris occurs on the groins, pubic area, genitals, perineum, or perianal skin/intergluteal cleft. Tinea facei, tinea corporis and tinea cruris typically present as patches with active erythematous, sometimes raised, sometimes scaly, sometimes papulovesiculopustular borders and central clearing. It should be noted that, with tinea cruris, the scrotum usually is not involved, whereas when the infecting agent is candidal, the scrotum is often involved.

Tinea pedis and tinea manuum

Overview   Tinea pedis and tinea manuum represent dermatophytic infections of the skin of the feet and hands, respectively.

Tinea pedis   Tinea pedis can present in three common patterns. First, there is the interdigital pattern, in which typically there are scaling, maceration and, sometimes, fissuring involving the interdigital or subdigital areas of the feet (usually between the fourth and fifth toes and/or between the third and fourth toes). In this type of tinea pedis, *Candida* and/or bacteria may secondarily involve the affected areas and add to the clinical manifestations produced by the dermatophytic infection of these areas.

Second, there is the so-called moccasin pattern of tinea pedis, in which case there is scaling, usually without significant erythema, involving one or both soles of the feet.

Third, there is the inflammatory pattern of tinea pedis, which presents as recurrent vesicles or vesicopustules, sometimes associated with scaling, involving one or both soles of the feet. The differential diagnosis of inflammatory tinea pedis includes dyshidrotic dermatitis (see Chapter 2); pustular psoriasis (see Chapter 4), which can be limited to the palms and/or soles; and bacterial pyoderma.

Inflammatory tinea pedis can produce what is called a dermatophytid reaction (also called an 'id' reaction), in which a sterile, vesicular eruption resembling dyshidrotic dermatitis occurs on, for example, one or both hands, as discussed in Chapter 2 in the discussion of dyshidrotic dermatitis. A dermatophytid reaction can be thought of as a localized hypersensitivity reaction to the presence of tinea elsewhere or as a manifestion of autosensitization resulting in autosensitization dermatitis. (Autosensitization and autosensitization dermatitis are discussed in Chapter 2.)

Tinea manuum   In my experience, tinea manuum typically presents as scaling with minimal erythema, or as vesicles, sometimes associated with minimal scaling and/or erythema, on one or both hands, usually the palmar aspect. The differential diagnosis of tinea manuum when vesicles are present includes dyshidrotic dermatitis (see Chapter 2) and a dermatophyid reaction (see above). Tinea manuum is frequently seen in association with tinea pedis, and when this occurs, one hand and both feet are frequently involved.

Tinea unguium

Overview   Tinea unguium is a dermatophytic infection of the nail. In contrast, onychomycosis refers to nail fungal infection due to a dermatophyte or to a non-dermatophyte. (Non-dermatophytic onychomycosis is discussed later in this chapter.) Tinea unguium can involve one or more toenails and/or fingernails. Toenails are involved more commonly than are fingernails.

Distal subungual tinea unguium   In my experience, tinea unguium usually begins as tinea pedis or tinea manuum that progresses to the skin of the distal, lateral and/or medial nail bed and extends on the nail bed under the nail plate as well as into the undersurface of the nail plate, from where it spreads through the thickness of the nail plate. As a result of this process, the nail plate can discolor and can separate from the underlying nail bed in association with the development of subungual debris. Separation of the nail plate from the nail bed is called 'onycholysis'. The subungual debris that can develop is composed of scaly, keratotic material. (The term 'keratotic' refers to keratin, which is the protein that makes up the dead, horny, outermost epidermal layer called the stratum corneum. The epidermis is the cutaneous layer that is located immediately above the dermis.) The infection process ultimately leads to nail plate deformity (which is called 'onychodystrophy'), typically manifested by thickening and friability of the nail plate. This pattern of development of tinea unguium is called distal subungual tinea unguium.

The differential diagnosis of this condition includes other causes of onychodystrophy such as psoriasis and damage to the nail matrix. (The nail matrix underlies the proximal nail fold and produces the nail plate. The proximal nail fold is the skin fold that is located at the proximal edge of the nail plate.)

Proximal white subungual tinea unguium   Tinea unguium can also occur when the dermatophyte infects the proximal nail fold, spreads under the cuticle, infects the proximal nail bed and produces white discoloration in the proximal portion of the nail plate (the surface of which is smooth and normal), from where this white discoloration can spread distally in the nail plate. This pattern of development of tinea unguium is called proximal white subungual tinea unguium, which is rare and occurs most commonly in patients infected with HIV.

White superficial tinea unguium   Lastly, tinea unguium can occur when the dermatophyte infects the nail plate from the surface of the nail plate, which becomes white, friable and rough. (In contrast, the surface of the nail plate in proximal white subungual tinea unguium is smooth and normal.) This pattern of development of tinea unguium is called white superficial tinea unguium, which involves the toenails more commonly than the fingernails.

Confirmation of the diagnosis of dermatophyte (tinea) infection

Overview of KOH preparations and fungal cultures   In order to confirm the diagnosis of a dermatophyte (tinea) infection, one must perform a potassium hydroxide (KOH) preparation and/or fungal culture of the involvement.

The results of a KOH preparation can be available in minutes, and whether or not a pathogenic fungus (i.e. a fungus that can cause skin, nail and/or hair disease) is present can be determined from examination of the KOH preparation. However, a fungus cannot be identified on the basis of KOH preparation results.

In contrast, it can take 4–6 weeks to obtain the final results of a fungal culture. However, if a fungus grows out, it can be specifically identified, and by its identity, one will know whether it is pathogenic with regard to skin (in which case it causes skin, nail and/or hair disease) or whether it is typically non-pathogenic with regard to skin (in which case it typically does not cause skin, nail and/or hair disease).

It should be noted that sometimes a KOH preparation will be positive when a fungal culture of the same specimen is negative (in which case the fungal culture result would be falsely negative) and vice versa, and sometimes a KOH preparation and a fungal culture of the same specimen can both be falsely negative (see below for further discussion regarding this).

If the health-care provider is not qualified to run the laboratory portion of these tests in his or her office, collected specimens can be sent to a clinical laboratory, which can run these tests.

Collection of specimens for KOH preparations and fungal cultures   For suspected tineas other than suspected tinea unguium, the health-care provider obtains the specimen by taking scrapings of the stratum corneum where there is involvement. (The stratum corneum is the dead, horny, outermost layer of the epidermis and is composed of the protein keratin. The epidermis is the cutaneous layer that is located immediately above the dermis.) This is done by scraping the scaling and, if vesicles and/or pustules are present, the vesicle and/or pustule roofs with a no. 15 scalpel, with its blade oriented perpendicularly to the skin surface, so that the collected specimen consists of the scaling and the vesicle and/or pustule roofs. If the involvement is in a hairy area, such as the scalp, the health-care provider also obtains plucked hairs, which can be plucked using a small hemostat with or without rubber tubing placed on its clamping arms. If the lesion is annular, the specimen as described above should be taken from the ring portion (which is the active, outer border) of the lesion.

If tinea unguium is suspected, the health-care provider obtains scrapings of the nail bed debris under the nail plate as proximally as possible. The tip of a no. 11 scalpel may be more effective in doing this than would be a no. 15 scalpel, and a 1-mm Fox-type curette, a 0 (0.5-mm) Heath-type curette, or a 000 (0.5-mm) Meyhoefer-type curette may be the most effective in doing this. (A Fox-type curette is a metal instrument with, at one end of the handle, a loop of metal with a cutting edge on one surface. A Heath-type curette is similar to but smaller than the Fox-type curette. A Meyhoefer-type curette is similar to the Fox- and Heath-type curettes, but instead of a loop at one end, the Meyhoefer-type curette has a cup.)

The health-care provider then places these scrapings (and, if the area of involvement is a hairy area such as the scalp, the plucked hairs) on a clean glass slide. He or she then places another clean glass slide on top of the first glass slide so that the specimen is held in place between the two glass slides, and the two glass slides are held together by wrapping paper tape around one or both ends of the slides. The health-care provider can write labeling information on the paper tape. He or she can then send the glass slides to a clinical laboratory for KOH preparation and/or fungal culture of the specimen that is between the two slides, and it should be specified that the specimen consists of skin scrapings (and, if appropriate, plucked hairs). Alternatively, the health-care provider can send the specimen to the clinical laboratory in a container (e.g. a sterile, urine specimen container) instead of between two glass slides.

An approach regarding false-negative KOH preparation and fungal culture results   As noted above, one can obtain false-negative KOH preparation and fungal culture results when testing for tinea. (This is especially the case with inflammatory tinea.)

If false-negative test results are suspected when dealing with possible tineas other than tinea unguium, the patient can be treated with a topical steroid of a potency that is appropriate for the area being treated (see Chapter 1), in which case the fungal testing should be repeated a week or two later, at which time the use of the topical steroid in the interval will make fungal testing more likely to show the presence of tinea if tinea is indeed present and therefore less likely to result in a false-negative test result for tinea. It should be noted that, if tinea is still strongly suspected despite negative test results for tinea, I treat the patient for tinea empirically.

Using the Wood's lamp for confirming the diagnosis of tinea capitis   It should be noted that tinea capitis can also be diagnosed by the presence of yellow-green fluorescence of actively growing hairs exposed to light from a Wood's lamp (which is a particular source of ultraviolet light), because some types of fungus that infect the actively growing hairs in tinea capitis can cause these hairs to fluoresce yellow-green when exposed to the light of a Wood's lamp. Since uninfected scales or crusts can also fluoresce when exposed to the light of a Wood's lamp, it is important to be sure that hairs and not just scales or crusts are fluorescing under the light of the Wood's lamp when one is using this method for diagnosing tinea capitis.

Testing pustules and pus for the presence of bacterial infection   If pus or pustules are present, obtaining a bacterial culture and sensitivities (C&S) of the pus or pustule contents as described for bacterial folliculitis in Chapter 17 should be considered in order to check for the presence of bacterial infection.

Treatment of dermatophyte (tinea) infections

Overview   In terms of treatment of dermatophyte (tinea) infections, the location of the infection has a bearing on the type of treatment used.

Treatment of tinea capitis   Tinea capitis generally does not respond to topical treatment, and oral griseofulvin is the treatment of choice for tinea capitis. For adults, the usual dose is 0.5–1 g/day of griseofulvin microsize (e.g. Grifulvin V® microsize tablets or oral suspension), and the pediatric dose is about 5 mg/pound per day of griseofulvin microsize (e.g. Grifulvin V microsize tablets or oral suspension), so that for children weighing 30–50 pounds, 125–250 mg daily is suggested, and for children weighing over 50 pounds, 250–500 mg daily is suggested. Optimal blood levels of griseofulvin should occur when it is taken with a fatty meal, which enhances absorption of the drug. Treatment is continued until the patient is clinically clear, and fungal testing is negative. This typically takes about 6 weeks.

When systemic griseofulvin is used to treat healthy patients for tinea capitis, it is generally not necessary to use routine laboratory monitoring to check for adverse effects due to griseofulvin. More specifically, I do not use routine laboratory monitoring for systemic griseofulvin therapy in healthy patients if the duration of the therapy is less than 3 months; if the duration of the therapy is more than 3 months in healthy patients, I obtain a complete blood count (CBC), liver function tests, creatinine and urinalysis at baseline and every 3 months thereafter while the patient is on systemic griseofulvin therapy.

Griseofulvin is contraindicated in patients with porphyria or hepatocellular failure and in pregnant patients. Women should not become pregnant until after one month following discontinuation of griseofulvin, and men should not father a child within at least six months following discontinuation of griseofulvin, according to the package insert. There is the possibility of cross-sensitivity with penicillin, but known penicillin-sensitive patients have been treated with griseofulvin without problems. Patients taking griseofulvin should be warned to avoid intense artificial or natural sunlight exposure, because photosensitivity reactions are occasionally associated with griseofulvin therapy. In terms of drug interactions, griseofulvin may affect the activity of warfarin-type anticoagulants, barbiturates usually depress griseofulvin activity, griseofulvin has been reported to decrease the efficacy of oral contraceptives, and may potentiate the effect of alcohol and thereby result in such effects as tachycardia and flushing.

Treatment of markedly inflamed tinea capitis   For patients who have markedly inflamed tinea capitis, a course of oral prednisone, if not otherwise unadvisable (for example, see discussion of systemic steroid therapy for severe non-specific dermatitis in Chapter 2), at a dose of 1 mg/kg every morning for the first 10–15 days of griseofulvin therapy may be beneficial in reducing symptoms and scarring.

Treatment of tinea barbae   As for tinea capitis, the treatment of choice for tinea barbae is oral griseofulvin, which is prescribed as it is for tinea capitis. However, for tinea barbae, the griseofulvin treatment is continued until 2–3 weeks after clinical clearing of the involvement.

Treatment of markedly inflamed tinea barbae   As with markedly inflamed tinea capitis (see above), a short course of prednisone, if not otherwise unadvisable, in addition to the griseofulvin therapy may be beneficial for patients with markedly inflamed tinea barbae.

Treatment of limited involvement of tinea facei (faciale), tinea corporis, tinea cruris, tinea pedis and tinea manuum   For limited involvement of tinea facei (faciale), tinea corporis, tinea cruris, tinea pedis and tinea manuum, topical treatment is my treatment of choice. I usually use clotrimazole (Lotrimin-AF®) cream, lotion, or solution twice daily to the involvement. [Clotrimazole is an over-the-counter, topical, imidazole-type, broad-spectrum antifungal agent. Broad-spectrum means it covers yeasts (i.e. *Candida*), the yeast/filamentous fungus *Malassezia furfur* and molds (i.e. dermatophytes).]

An alternative, commonly used, over-the-counter, topical, imidazole-type, broad-spectrum antifungal agent is miconazole (Micatin®) cream, which, when I prescribe it, I have the patient use twice daily.

Topical, imidazole-type, broad-spectrum antifungal agents that require prescriptions include ketoconazole (Nizoral®) cream, which I have not found to be superior to clotrimazole or miconazole, and econazole (Spectazole®) cream, which in my experience is sometimes more effective than are the other topical imidazole-type antifungal agents but sometimes is more irritating, particularly when used for tinea cruris or tinea facei (faciale). When I prescribe Nizoral cream or Spectazole cream, I have the patient use it twice daily.

When I have a patient use a topical imidazole-type antifungal agent for a dermatophyte infection, I usually expect to see improvement within about 4 weeks of therapy.

If a patient is not able to use a topical imidazole-type antifungal agent (for example, if a patient is allergic to such agents), I instead try the broad-spectrum, ethanolamine-type, topical antifungal agent ciclopirox olamine (Loprox®) cream or lotion, which requires a prescription. I have the patient use this twice daily, and I usually expect to see improvement within about 4 weeks of therapy.

Terbinafine (Lamisil AT) cream is available as an over-the-counter, topical, allylamine-type antifungal agent that can be used for the treatment of tinea facei (faciale), tinea corporis, tinea cruris, tinea pedis and tinea manuum. For tinea facei (faciale), tinea corporis and tinea cruris, it can be used once daily for 1 week; for tinea pedis between the toes, it can be used twice daily for 1 week; for tinea pedis on the soles or sides of the feet, it can be used twice daily for 2 weeks; and for tinea manuum, I would recommend using it twice daily for 2 weeks. Lamisil AT cream is recommended for patients 12 years of age and older. Improvement with terbinafine cream should be expected to occur within 2 weeks for tinea facei (faciale), tinea corporis and tinea cruris and within 4 weeks for tinea pedis and tinea manuum. (In patients treated for tinea with terbinafine cream there can be continued improvement during the 2–6 weeks after the terbinafine cream has been discontinued.) I have generally not found the need to prescribe terbinafine cream, because I have generally obtained good results with the other above-described topical antifungal agents.

Special considerations regarding the treatment of interdigital tinea pedis   Special mention should be made regarding the treatment of interdigital tinea pedis because, in this type of dermatophytic infection, *Candida* and/or bacteria not uncommonly secondarily involve the affected areas. The above-described broad-spectrum topical antifungal agents should cover *Candida* as well as dermatophytes, but should not be expected to have much effect on bacteria that are present. (Treatment of *Candida* is not a label indication for Lamisil AT cream, which is not considered to be a broad-spectrum antifungal agent.)

I usually find that, when interdigital tinea pedis does not respond to clotrimazole cream, it frequently will respond to econazole cream.

Frequently, if bacteria are secondarily involved, *Pseudomonas* is present (particularly if the affected area has a greenish discoloration), and adding topical gentamycin cream twice daily to the topical antifungal agent will result in clearing of the involvement. However, sometimes it may be necessary to obtain a bacterial C&S of the affected areas and add an appropriate oral antibiotic (based on the bacterial C&S results) to the therapy with the topical broad-spectrum antifungal agent. If a bacterial C&S are not obtained, I would empirically add a course of oral erythromycin 500 mg every 6 h or a course of cephalexin (Keflex®) 500 mg every 6 h in adults, if not otherwise unadvisable, to the therapy with the topical broad-spectrum antifungal agent.

Treatment of extensive, severe, or unresponsive involvement of tinea facei (faciale), tinea corporis, tinea cruris, tinea pedis and tinea manuum   If the involvement of tinea facei (faciale), tinea corporis, tinea cruris, tinea pedis, or tinea manuum is extensive, severe, or unresponsive to topical therapy as described above, systemic therapy with griseofulvin (see the discussion regarding griseofulvin in the treatment of tinea capitis section above) should be considered. For example, griseofulvin microsize tablets or microsize oral suspension (e.g. Grifulvin V) 0.5–1 g daily with a fatty meal (for maximal absorption) for adults and approximately 5.5 mg/pound per day for children, if not otherwise unadvisable (see above discussion of systemic griseofulvin for the treatment of tinea capitis), until clearing, can be used for tinea facei (faciale), tinea corporis and tinea cruris. (At approximately 5.5 mg/pound per day, the suggested griseofulvin microsize dosage for children weighing 30–50 pounds would be 125–250 mg daily, and the suggested dosage for children weighing over 50 pounds would be 250–500 mg daily.) In children and adults, clearing of these types of tinea involvement with the griseofulvin microsize therapy may take about 2–4 weeks. For tinea pedis and tinea manuum, which can be more difficult to eradicate, the dosage of griseofulvin microsize for adults should be about 1 g daily, until clearing, and for children, in whom I personally have almost never seen tinea pedis or tinea manuum, the griseofulvin microsize dosage that I would use would be that which is described above for children for tinea facei (faciale), tinea corporis and tinea cruris, until clearing. (Clearing of tinea pedis and tinea manuum with the griseofulvin microsize therapy may take about 4–8 weeks.)

As is the case with systemic griseofulvin treatment of tinea capitis, it is generally not necessary to use routine laboratory monitoring to check for adverse effects due to griseofulvin when systemic griseofulvin is used to treat healthy patients for tinea facei (faciale), tinea corporis, tinea cruris, tinea pedis and tinea manuum. More specifically, I do not use routine laboratory monitoring for systemic griseofulvin therapy in healthy patients if the duration of the therapy is less than 3 months; if the duration of the therapy is more than 3 months in healthy patients, I obtain a CBC, liver function tests, creatinine and urinalysis at baseline and every 3 months thereafter while the patient is on systemic griseofulvin therapy.

Although the systemic, imidazole-type, oral, antifungal agent ketoconazole (Nizoral) tablets are approved for the treatment of severe, recalcitrant, cutaneous, dermatophytic infections in patients who have not responded to topical therapy or oral griseofulvin, or who are unable to take griseofulvin, I generally avoid prescribing oral ketoconazole for such patients because I am aware of instances in which single doses of oral ketoconazole apparently caused severe idiosyncratic liver reactions.

Treatment of tinea unguium Traditionally, the treatment of choice for tinea unguium has been oral griseofulvin (see the discussion regarding griseofulvin in the treatment of tinea capitis section above). For example, griseofulvin microsize (e.g. Grifulvin V) 1 g daily, if not otherwise unadvisable, was used for the treatment of tinea unguim in healthy adults, and this treatment was continued until clearing. When systemic griseofulvin is used to treat healthy patients for tinea unguium, routine griseofulvin laboratory monitoring consisting of a CBC, liver function tests, creatinine and urinalysis is carried out at baseline and every 3 months thereafter while the patient is on systemic griseofulvin therapy. (I have virtually never seen tinea unguium in children.) Clearing of tinea unguium with griseofulvin therapy may take at least 4 months for fingernails and at least 6 months for toenails and occurs as the result of outgrowth of healthy new nail.

The newer oral antifungal agents terbinafine (Lamisil®) tablets and itraconazole (Sporanox®) capsules are much more effective than is griseofulvin in treating tinea unguium and have therefore replaced griseofulvin with regard to the treatment of tinea unguium.

Lamisil tablets should not be used in patients with pre-existing liver disease or renal impairment (creatinine clearance ≤ 50 ml/min) and should not be used in pregnant or breast-feeding patients. Rare cases of liver failure, which in some cases led to death or liver transplant, have occurred in patients with and without pre-existing liver disease when they were treated with Lamisil tablets for onychomycosis. If clinical or biochemical evidence of liver injury develops, Lamisil tablets should be discontinued. Serious skin reactions (e.g. toxic epidermal necrolysis and Stevens-Johnson syndrome) have been reported with Lamisil therapy. Treatment with Lamisil should be discontinued if progressive skin rash occurs.

The dosage for adults of Lamisil tablets for the treatment of fingernail tinea unguium is 250 mg orally daily for 6 weeks, and the dosage for adults for the treatment of toenail tinea unguium is 250 mg orally daily for 12 weeks. The optimal clinical effect of oral Lamisil treatment of tinea unguium is seen months after Lamisil therapy is discontinued and occurs as the result of outgrowth of healthy new nail.

For patients who are going to be on Lamisil tablets for only 6 weeks, I generally check a CBC, liver function tests and creatinine to confirm that the results of these tests are satisfactory before I start treatment.

For patients who are going to be on Lamisil tablets for 12 weeks, I obtain a baseline CBC, liver function tests and creatinine, and I repeat the CBC and liver function tests at 6 weeks.

I have patients on Lamisil tablets discontinue the treatment and notify me immediately if they develop any signs or symptoms of hepatic dysfunction (such as fatigue, anorexia, persistent nausea, vomiting, jaundice, right upper abdominal pain, dark urine, and/or pale stools), at which time I obtain liver function tests and proceed accordingly.

If the patient develops clinical evidence of other infection while on Lamisil therapy, a CBC should be obtained, and if the neutrophil count is ≤ 1000 cells/mm³, Lamisil should be discontinued, and supportive treatment should be initiated.

The safety and efficacy of Lamisil tablets have not been established in pediatric patients.

Sporanox is contraindicated for the treatment of onychomycosis in patients with evidence of ventricular dysfunction such as congestive heart failure (CHF) or a history of CHF. Also as onychomycosis is not a serious condition, Sporanox should not be used for the treatment of onychomycosis in patients with risk factors for CHF. Sporanox therapy should be stopped immediately if signs or symptoms of CHF develop (all patients taking Sporanox should be instructed as to the signs and symptoms of CHF).

Sporanox is contraindicated for the treatment of onychomycosis in pregnant patients and in women contemplating pregnancy. Sporanox should not be given to women of childbearing potential for the treatment of onychomycosis unless they are taking effective measures to prevent pregnancy and unless they begin Sporanox therapy on the second or third day following the onset of menses. Effective contraception should be continued throughout Sporanox therapy and for 2 months following the end of treatment.

The use of Sporanox with cisapride, oral midazolam, pimozide, quinidine, dofetilide and triazolam is contraindicated, as is use of Sporanox with HMG CoA-reductase inhibitors metabolized by CYP3A4, such as lovastatin and simvastatin. Since Sporanox has the potential for drug interactions with many other drugs, it is especially important that the package insert for Sporanox be consulted for potential drug interactions before Sporanox is prescribed for a patient taking any other medication(s). Patients on Sporanox should be instructed to contact their health care provider before taking any medications concomitantly with Sporanox, so that potential drug interactions with Sporanox can be avoided.

Sporanox has been associated with rare cases of serious hepatotoxicity, including hepatic failure and death, and in some of these cases there were no pre-existing liver disease and no serious underlying medical condition. Some cases of serious hepatotoxicity occurred within the first week of treatment. Since onychomycosis is not a serious condition, Sporanox should not be initiated for the treatment of onychomycosis in patients who have elevated liver enzymes or active liver disease or who have had liver toxicity with other medications. Monitoring of liver function tests should be considered for all patients receiving Sporanox. I recommend obtaining liver function tests at baseline and then monthly while the patient is on Sporanox therapy. Sporanox therapy should be stopped immediately and liver function testing should be performed if signs or symptoms suggestive of liver dysfunction develop (all patients taking Sporanox should be instructed to report any unusual fatigue, anorexia, nausea and/or vomiting, jaundice, dark urine, or pale stools).

Sporanox therapy should not be used for the treatment of onychomycosis in breast-feeding patients.

The safety and efficacy of Sporanox have not been established in pediatric patients.

Sporanox therapy for tinea unguium of the fingernails in adults consists of two pulses of Sporanox capsules, with each pulse consisting of 200 mg orally twice daily with meals (meals enhance the absorption of the Sporanox) for 1 week, with a period of 3 weeks off Sporanox between the two pulses of Sporanox.

The recommended Sporanox capsule dosage for adults with tinea unguium of the toenails is 200 mg orally daily with meals for 12 consecutive weeks. However, for adults with tinea unguium of the toenails, many dermatologists instead use three pulses of Sporanox capsules, with each pulse consisting of 200 mg orally twice daily with meals for 1 week, with a period of 3 weeks off Sporanox between each of the three pulses of Sporanox.

It should be noted that Sporanox capsules are available in the Sporanox PulsePak, which facilitates prescribing Sporanox pulse therapy as described above.

As is the case with Lamisil treatment of tinea unguium, the optimal clinical effect of Sporanox treatment of tinea unguium is seen months after Sporanox therapy is discontinued and occurs as the result of outgrowth of healthy new nail.

Mention should be made of Penlac Nail Lacquer® (ciclopirox topical solution 8%), which requires a prescription and is indicated – as a component of a comprehensive management program (see below) – for the topical treatment of mild to moderate tinea unguium of fingernails and toenails without lunula involvement in immunocompetent patients.

An *in vitro* study showed that the ciclopirox in Penlac Nail Lacquer penetrated up to a depth of approximately 0.4 mm into onychomycotic toenails after topical application, and nail plate concentrations decreased as a function of nail depth. Nail bed concentrations were not determined. In clinical studies, less than 12% of patients treated with Penlac Nail Lacquer for tinea unguium achieved either a completely clear or almost clear nail, where an almost clear nail meant that there was 10% or less residual nail involvement.

The regimen for treatment of tinea unguium with Penlac Nail Lacquer is as follows: removal of unattached, infected nail (as frequently as monthly), trimming of onycholytic nail (i.e. nail that is unattached to the nail bed) and filing of excess horny material by a professional trained in the treatment of nail disorders. Every 7 days, the patient should file away (with an emery board) loose nail material and trim the nail (as required) after Penlac Nail Lacquer is removed with alcohol. Penlac Nail Lacquer should be applied by the patient once daily to all affected nails with the applicator brush provided. (The Penlac Nail Lacquer should be applied evenly over the entire nail plate and 5 mm of surrounding skin and, if possible, it should be applied to the nail bed, hyponychium and the undersurface of the nail plate when it is free of the nail bed. Contact with the surrounding skin may produce mild, transient irritation.) The Penlac Nail Lacquer should not be removed on a daily basis; daily applications should be made by the patient over the previous coat and removed with alcohol every 7 days. This cycle should be repeated throughout the duration of therapy. Up to 48 weeks of this therapy are considered the full treatment period needed to achieve a clear or almost clear nail, where an almost clear nail indicates that there is 10% or less residual nail involvement. Six months of this therapy may be required before initial improvement is noticed. The patient should not use nail polish or other nail cosmetic products on the treated nails, and the patient should keep Penlac Nail Lacquer away from heat or an open flame, because it is flammable. The patient should be made aware that clinical studies have shown that, with this therapeutic regimen, less than 12% of patients were able to achieve either a completely clear or almost clear nail.

Since it is not known whether ciclopirox might reduce the effectiveness of systemic antifungal agents with regard to the treatment of tinea unguium, the concomitant use of Penlac Nail Lacquer and systemic antifungal agents is not recommended for the treatment of tinea unguium. The risk of removal of unattached, infected nail by the health-care provider and trimming by the patient should be carefully considered before prescribing the above-described Penlac Nail Lacquer treatment regimen for patients who have a history of insulin-dependent diabetes mellitus or diabetic neuropathy.

Pityriasis versicolor

Overview

Pityriasis versicolor is also known as tinea versicolor, but the latter name should not be used because, strictly speaking, the term tinea should be used only when referring to dermatophytic infections (see above), and pityriasis versicolor (tinea versicolor) is not due to a dermatophytic infection.

Pityriasis versicolor is due to the dimorphic fungus *Malassezia furfur*, which, in its non-pathogenic yeast form, is part of the normal flora of the stratum corneum. (The stratum corneum is the dead, horny, outermost layer of the epidermis and is composed of the protein keratin. The epidermis is the cutaneous layer that is located immediately above the dermis.) For not always clear reasons, this non-pathogenic yeast form converts to the pathogenic mycelial (filamentous) form, which produces the clinical changes characteristic of pityriasis versicolor.

Patients with pityriasis versicolor typically present with usually asymptomatic hyperpigmented and/or hypopigmented, scaly macules and/or patches usually on the trunk and proximal extremities. (Macules are small, non-raised, non-palpable lesions. Patches are large, non-raised, non-palpable lesions.) I have virtually never seen pityriasis versicolor in pediatric patients.

Confirmation of the diagnosis of pityriasis versicolor

The diagnosis of pityriasis versicolor is confirmed via a KOH preparation of scrapings from lesions. (See the discussion earlier in this chapter regarding KOH preps.) When the typical findings of clusters of yeasts (single-celled fungal forms) and short, septate hyphae (filamentous fungal forms), comprising the so-called 'spaghetti and meatballs' pattern, are seen on KOH preparations of scrapings from lesions, the diagnosis of pityriasis versicolor is confirmed. Because these KOH preparation findings are characteristic, fungal cultures are not necessary.

Also, the lesions of pityriasis versicolor may fluoresce a yellowish color when exposed to the ultraviolet light of a Wood's lamp.

Treatment of pityriasis versicolor

Selenium sulfide lotion   I usually treat pityriasis versicolor by having the patient apply selenium sulfide lotion 2.5% (Selsun Lotion®) to the trunk and involved extremities and having the patient wash it off 10 min later. I have the patient repeat this sequence daily for 7 days.

In order to prevent recurrence, some dermatologists recommend subsequently applying and then washing off this medication 10 min later once or twice per month.

Under ordinary circumstances, this medication should not be used for the treatment of pityriasis versicolor in pregnant patients. Safety and efficacy of this medication in infants have not been established.

Imidazole-type and ethanolamine-type topical antifungal agents   Alternatively, pityriasis versicolor can be treated with topical imidazole-type broad-spectrum antifungal agents, such as clotrimazole (Lotrimin-AF) cream, lotion, or solution to the affected areas twice daily for 2–4 weeks, or with the topical ethanolamine-type broad-spectrum antifungal agent ciclopirox olamine (Loprox) cream or lotion to the affected areas twice daily for 2–4 weeks. The safety and efficacy of Loprox cream and lotion have not been established in patients younger than 10 years of age.

Ketoconazole (Nizoral) tablets   Although it has not been approved by the FDA for the treatment of pityriasis versicolor, some dermatologists have used the systemic, imidazole-type, oral, antifungal agent ketoconazole (Nizoral) tablets for the treatment of pityriasis versicolor. However, I do not recommend the use of these tablets, because, as noted previously, I am aware of instances in which single doses of oral ketoconazole apparently caused severe idiosyncratic liver reactions, and it does not seem reasonable to me to take such a risk when treating such a basically benign condition as pityriasis versicolor.

Ketoconazole (Nizoral) 2% Shampoo   For the treatment of pityriasis versicolor, a single application of Nizoral (ketoconazole 2%) Shampoo is applied to the involvement and to a wide margin surrounding the involvement and is then washed off 5 mins later. I feel that this medication should not be used in pregnant or breast-feeding patients unless its use is approved by the patient's obstetrician or breast-fed baby's pediatrician, respectively. Safety and efficacy of this medication in children have not been established.

Special considerations regarding treatment of pityriasis versicolor

It should be noted that, after pityriasis versicolor has been adequately treated, the hyperpigmented and hypopigmented discoloration of the condition can persist for a while before fading. Adequate treatment can be confirmed by the presence of a negative KOH preparation result following treatment. Also, after adequate treatment, scaling is no longer present.

It should be noted that, before adequate treatment of pityriasis versicolor is completed, sun exposure can exacerbate the appearance of the hyper-pigmented and hypopigmented changes of the condition. Sun exposure can make the hyperpigmented changes darker and can darken (i.e. tan) the uninvolved skin without darkening the involved hypopigmented areas, thereby making the contrast between the involved and uninvolved skin greater. After completion of adequate treatment, these effects of sun exposure do not occur.

'Off label' use of Sporanox capsules for the treatment of tineas and pitryriasis versicolor

The more recent systemic antifungal agents Sporanox (itraconazole) capsules (a triazole-type antifungal agent) and Lamisil (terbinafine) tablets (an allylamine-type antifungal agent) have not been approved by the FDA for the treatment of superficial fungal infections other than tinea unguium.

However, some dermatologists have used Sporanox capsules as follows. For the treatment of dermatophytic infections of the skin where there are sebaceous glands (e.g. tinea capitis, tinea barbae, tinea facei (faciale), tinea corporis and tinea cruris) and for the treatment of pityriasis versicolor, which is due to a non-dermatophytic superficial fungus (see above) and occurs on skin where there are sebaceous glands, Sporanox capsules 200 mg orally once daily with meals (meals enhance the absorption of the Sporanox) are prescribed for 1 week for adults. For the treatment of der-matophytic infections of the skin where there are no sebaceous glands (e.g. for tinea pedis and tinea manuum), Sporanox capsules 200 mg orally twice daily with meals are prescribed for 1 week for adults.

Sporanox is contraindicated for the treatment of these tineas and pityriasis versicolor in patients with evidence of ventricular dysfunction such as CHF or a history of CHF. Also, Sporanox should not be used for the treatment of these tineas and pityriasis versicolor in patients with risk factors for CHF. Sporanox therapy should be stopped immediately if signs or symptoms of CHF develop (all patients taking Sporanox should be instructed as to the signs and symptoms of CHF).

Sporanox is contraindicated for the treatment of these tineas and pityriasis versicolor in pregnant patients and in women contemplating pregnancy. Sporanox should not be given to women of childbearing potential for the treatment of these tineas and pityriasis versicolor unless they are taking effective measures to prevent pregnancy and unless they begin Sporanox therapy on the second or third day following the onset of menses. Effective contraception should be continued throughout Sporanox therapy and for 2 months following the end of treatment. Sporanox therapy should not be used for the treatment of these tineas and pityriasis versicolor in breast-feeding patients. For additional details on side-effects and precautions/warning regarding Sporanox therapy, see *Tinea unguium treatment* in this Chapter.

Superficial cutaneous candidal infections (candidiasis), excluding chronic mucocutaneous candidiasis

Overview of intertriginous candidiasis

Superficial cutaneous candidal infections (e.g. superficial cutaneous candidiasis) are typically due to the species *Candida albicans* and usually involve intertriginous (i.e. skin-fold) areas (such as the groins, inframammary areas, axillae, etc.), in which case the condition is manifested by erythema and maceration, typically with erythematous satellites and vesicopustules that are beyond the borders of the main involvement. The vesicopustules break, leaving behind erythematous macules with necrotic epidermal collarettes that are minimally adherent.

Predisposing factors include obesity and diabetes mellitus.

Overview of candidal balanitis

Candidal balanitis consists of erythema and small papules or papulopustules involving the glans penis and/or the coronal sulcus. The papulopustules can break, leaving behind erythematous macules with collarettes of scale. Candidal infection may also involve the scrotum (unlike tinea, which usually spares the scrotum) as well as the groins.

Diabetes mellitus, lack of circumcision and a vaginal candidal infection in a sexual partner are predisposing factors for genital candidiasis in males.

Overview of candidal paronychia

Candidal infection of the proximal and/or lateral nail fold(s) (i.e. candidal paronychia) is the usual cause of chronic paronychia, is typically manifested by erythema and swelling of the proximal and/or lateral nail fold(s), usually develops slowly and typically follows excessive exposure of the proximal and lateral nail folds to water. Sometimes pus can be expressed from the area between the skin of the proximal and/or lateral nail fold(s) and the underlying nail plate. (The proximal nail fold is the skin fold that is located at the proximal edge of the nail, and the lateral nail folds are the skin folds that are adjacent to the sides of the nail. Paronychia is a term that is used to refer to inflammation of the proximal and/or lateral nail fold(s).)

Special considerations regarding candidal paronychia

Candidal infection of the proximal and/or lateral nail fold(s) (i.e. candidal paronychia), which is the usual cause of chronic paronychia, needs to be distinguished from bacterial infection of the proximal and/or lateral nail fold(s) (i.e. bacterial paronychia), which is the usual cause of acute paronychia.

Like candidal paronychia, bacterial paronychia is typically manifested by erythema and swelling of the proximal and/or lateral nail fold(s), and sometimes pus can be expressed from the area between the skin of the proximal and/or lateral nail fold(s) and the underlying nail plate. However, bacterial paronychia usually develops acutely and typically follows injury to the cuticle or proximal or lateral nail fold, whereas candidal paronychia usually develops slowly and typically follows excessive exposure of the proximal and lateral nail folds to water. Also, in my experience bacterial paronychia tends to be more acutely tender and painful than is candidal paronychia, and pus tends to be more commonly present with bacterial paronychia than it is with candidal paronychia. The evaluation and treatment of bacterial paronychia are further discussed in Chapter 17.

It should be noted that the presence of concomitant bacterial infection can sometimes complicate the presentation of candidal paronychia.

Patients who do not have the condition known as chronic mucocutaneous candidiasis but do have candidal paronychia that is chronic can subsequently secondarily develop onycholysis (separation of the nail plate from the nail bed) and/or onychodystrophy (nail deformity) of the corresponding nail, whereas *Candida albicans* invades the nail directly and produces onychodystrophy only in patients with chronic mucocutaneous candidiasis. Chronic mucocutaneous candidiasis, which is briefly discussed later in this chapter, refers to a group of syndromes in which patients who have particular immunological defects develop chronic candidal infections of the skin, oropharynx, and nails.

Overview of facial candidiasis

I have seen candidiasis consisting of moist erythema, sometimes with small papules and/or papulopustules, involving facial skin around the mouth and on the cheeks, particularly in infants.

Overview of so-called 'diaper candidiasis'

So-called 'diaper candidiasis' is related to the occlusive nature of diapers in conjunction with the presence of *Candida* in the gastrointestinal tract. (For discussion of so-called 'diaper dermatitis', see Chapter 2.) Diaper candidiasis typically begins as erythema involving the perianal area. The involvement spreads from there to the perineum, inguinal regions and adjacent areas, and generally consists of erythema, typically with erythematous satellites and vesicopustules that are beyond the borders of the main involvement. The vesiclopustules break, leaving behind erythematous macules with necrotic epidermal collarettes that are minimally adherent.

Confirmation of the diagnosis of candidiasis

KOH preparations and fungal cultures   When suspected clinically, the diagnosis of superficial cutaneous candidiasis can be confirmed by obtaining a KOH preparation and/or a fungal culture of skin scrapings of the involvement. (See the discussion earlier in this chapter regarding KOH preps and fungal cultures.) In the case of candidal paronychia, KOH preps and fungal cultures are commonly falsely negative, and the diagnosis is therefore generally made on the basis of the typical clinical presentation of candidal paronychia in contrast to that of bacterial paronychia, as described above.

It should be noted that, if an organism from the genus *Candida* is isolated on fungal culture, the species needs to be identified in order to determine whether or not the patient does indeed have a candidal infection, because most species in the genus *Candida* are non-pathogenic skin colonizers and do not cause disease in healthy humans.

Testing pus and pustules for the presence of bacterial infection   If pus or pustules are present, or if secondary bacterial infection is suspected, a bacterial C&S of the involvement should be obtained, with a course of appropriate oral antibiotic therapy prescribed, depending on the bacterial C&S results.

Treatment of superficial cutaneous candidal infections

Non-specific/indirect treatment of candidiasis   In treating superficial cutaneous candidiasis, the health care provider should correct any predisposing factors that can be corrected. Patients with diabetes mellitus should have their diabetes mellitus under good control. Patients with obesity should lose weight.

Patients with candidiasis of intertriginous areas should keep the areas as dry as possible, should in general wear loose-fitting clothing, should preferably wear clothing made of cotton, and should avoid wearing nylon, other synthetic fabrics and wool. More specifically, women should wear brassieres that give adequate support and cotton underpants and should avoid wearing pantyhose and nylon underpants, and men should wear cotton boxer shorts and should avoid wearing briefs. To facilitate keeping the intertriginous areas dry and thereby help prevent recurrence of intertriginous candidiasis once it has been effectively treated and has resolved, patients should be advised to use an absorbent powder such as Zeasorb® powder in the intertriginous areas. (When an absorbent powder such as Zeasorb powder is applied, it should always be applied to a clean, dry surface because it otherwise builds up and becomes doughy and 'caked on'.)

Patients who have candidal paronychia should as much as possible avoid exposing their nail folds to water. If the involvement occurs on the fingers (which is typically the case with candidal paronychia), the patients should be advised to avoid excessive hand washing and should be told to wear white cotton gloves under plastic (i.e. vinyl) gloves whenever their hands are exposed to water for prolonged periods of time (e.g. when washing dishes, washing cars, etc.) and whenever they are engaged in activities that would otherwise require them to wash their hands afterward. White cotton gloves and plastic (i.e. vinyl) gloves can be obtained through pharmacies. The white cotton gloves are worn to absorb the excessive sweat that would otherwise accumulate as a result of the plastic gloves being worn. The presence of the excessive sweat that would otherwise accumulate would make it as though the patients' hands were immersed in water.

For patients with diaper candidiasis, the involved areas should be kept meticulously dry. This can be facilitated by changing diapers as soon as they become soiled, by avoiding the use of occlusive (e.g. plastic) coverings over the diapers, and by the use of an absorbent powder such as Zeasorb powder. When an absorbent powder such as Zeasorb powder is applied, it should always be applied to a clean, dry surface because it otherwise builds up and becomes doughy and 'caked on'.

Specific/direct treatment of candidiasis   For specific/direct treatment of candidiasis, any broad-spectrum, topical antifungal lotion should be used. In patients who are not allergic to imidazole-type antifungal agents, I prescribe a broad-spectrum, topical imidazole-type antifungal agent such as clotrimazole (Lotrimin-AF) lotion twice daily to the involvement until it clears. In patients who are allergic to imidazole-type antifungal agents, I prescribe the topical, broad-spectrum, ethanolamine-type antifungal agent ciclopirox olamine (Loprox) lotion twice daily to the involvement until it clears.

Specific/direct antifungal treatment of candidal paronychia involves the use of the broad-spectrum topical imidazole-type antifungal agent clotrimazole (Lotrimin-AF) solution, which is applied twice daily to the involved nail fold, including the area that is at the juncture of the skin of the nail fold and the corresponding nail plate. Treatment is continued until the condition clears. If the patient is allergic to imidazole-type antifungal agents, the ethanolamine-type, broad-spectrum, topical antifungal agent ciclopirox olamine (Loprox) lotion should be used in place of the clotrimazole solution. If chronic candidal paronychia is associated with a corresponding secondarily dystrophic nail, the nail should generally begin to grow out normally once the chronic paronychia clears.

If a bacterial C&S (see above) isolates pathogenic bacteria, appropriate oral antibiotic therapy should be prescribed accordingly.

Chronic mucocutaneous candidiasis

Overview

Chronic mucocutaneous candidiasis refers to a group of syndromes in which patients who have particular immunological defects develop chronic candidal infections of the skin, oropharynx and nails. In my experience, chronic mucocutaneous candidiasis is rare.

Treatment of chronic mucocutaneous candidiasis

Because this problem has traditionally been notoriously difficult to treat and since optimal current treatment of this condition involves immune deficiency correction along with the use of antifungal drugs, patients with chronic mucocutaneous candidiasis should be referred to a dermatologist and/or an infectious disease specialist.

Non-dermatophytic onychomycosis

Overview

As noted above, fungi other than dermatophytes can infect toenails and/or fingernails and cause onychomycosis. These fungi, which can be molds or yeasts, are usually considered to be non-pathogenic but can sometimes infect the nail and be pathogenic.

When a non-dermatophytic fungus is isolated on fungal culture of a dystrophic nail, it can be difficult to determine whether the fungus is merely a contaminant colonizing the dystrophic nail or is truly infecting the nail. Onychomycosis due to non-dermatophytes seems to occur more commonly in already abnormal nails or in nails of older individuals and usually occurs in toenails rather than fingernails.

The non-dermatophytic fungus *Candida albicans* (which is a yeast) invades the nail directly and produces onychodystrophy only in patients with chronic mucocutaneous candidiasis. Chronic mucocutaneous candidiasis, which was briefly discussed previously in this chapter in the discussion of candidiasis, refers to a group of syndromes in which patients who have particular immunological defects develop chronic *Candida* infections of the skin, oropharynx and nails. Onychodystrophy occurring with direct candidal invasion of the nail in patients with chronic mucocutaneous candidiasis should be distinguished from the situation in which patients who do not have chronic mucocutaneous candidiasis develop candidal paronychia that is chronic and subsequently secondarily develop onycholysis and/or onychodystrophy of the corresponding nail, as discussed previously in this chapter. Candidal paronychia is a candidal infection of the proximal and/or lateral nail fold(s) and was discussed previously in this chapter in the discussion of candidiasis.

Treatment of non-dermatophytic onychomycosis

Non-dermatophytic onychomycosis can be difficult to treat. There is no specific uniformly effective antifungal medication approved for the treatment of this condition.

It is felt that itraconazole (Sporanox) capsules, which are approved and indicated for the treatment of tinea unguium (i.e. dermatophytic onychomycosis), as discussed previously in this chapter, can be beneficial in the treatment of non-dermatophytic onychomycosis, and it is felt that this medication is more beneficial in this regard than are terbinafine (Lamisil) tablets, which are also approved and indicated for the treatment of tinea unguium, as discussed previously in this chapter, although neither drug is approved for the treatment of non-dermatophytic onychomycosis.

Other methods of treatment for non-dermatophytic onychomycosis involve avulsion of affected nails.

INTERTRIGO

Overview

I think of intertrigo as inflammation due to irritation (resulting, for example, from friction and moisture) involving intertriginous skin (i.e. skin-fold areas) without primary fungal or bacterial infection, although fungi (e.g. *Candida*) and/or bacteria may or may not secondarily infect the involvement, which typically clinically consists of erythema and, sometimes, maceration involving intertriginous areas.

This condition tends to be more common in obese individuals and in women with pendulous breasts, probably because the skin folds in question tend to be more exaggerated in these individuals.

A KOH preparation and/or fungal culture of skin scrapings from involved areas can be performed to test for the presence of fungi, and a bacterial C&S of affected areas can be performed to test for the presence of bacteria. (See the discussion of KOH preps and fungal cultures earlier in this chapter.)

Treatment of intertrigo

Since fungal testing can be falsely negative, the broad-spectrum, topical, imidazole-type antifungal agent clotrimazole (Lotrimin-AF) lotion or, if the patient is allergic to imidazole-type antifungal agents, the broad-spectrum, topical ethanolamine-type antifungal agent ciclopirox olamine (Loprox) lotion can be empirically used twice daily to the involvement in addition to hydrocortisone lotion 1% twice daily until the condition clears, in order to treat active disease in adults. In pediatric patients, I would use hydrocortisone 0.5% in place of hydrocortisone 1%.

If a bacterial C&S reveals pathogenic bacteria, a course of an appropriate oral antibiotic should also be prescribed.

To hasten the resolution of active disease and to prevent recurrence of the problem once it has resolved, the involved areas should be kept meticulously dry. This can be facilitated by the use of an absorbent powder such as Zeasorb powder. (When an absorbent powder such as Zeasorb powder is applied, it should always be applied to a clean, dry surface because it otherwise builds up and becomes doughy and 'caked on'.) Other beneficial measures include the wearing of loose-fitting clothing, preferably made of cotton, and the wearing of nylon, other synthetic fabrics and wool should be avoided. More specifically, women should wear brassieres that give adequate support and cotton underpants and should avoid wearing pantyhose and nylon underpants, and men should wear cotton boxer shorts and should avoid wearing briefs.

PERLECHE

Overview

I think of perleche (angular cheilitis, angular stomatitis), which presents as inflammation typically consisting of erythema and, sometimes, whitish maceration and/or fissuring involving the skin adjacent to the corners of the mouth, as being, depending on the situation, a variant of intertrigo (primary irritant inflammation of a skin-fold area with or without secondary fungal and/or bacterial infection); a variant of intertriginous candidiasis (primary candidal infection of a skin-fold area); a result and manifestation of riboflavin deficiency with or without secondary candidal infection; or a result and manifestation of zinc deficiency with or without secondary candidal and/or bacterial infection.

Intertrigo-like and intertriginous candidiasis-like types of perleche

In the case of the intertrigo-like and intertriginous candidiasis-like types of perleche, the patients tend to have exaggerated skin folds at the corners of the mouth. These exaggerated skin folds can be due to laxity of skin associated with aging and/or due to edentulousness, improperly fitting dentures, or malocclusion. In this situation, saliva is retained in the skin folds and maceration occurs. Analogous to intertrigo, this can ultimately lead to the development of inflammation due to irritation, in which case secondary fungal (e.g. candidal) and/or bacterial infection may or may not be present.

Alternatively, analogous to intertriginous candidiasis, primary candidal infection can occur in these skin fold areas.

Riboflavin and zinc deficiency types of perleche

In the types of perleche with riboflavin and zinc deficiency, the clinical changes of perleche are due to deficiencies of these nutrients. Scrapings for KOH preparation and fungal culture (see earlier discussion regarding KOH preps and fungal cultures) and a bacterial C&S can be obtained to test for *Candida* and pathogenic bacteria, respectively (candidal and/or bacterial infection can be present secondarily).

The presence of other characteristic features of riboflavin or zinc deficiency suggests riboflavin or zinc deficiency as the cause of a patient's perleche.

Riboflavin deficiency is usually accompanied by deficiency of other B complex vitamins, may accompany Plummer–Vinson syndrome, and also results in integumentary manifestations other than perleche. Plummer–Vinson syndrome includes sideropenic anemia and epithelial lesions, may be accompanied by deficiency of other B complex vitamins and iron, and has a relationship to postcricoid carcinoma. Other integumentary manifestations of riboflavin deficiency include seborrheic dermatitis-like greasy scaling involving the nasolabial folds of the face, the alae of the nose, the vestibule of the nose, and, sometimes, the ears and the canthi (corners) of the eyelids; vertical fissuring involving the vermilion borders of the lips; smooth, magenta-colored glossitis; changes similar to non-specific dermatitis involving the vulva, scrotum and, sometimes, the shaft of the penis or the medial (inner) aspects of the thighs; and, rarely, interstitial keratitis and vascularization of the corneas. (See Chapter 2 regarding seborrheic dermatitis and non-specific dermatitis.)

Manifestations of zinc deficiency other than perleche typically include acral and anogenital non-specific dermatitis-like changes, alopecia and diarrhea. (Acral areas are peripheral – i.e. the face, hands and feet. See Chapter 2 regarding non-specific dermatitis.)

Treatment of perleche

Treatment of intertrigo-like and intertriginous
candidiasis-like perleche

A component of the treatment and prevention of the intertrigo-like and intertriginous candidiasis-like perleche should be geared toward keeping the areas where involvement is present or occurs dry. Also, the patient can be referred to his or her dentist for correction of edentulousness, improperly fitting dentures, or malocclusion.

The topical, broad-spectrum, imidazole-type antifungal agent clotrimazole (Lotrimin-AF) lotion or, if the patient is allergic to imidazoles, the topical, broad-spectrum, ethanolamine-type antifungal agent ciclopirox olamine (Loprox) lotion can be used twice daily, until the condition clears, if candidal infection is present, and a course of an oral antibiotic chosen on the basis of bacterial C&S results can be prescribed if bacterial infection is present.

For intertrigo-like perleche, where the problem is not primary candidal infection, hydrocortisone lotion 1% can be used twice daily for the inflammation, until it clears, in adults. In pediatric patients, I would use hydrocortisone 0.5%.

The way I generally approach intertrigo-like and intertriginous candidiasis-like perleche is to prescribe empirically clotrimazole (Lotrimin-AF) lotion or ciclopirox olamine (Loprox) lotion (KOH preps and fungal cultures can be falsely negative) followed by hydrocortisone lotion 1% followed by Polysporin Ointment® (polymyxin B sulfate/bacitracin zinc) twice daily, until the condition clears, in adults. (It is immaterial whether the antifungal lotion or the hydrocortisone lotion is applied first or second in the sequence, but the Polysporin Ointment should always be applied third.) In pediatric patients, I would use hydrocortisone lotion 0.5% in place of the hydrocortisone lotion 1%.

If the intertrigo-like perleche keeps recurring, Vaseline Petroleum Jelly® (white petrolatum) or Aquaphor Ointment® (petrolatum in a more water-miscible form) can be tried as a thin protectant film applied to the areas where involvement occurred in order to try to prevent recurrence of the problem after clearing has been achieved.

Treatment of perleche due to zinc and riboflavin deficiency

If it is determined that a patient's perleche is due to zinc or riboflavin deficiency, the approach to the problem includes correcting the deficiency.

19

Pseudofolliculitis barbae

OVERVIEW

Pseudofolliculitis barbae (also known as pili incarnati) is a condition in which, typically, curly hairs grow into the skin (producing ingrown hairs) as a result of shaving. This results in a foreign-body type inflammatory reaction to the hair, producing erythematous papules. In addition there may be pustules in association with the papules. This condition is not due to infection, but is due to an inflammatory reaction. Pseudofolliculitis barbae occurs most commonly in blacks.

SPECIAL CONSIDERATIONS REGARDING PSEUDOFOLLICULITIS BARBAE

The common differential diagnosis of pseudofolliculitis barbae includes bacterial folliculitis (see Chapter 17), tinea barbae (see Chapter 18) and acne (see Chapter 9).

Bacterial culture and sensitivities (C&S) of pustule contents should be negative in patients with pseudofolliculitis barbae and should reveal pathogenic bacteria in patients with bacterial folliculitis, but be aware that false-negative bacterial C&S results can occur in cases of bacterial folliculitis. (Pustule contents can be accessed by piercing pustule roofs with a 20-gauge needle or a no. 11 scalpel.) Bacterial C&S of pustule contents should also be negative in patients with acne, but patients with acne should also have comedones. A potassium hydroxide (KOH) preparation and/or fungal culture of scrapings and plucked hairs of involved areas should reveal evidence of a dermatophytic fungus in patients with tinea barbae, but be aware that false-negative KOH preparation and fungal culture results can occur in cases of tinea barbae (see Chapter 18 for discussion of KOH preps, fungal cultures and tinea barbae). Rosacea, perioral dermatitis and possibly steroid dependent facial dermatosis (see Chapter 10) might also be considered in the differential diagnosis.

TREATMENT OF PSEUDOFOLLICULITIS BARBAE

The best treatment for pseudofolliculitis barbae is for the patient to stop shaving and allow the hair to grow out. When this is done, the hairs that have curled into the skin (thereby resulting in a foreign body-type reaction producing erythematous papules and pustules) continue to grow, and, as they grow, they pop out of the skin, and the erythematous papules and pustules resolve.

Patients for whom allowing the hair to grow out is unacceptable should be instructed not to try to achieve an extremely close shave, not to pull the skin taught when shaving, to shave in the direction of the grain of the hairs and not against the grain of the hairs and to shave every other day. When using a safety razor, patients should use a shaving gel (gels seem to be better than creams or foams), and should consider using the Bumpfighter Razor®, which is a brand of safety razor that is specially designed for patients with pseudofolliculitis barbae. If an electric razor is used, it should be an adjustable razor that is at the setting that provides the least close shave.

An alternative to shaving is the use of a chemical depilatory (these are available over the counter).

For unclear reasons, the use of topical tretinoin (Retin-A®) seems to provide beneficial results in patients with pseudofolliculitis barbae who shave. When I prescribe Retin-A for pseudofolliculitis barbae, I generally start out having the patient use Retin-A cream 0.025% nightly at bedtime as described for acne in Chapter 9, and I have the patient also follow the shaving recommendations as described above.

Careful intralesional injection of injectible Kenalog® (triamcinolone) suspension as described in Chapter 9 for inflammatory acne nodules may be beneficial for inflammatory papular lesions of pseudofolliculitis barbae. Likewise, if any of the lesions are hypertrophic or keloidal scars (these are typically firm), careful intralesional injections of injectible Kenalog (triamcinolone) suspension as described for hypertrophic scars and keloids in Chapter 8 may be beneficial.

20

Pseudomonas nail infection, idiopathic distal onycholysis and pigmented nail streaks

PSEUDOMONAS NAIL INFECTION

Overview

In my experience, *Pseudomonas* nail infection typically presents as distal onycholysis (separation of the nail plate from the nail bed) with associated greenish discoloration. There may also be associated colonization of *Candida*.

Treatment of *Pseudomonas* nail infection

In treating this problem, I trim the onycholytic portion of the nail as far back as is comfortably possible, and I have the patient continue to do this. I also have the patient carry out vinegar and water soaks (for which one part of vinegar is mixed with four parts of water) of the affected nail for 5–10 min followed by dropping clotrimazole (Lotrimin-AF®) topical solution between the nail plate and nail bed twice daily until all greenish discoloration has resolved and new, attached nail has grown out completely. (The vinegar and water soaks are used to treat the *Pseudomonas* infection, and the clotrimazole topical solution is used to treat a possible candidal component.) If the patient is allergic to imidazole-type antifungal agents, I have the patient use ciclopirox olamine (Loprox®) topical lotion, which is an ethanolamine-type antifungal agent, in place of the clotrimazole solution.

IDIOPATHIC DISTAL ONYCHOLYSIS

Overview

I think of idiopathic distal onycholysis as being a condition in which there is separation of the nail plate from the nail bed occurring distally in the nail plate/nail bed unit and as being a condition that is not due to a primary *Pseudomonas* infection, primary fungal infection (although, in my experience, secondary colonization of *Candida* may be present), specific skin disorder, such as psoriasis, neoplasm, drug reaction, or metabolic problem. Primary fungal infection is ruled out via potassium hydroxide (KOH) preparation and fungal culture of scrapings from involved nail beds. See Chapter 18 for discussion of KOH preparations, fungal cultures and fungal infections of nails. For discussion of psoriasis, see Chapter 4. With regard to metabolic problems and onycholysis, thyrotoxicosis, for example, can produce a characteristic type of onycholysis known as Plummer's nail, in which the free edge of the nail curves upward.

In my experience, most patients presenting with idiopathic distal onycholysis are women with long fingernails, and in this situation the condition may be due to frequent, minor, inadvertent trauma (of which the patient is unaware) to long nails, thereby traumatically causing distal separation of the nail plate from the nail bed.

Treatment of idiopathic distal onycholysis

In the treatment of this condition, I trim back the onycholytic portion of the nail as far as is comfortably possible, and I have the patient continue to do this. I also have the patient carry out vinegar and water soaks (for which one part of vinegar is mixed with four parts of water) of the affected nail for 5–10 min followed by dropping clotrimazole (Lotrimin-AF) topical solution between the nail plate and nail bed twice daily until normal, attached nail grows out completely. The vinegar and water soaks are used to treat a possible *Pseudomonas* component that may be present subclinically, in which case there is no visible greenish discoloration. The clotrimazole topical solution is used to treat a possible candidal component, even if KOH preparation and fungal culture results are negative for *Candida* because these test results can be falsely negative. If the patient is allergic to imidazole-type antifungal agents, ciclopirox olamine (Loprox) topical lotion, which is an ethanolamine-type antifungal agent, can be used in place of the clotrimazole solution.

PIGMENTED NAIL STREAKS

Pigmented nail streaks are typically brown streaks that are oriented longitudinally in the nail plate and extend from the proximal nail fold to the distal edge of the nail. (The proximal nail fold is the skin fold that is located at the proximal edge of the nail plate.) Pigmented nail streaks can be solitary or multiple and can involve a single nail or multiple nails. Pigmented nail streaks can be due to lentigo simplex lesions or melanocytic nevi in the nail matrix; they can be due to malignant melanoma in the nail matrix; or they can be due to drugs (e.g. minocycline (Minocin®)). Lentigo simplex lesions can be considered to be precursors to junctional melanocytic nevi. The nail matrix is located under the proximal nail fold and produces the nail plate. See Chapter 24 for discussion of lentigo simplex lesions and melanocytic nevi and see Chapter 26 for discussion of malignant melanoma.

Benign pigmented nail streaks are seen not uncommonly in Black individuals, who nonetheless can have pigmented nail streaks that are due to malignant melanoma in the nail matrix.

Patients with pigmented nail streaks, especially patients with pigmented nail streaks that have features that make one suspect the presence of malignant melanoma in the nail matrix, should be referred to a dermatologist for evaluation and consideration of doing a nail matrix biopsy to rule out the presence of malignant melanoma in the nail matrix. (Biopsy of the nail matrix involves temporarily reflecting back the proximal nail fold as a flap in order to gain access to the underlying nail matrix.) Pigmented nail streak features that make one suspect the presence of malignant melanoma in the nail matrix include a solitary streak (if there are multiple streaks, they are not likely to be due to malignant melanoma because it is not likely for a patient to have multiple malignant melanomas in multiple nail matrices at one time); a streak in a White patient; a streak that is irregular in any patient (e.g. a streak that has different shades of color and/or has edges that are not sharply demarcated in that the pigment trails off, fades, or leaches into the adjacent normal nail and does not stop sharply and abruptly at the juncture with the adjacent normal nail); a streak that is changing in any patient; a streak that is very dark in any patient; a streak that is very wide in any patient; and a streak that is associated with pigment involving the skin of the proximal nail fold in any patient (this is called Hutchinson's sign and is a late finding of malignant melanoma involving the nail matrix).

Lastly, if there is any uncertainty at all as to the cause of a pigmented nail streak, the patient should be referred to a dermatologist.

21

Urticaria/angioedema, urticarial vasculitis and pruritus without rash

URTICARIA/ANGIOEDEMA

Overview

Urticaria (hives) typically presents as an eruption of usually itchy wheals that can be flesh colored, erythematous or blanched. A wheal is a circumscribed area of edema involving the superficial portion of the dermis, which is the cutaneous layer that is located immediately below the epidermis, which is the superficial cutaneous layer. (An example of a wheal is what typically forms as the result of a superficial intradermal injection.) When the edema extends into the deep dermis and/or subcutaneous or submucosal tissue, thereby producing an area of deep swelling, the condition is called angioedema rather than urticaria.

Typically, individual lesions are evanescent and spontaneously resolve within 24–48 h, and patients continue to develop new lesions for an indefinite period of time.

If the overall condition has been present for less than 6–8 weeks, it is considered acute; if it has been present for a period of time longer than that, it is considered chronic.

Urticaria and angioedema can be present alone or in combination.

From this point on, when the discussion applies to both entities, I will use the term urticaria/angioedema, and when the discussion applies only to one or the other entity, I will use the appropriate term (either urticaria or angioedema, depending on the situation).

Urticaria/angioedema can be associated with systemic (such as respiratory and gastrointestinal) manifestations.

Type I hypersensitivity reaction to specific antigen

A common presentation of urticaria/angioedema is as a type I hypersensitivity reaction to specific food antigens (e.g. nuts, chocolate, shellfish), drugs (especially the penicillins), venom from arthropods (e.g. bees, wasps), or inhaled antigens. This type of reaction involves mast cell degranulation mediated by IgE.

Urticaria/angioedema associated with intestinal worm infestation

Sometimes infestation with intestinal worms can be associated with urticaria/angioedema. It is not clear as to whether or not this involves an IgE-mediated reaction.

Dermatographism

Another common presentation of urticaria is dermatographism (or dermographism), which is the condition wherein scratching of the skin results in the formation of a wheal at the site where the skin was scratched. Patients with dermatographism can present with episodes of itching of normal-looking skin on which wheals develop when and where the patient scratches.

Pressure urticaria

Pressure urticaria is the condition in which deep edema with erythema develops at sites where constant cutaneous pressure has been applied.

Vibratory angioedema

Vibratory angioedema is angioedema that occurs as a result of exposure to vibration.

Cold urticaria

Cold urticaria results from exposure to cold, which can be in the form of ambient temperature, ingestion of cold food or drink, or application of a cold object (e.g. an ice cube) to the skin surface.

Rarely, cold urticaria can be associated with cold agglutininemia, cryofibrinogenemia, cryoglobulinemia and cold hemolysinemia.

Heat urticaria

Patients with the rare condition of heat urticaria develop wheals at cutaneous sites shortly after heat is applied locally to the sites.

Solar urticaria/angioedema

Solar urticaria/angioedema is the condition in which patients develop urticaria (and occasionally angioedema, bronchospasm and syncope) shortly after exposure to sunlight or certain wavelengths of artificial light.

This condition can sometimes be associated with systemic lupus erythematosus or erythropoietic protoporphyria.

Cholinergic urticaria/angioedema

In patients with cholinergic urticaria/angioedema, urticaria and sometimes angioedema develop as a result of an increase in body temperature resulting from physical exertion, fever, or a warm shower or bath. Systemic (such as respiratory and gastrointestinal) symptoms and signs may also develop.

Adrenergic urticaria

Patients who develop urticaria as a result of emotional stress can be said to have adrenergic urticaria.

Aquagenic urticaria and aquagenic pruritus

Aquagenic urticaria is urticaria that develops following cutaneous exposure to water of any temperature. (In comparison, in aquagenic pruritus the water exposure results in pruritus without urticaria. Aquagenic pruritus can sometimes be associated with Hodgkin's disease, polycythemia vera, the hypereosinophilic syndrome and the myelodysplastic syndrome, so patients with aquagenic pruritus should be evaluated and followed for such conditions.)

Latex-associated urticaria

Urticaria (and sometimes systemic manifestations, including shock) can occur as a result of cutaneous or mucosal contact with natural latex antigens (e.g. in latex gloves) and inhalation of latex antigens (which, for example, can be released into the air with powder from latex gloves).

Urticaria/angioedema due to direct mast cell degranulation

It should be noted that some chemicals (such as opiates and radiocontrast media) can cause direct mast cell degranulation, thereby resulting in urticaria/angioedema.

Urticaria/angioedema due to arachidonic acid metabolism abnormalities

Ingestion of aspirin or other non-steroidal anti-inflammatory drugs can result in the development of urticaria/angioedema, allergic rhinitis, and/or asthma relating to arachidonic acid metabolism abnormalities.

Hereditary angioedema

Hereditary angioedema is a condition in which patients develop recurrent angioedema involving the skin, mucous membranes, gastrointestinal tract and upper respiratory tract as a result of an inherited deficiency of the inhibitor of activated C1 (the first component of the complement system).

Angioedema associated with acquired deficiency of the inhibitor of activated C1

There are two types of recurrent angioedema associated with acquired deficiency of the inhibitor of activated C1. One type is associated with malignancies (particularly B-cell lymphomas) and autoantibody to a para-protein, and the other type is associated with an autoantibody to the inhibitor of activated C1. The recurrent angioedema involves the skin, gastrointestinal tract and upper respiratory tract.

Urticaria/angioedema associated with angiotensin-converting enzyme inhibitors

Angioedema (and, rarely, urticaria) can occur with therapy with angiotensin-converting enzyme inhibitors as a result of an unclear mechanism.

Urticaria as a manifestation of serum sickness and as an adverse reaction to administration of blood products

Urticaria can be a manifestation of serum sickness and can also represent an adverse reaction to administration of blood products (e.g. whole blood, plasma, or immunoglobulin). Serum sickness refers to a constellation of adverse symptoms and signs that can occur following administration of heterologous serum or certain drugs.

Urticaria associated with underlying medical problems

Traditionally it has been felt that some cases of urticaria can be caused by underlying bacterial infection, viral infection, fungal infection, juvenile rheumatoid arthritis, or malignancy.

Chronic idiopathic urticaria/angioedema

In the majority of cases of chronic urticaria/angioedema, the cause is unknown, in which case the condition is referred to as chronic idiopathic urticaria/angioedema, the diagnosis of which is made by excluding other possible causes of urticaria/angioedema.

Evaluation of patients with urticaria and/or angioedema

Evaluation of patients with urticaria and/or angioedema involves taking a thorough history, performing a physical examination, performing routine screening laboratory testing, and performing appropriate specific laboratory testing based on the findings of the history and physical examination. All of this is to try to determine the cause of the patient's urticaria and/or angioedema.

If no cause is found from the history, physical examination and laboratory evaluation, it is useful to have the patient keep a diary in which he or she keeps track of activities, his or her location and what is eaten, in conjunction with the corresponding dates and times, along with the dates and times when the urticaria and/or angioedema is present, absent, better and worse, in order to try to detect correlations that might lead to the cause of the patient's urticaria and/or angioedema.

If urticarial vasculitis (see below) is suspected, skin biopsy of a lesion is confirmatory.

Treatment of urticaria and angioedema

Treatment of urticaria and angioedema involves eliminating the underlying cause, when known.

Symptomatic treatment of typical urticaria/angioedema involves the use of an H1-type antihistamine. I usually first try the sedating H1-type antihistamine hydroxyzine (Atarax®) 10 mg one to three pills every 4–6 h as required for itching or rash in adults. I have the patient start out at the lowest dose and frequency and adjust the dose and frequency according to response and adverse effects. I warn the patient regarding the medication's potential for sedation (excessive drowsiness can be transitory and may disappear in a few days of continued therapy or upon dosage reduction) and its potential for increasing the effects of alcohol. The prescriber should take into consideration that hydroxyzine potentiates the effect of other central nervous system depressants, and the patient should be warned about this. Because of hydroxyzine's potential for sedation, patients taking hydroxyzine should be warned regarding driving vehicles or operating dangerous machinery. Dosage for pediatric patients is as described in the package insert. Hydroxyzine is contraindicated in early pregnancy and should not be given to breast-feeding patients.

If the patient is not having a problem with excessive sedation but the hydroxyzine is not satisfactorily controlling the urticaria/angioedema, I then switch to a trial of the sedating H1-type antihistamine diphenhydramine (Benadryl®) 25 mg one to two pills every 4–6 h as required for itching or rash in adults. I have the patient start out at the lowest dose and frequency and adjust the dose and frequency according to response and adverse effects. I warn the patient regarding diphenhydramine's potential for sedation and its additive effect with alcohol. The prescriber should take into consideration that diphenhydramine has additive effects with other central nervous system depressants, and the patient should be warned about this. Because of diphenhydramine's potential for sedation, patients taking diphenhydramine should be warned regarding activities requiring mental alertness, such as driving vehicles, operating machinery, etc. When prescribing diphenhydramine, the prescriber should be aware that monoamine oxidase inhibitors prolong and intensify the anticholinergic effects of diphenhydramine. Dosage for pediatric patients is as described in the package insert (particularly in young pediatric patients, diphenhydramine, like other antihistamines, may cause excitation). In elderly patients (e.g. 60 years of age or older), diphenhydramine, like other antihistamines, is more likely to cause dizziness, sedation and hypotension. Diphenhydramine is contraindicated in neonates, premature infants and breast-feeding patients. It is not contraindicated in pregnant patients, in whom it should be used only if clearly needed. Diphenhydramine, like other antihistamines, should be used with particular caution in patients with narrow-angle glaucoma, stenosing peptic ulcer, pyloroduodenal obstruction, symptomatic prostatic hypertrophy or bladder-neck obstruction. Diphenhydramine should also be used with caution in patients with asthma, increased intraocular pressure, hyperthyroidism, cardiovascular disease, hypertension, or lower respiratory disease.

I have not found cetirizine (Zyrtec®), which is a human metabolite of hydroxyzine, to be particularly superior to hydroxyzine.

If a patient is having a problem with antihistamine-associated sedation, I switch the antihistamine to the non-sedating H1-type antihistamine loratadine (Claritin®) 10 mg once daily for patients 6 years of age and older. For children 2 to 5 years of age, the recommended dose is Claritin Syrup 5 mg (1 teaspoonful) once daily. In patients 6 years of age and older with liver failure or renal insufficiency (glomerular filtration rate less than 30 ml/min), the starting dose should be 10 mg every other day. In children 2 to 5 years of age with liver failure or renal insufficiency, the starting dose should be Claritin Syrup 5 mg (1 teaspoonful) every other day. Loratadine should be used during pregnancy only if clearly needed and should not be administered to a breast-feeding patient.

I have not found the non-sedating H1-type antihistamine fexofenadine (Allegra®) to be superior to loratadine.

Patients with hereditary angioedema associated with an inherited deficiency of the inhibitor of activated C1 or with angioedema associated with an acquired deficiency of the inhibitor of activated C1 should be evaluated, treated and followed in conjunction with a dermatologist.

URTICARIAL VASCULITIS

Overview

Urticarial vasculitis is a condition in which cutaneous necrotizing venulitis produces lesions of urticaria, sometimes in combination with angioedema, with or without systemic involvement, which can include involvement of the gastrointestinal tract, kidneys, lungs, eyes and/or central nervous system. (More typical lesions of cutaneous necrotizing venulitis include purpura (cutaneous extravasated blood), vesicles, pustules, necrosis and ulcers.)

Urticarial vasculitis can be idiopathic or can be associated with such factors as connective tissue disorders, serum sickness, infections (e.g. hepatitis B, hepatitis C, infectious mononucleosis), colon cancer and medications (e.g. Prozac® (fluoxetine), non-steroidal anti-inflammatory agents, potassium iodide).

Differentiating urticarial vasculitis from typical urticaria

Lesions of urticarial vasculitis can be itchy, burning, or painful, whereas lesions of typical urticaria are usually just itchy. Individual lesions of urticarial vasculitis spontaneously resolve more slowly than do those of typical urticaria. (Although lesions of urticarial vasculitis can resolve within 24–48 h, they often can persist for 3–5 days. Lesions of typical urticaria usually spontaneously resolve within 24–48 h.) Wheals with foci of purpura within them and blisters may be present in urticarial vasculitis, which is not the case with typical urticaria. Although lesions of urticarial vasculitis usually leave behind normal skin when they resolve, the lesions in some patients leave behind hyperpigmentation, whereas lesions of typical urticaria always leave behind totally normal skin when they resolve. Biopsy of lesions of urticarial vasculitis reveals necrotizing venulitis, whereas biopsy of lesions of typical urticaria reveals edema without vasculitis.

Treatment of urticarial vasculitis

Patients with urticarial vasculitis should be evaluated, treated and followed in conjunction with a dermatologist.

PRURITUS WITHOUT RASH

Overview

Pruritus without rash presents as pruritus without any associated clinically observed physical changes involving the skin.

A sort of pseudopruritus without rash condition occurs when a patient has unobserved dryness of the skin (xerosis) causing pruritus. (For discussion of cutaneous xerosis, see Chapter 14).

True pruritus without rash can be caused by such internal disorders as hyperthyroidism, hyperparathyroidism, renal insufficiency, hepatobiliary disease, internal malignancy (most commonly leukemia and lymphoma, including Hodgkin's disease), and possibly diabetes mellitus. Contradicting previous assertions, a recent controlled study showed that the incidence of generalized pruritus without rash in diabetic patients was no greater than that in non-diabetic patients. Aquagenic pruritus (pruritus that follows cutaneous contact with water) can sometimes be associated with Hodgkin's disease, polycythemia vera (a marker for polycythemia rubra vera is pruritus associated with bathing), the hypereosinophilic syndrome and the myelo-dysplastic syndrome.

Management of pruritus without rash

If there is xerosis causing the pruritus, the xerosis should be evaluated and treated as discussed in Chapter 14. In patients who have true pruritus without rash, evaluation for and treatment of an underlying causative disorder should be performed.

Symptomatic treatment of true pruritus without rash includes the use of systemic antihistamines as discussed previously in this chapter in the section dealing with the treatment of urticaria and angioedema. Non-prescription topical preparations such as Prax® (pramoxine) lotion and Sarna® (camphor and menthol) lotion can be beneficial. Also, the prescription topical preparation Eurax® (crotamiton) lotion or cream can be effective.

(I use crotamiton in pregnant patients only if its use is approved by the patient's obstetrician. Safety and effectiveness of this medication in children have not been established.) Tub soaks using Aveeno® bath powder or Aveeno-Oilated® bath powder (both of which are non-prescription) mixed in tepid water as described for non-specific dermatitis in Chapter 2 can be beneficial and soothing.

For patients with pruritus due to chronic renal disease, the patient can be referred to a dermatologist who can arrange for phototherapy consisting of exposure to ultraviolet B light, which can be effective in the treatment of pruritus due to chronic renal disease.

22

Liquid nitrogen treatment of appropriate skin lesions

LESIONS THAT CAN BE TREATED USING LIQUID NITROGEN

Certain benign skin lesions can be effectively treated by the application of liquid nitrogen, and these lesions include verrucae (warts due to human papilloma virus), mollusca contagiosa (growths due to a pox virus), acrochordons (skin tags, soft fibromas, fibroepithelial polyps), seborrheic keratoses and solar lentigines. Verrucae, mollusca contagiosa, acrochordons and seborrheic keratoses are benign lesions that are discussed in Chapter 23. Solar lentigines are benign lesions that are discussed in Chapter 24.

The common premalignant lesions called actinic (or solar) keratoses can also be effectively treated by the application of liquid nitrogen. Actinic (or solar) keratoses are discussed in Chapter 25 and have the potential for the development of squamous cell carcinoma within them. Squamous cell carcinoma is discussed in Chapter 26.

LESIONS THAT SHOULD NEVER BE TREATED USING LIQUID NITROGEN

Melanocytic nevi (see Chapter 24) should never be treated using liquid nitrogen, because malignant melanoma (see Chapter 26) can be associated with melanocytic nevi, and therefore removal of melanocytic nevi should always be done in such a way that the specimen can be sent for histopathologic examination (biopsy) and should never be done by destruction (as is the case with liquid nitrogen treatment).

Also, partially removed or partially destroyed melanocytic nevi can recur and can clinically and histopathologically look like malignant melanoma but not be malignant melanoma (this condition can be called 'pseudo-melanoma'), and this can be confusing and cause problems in patients for whom no prior biopsy to confirm the benignity of the original lesion was performed.

PRECAUTIONS REGARDING LIQUID NITROGEN AND LIQUID NITROGEN TREATMENT

One must be very careful in the handling and use of liquid nitrogen because contact with it can cause severe frostbite at the site of contact. This is due to the extremely low temperature of liquid nitrogen. Also, liquid nitrogen should be placed only in containers made of appropriate material (e.g. polystyrene cups) or in containers with linings made of appropriate material (e.g. special, Thermos®-like, lined vessels), and liquid nitrogen should never be kept in a closed container without appropriate venting (otherwise, pressure can build up in the container to the point where a pressure explosion occurs).

Because of the potential for poor wound healing, liquid nitrogen treatment should not be done anywhere there is impaired circulation and/or sensation, which occur(s) in patients with such conditions as peripheral vascular disease, diabetes mellitus, and Buerger's disease (thromboangiitis obliterans). In patients with Raynaud's phenomenon, liquid nitrogen treatment should not be used on the distal lower or upper extremities. In patients with such conditions as cryoglobulinemia, cryofibrinogenemia, cold agglutininemia and cold urticaria (see Chapter 21), liquid nitrogen treatment should not be used at all.

Excessive or aggressive liquid nitrogen treatment can damage underlying structures. One must be very careful when doing liquid nitrogen treatment of lesions involving the proximal nail folds because, if the freeze goes too deeply, the nail matrix (which forms the nail plate and underlies the proximal nail fold) can be damaged by the liquid nitrogen treatment, and this can result in the development of nail deformity, which can be permanent.

Also, one must be particularly careful using liquid nitrogen treatment at sites where nerves are relatively close to the surface of the skin (such as on the sides of the digits, at the elbows, at the angle of the mandible) because, if the liquid nitrogen treatment is excessive and goes too deeply, damage to the underlying nerve can occur.

In addition, particular care needs to be taken when lesions on the genitalia are being treated with liquid nitrogen.

ADVERSE SEQUELAE OF LIQUID NITROGEN TREATMENT

Adverse sequelae of liquid nitrogen treatment include post-inflammatory pigmentary alteration (hypopigmentation/depigmentation, hyperpigmentation), especially in dark-skinned patients, as well as scarring (if scarring develops, it has the potential of being hypertrophic or keloidal, especially in dark-skinned patients). For discussion of post-inflammatory pigmentary alteration, see Chapter 7. For discussion of hypertrophic scars and keloids, see Chapter 8. Obviously, the more vigorous the liquid nitrogen treatment, the greater the likelihood of adverse sequelae; and the less vigorous the liquid nitrogen treatment, the greater the chance that the lesion will not be completely destroyed (thereby leaving behind residual lesion that needs to be treated again).

TWO GOOD METHODS OF LIQUID NITROGEN TREATMENT

One way of performing liquid nitrogen treatment involves the use of a cotton-tipped applicator with liquid nitrogen placed in a Styrofoam cup. The cotton-tipped applicator should have a solid wooden handle, because liquid nitrogen spurts from the hollow channel in cotton-tipped applicators with hollow plastic handles and because the plastic of cotton-tipped applicators with plastic handles can crack when such cotton-tipped applicators are placed in liquid nitrogen.

A cotton-tipped applicator with a solid wooden handle can be made in various sizes in order to correspond to the size of the lesion being treated in order to provide greater precision when treating the lesion. This is done by breaking off the end of a cotton-tipped applicator's solid wooden handle so that jagged edges are produced. A cotton-tipped applicator of the desired size is then produced by twirling an appropriate amount of cotton on the jagged edge of the wooden handle (where the tip was broken off).

When treating a lesion with liquid nitrogen placed in a Styrofoam cup and a cotton-tipped applicator, the cotton-tipped applicator is dipped in the liquid nitrogen and then applied to the lesion for a moment, and this sequence is repeated until the lesion and a narrow (e.g. 1 mm) rim of normal skin around the lesion are white from the freezing. It is important to note that, when the liquid nitrogen-soaked cotton-tipped applicator is touched to the lesion with greater pressure, the warm blood in the cutaneous blood vessels associated with the lesion is 'pushed away', so that less heat can be transferred from the warm blood to the site of the liquid nitrogen treatment. As a result of this, this site of liquid nitrogen treatment gets colder, and therefore the freezing effect (freezing destruction) is greater than when less pressure is applied to the lesion through contact with the liquid nitrogen-soaked cotton-tipped applicator.

Another liquid nitrogen treatment method that I have found to be very useful involves the use of metal forceps in place of the above-described cotton-tipped applicator. With this method, liquid nitrogen is placed in a Styrofoam cup, and the handle portion of metal, non-toothed forceps is then held between the thumb and index finger. The tips of the forceps are then dipped for a second or two into the liquid nitrogen in the Styrofoam cup, after which the lesion to be destroyed is 'pinched' between the tips of the forceps until the lesion turns white from freezing. Sometimes this needs to be done to the point where there is a narrow (e.g. 1 mm), white rim of frozen normal skin around the lesion. Also, it is sometimes necessary to repeat this sequence (i.e. dipping the forceps into the liquid nitrogen followed by 'pinching' the lesion) multiple times, in order to achieve the desired degree of freezing described above. Smaller forceps with smaller tips work better for smaller lesions, and larger forceps with larger tips work better for larger lesions. To insulate the fingers from cold forceps handles that become cold from repeated dipping into the liquid nitrogen, gloves can be worn, or rubber tubing can be placed around the forceps handles, if necessary. (This is generally not necessary when large, long forceps are used.) This technique is particularly effective for exophytic, non-broad lesions. Exophytic lesions are lesions that rise above the skin surface. Non-broad lesions do not have large diameters.

CLINICAL CHANGES FOLLOWING LIQUID NITROGEN TREATMENT

Within a day or so after the liquid nitrogen treatment, the development of blistering and crusting may occur, with the lesion subsequently falling off. Alternatively, the lesion may darken within a day or so and then fall off. The liquid nitrogen treatment site may normally be somewhat erythematous, tender and/or painful, but not excessively so, and it may be slightly swollen, depending on how vigorously the liquid nitrogen treatment was performed.

WOUND CARE FOLLOWING LIQUID NITROGEN TREATMENT

I generally do not have patients avoid exposing the wound to water or carry out wound care following liquid nitrogen treatment. However, if I am concerned that the patient might be a candidate for poor wound healing, I will have the patient avoid exposing the wound to water, and I will have him or her clean the wound with hydrogen peroxide-soaked cotton-tipped applicators followed by drying with gauze followed by the application of

Polysporin Ointment® (polymyxin B sulfate/bacitracin zinc) with a fresh cotton-tipped applicator, with this sequence being performed twice daily until the wound heals.

Whether or not wound care is being carried out, I always have the patient leave liquid nitrogen treated wounds open to the air.

DEVELOPMENT OF BACTERIAL INFECTION FOLLOWING LIQUID NITROGEN TREATMENT

Manifestations of bacterial infection include the presence of pus, greater than expected pain or tenderness, greater than expected erythema and greater than expected swelling. (It should be remembered that pus is a cloudy exudate, whereas blister fluid or serum, the presence of which is normal following liquid nitrogen treatment, may be yellow but is clear.)

If the development of bacterial infection (which I have found to be very rare following liquid nitrogen treatment) is suspected, a bacterial culture and sensitivities (C&S) of the involvement should be obtained, and the patient should be started empirically on a course of an oral antibiotic such as cephalexin (Keflex®) 250–500 mg every 6 h (or, if the patient is unable to take cephalexin, erythromycin 250–500 mg every 6 h) in adults, if not otherwise unadvisable, with the antibiotic being modified according to patient response and C&S results. Pediatric dosage is as described in the package inserts.

ALLERGY TO TOPICAL ANTIBIOTIC

Allergy to Polysporin Ointment, or to any other topical preparation, can be manifested by the development of increased inflammation or by non-healing of a wound without associated increased inflammation.

If a patient is allergic to Polysporin Ointment and not allergic to iodine, I have the patient use brown Betadine Ointment® (povidone-iodine) instead of Polysporin Ointment. Clear Betadine Ointment should not be used in this situation, because it contains the same active ingredients that Polysporin Ointment contains.

It should be noted that, if a patient is using a topical antibiotic for wound care, the clinical findings (i.e. increased inflammation) of an allergic reaction to the topical antibiotic being used can mimic some of the clinical findings of bacterial infection (although, in general, an allergic reaction to the topical antibiotic would tend to be itchy whereas a bacterial infection of the wound would tend to be painful and/or tender, and pus may be present).

Therefore, when a bacterial infection of a wound for which a topical antibiotic is being used for wound care is suspected, an allergic reaction to the topical antibiotic being used should also be considered.

BILLING FOR LIQUID NITROGEN TREATMENT

Liquid nitrogen treatment of verrucae, mollusca contagiosa, acrochordons, seborrheic keratoses and solar lentigines, which are benign lesions, and of actinic (solar) keratoses, which are premalignant lesions, is billed using the category 'destruction of benign or premalignant skin lesion(s)'.

WHEN TO REFER

If there is any doubt regarding a lesion, site, or patient being appropriate for liquid nitrogen treatment, liquid nitrogen treatment should not be performed, and the patient should be referred to a dermatologist.

Also, if a liquid nitrogen-treated lesion does not resolve completely as expected, or if it recurs unexpectedly, the patient should be referred to a dermatologist for consultation.

23

Common benign non-melanocytic skin lesions

SEBORRHEIC KERATOSES

Overview

Seborrheic keratoses are benign, keratotic, raised lesions with a 'stuck-on' appearance. The term keratotic is used because seborrheic keratoses are made up of keratinocytes and contain the protein keratin. Keratinocytes are the cells that make up the bulk of the epidermis and produce keratin, which is the substance of which hair, nails and the stratum corneum are composed. The stratum corneum is the dead, horny, most superficial layer of the epidermis, which is the superficial cutaneous layer that is located immediately above the dermis. When it is said that seborrheic keratoses have a 'stuck-on' appearance, it is meant that seborrheic keratoses typically look as though they were 'stuck on' to the surface of the skin. Seborrheic keratoses may be flesh colored or any shade of brown and may sometimes even be black.

Horn pseudocysts

A characteristic feature of many seborrheic keratoses is the presence of horn pseudocysts on the surfaces of the lesions. Horn pseudocysts are invaginations on the surface of a seborrheic keratosis and are seen as small holes on the surface of the lesion. These small surface holes, which are characteristic of seborrheic keratoses and which, when present, are very useful in diagnosing a lesion as a seborrheic keratosis, are more easily visualized with the aid of a magnifying hand lens. The small surface holes of horn pseudocysts are also more easily visualized by briefly, lightly touching the surface of the lesion with a liquid nitrogen-soaked cotton-tipped applicator (i.e. a cotton-tipped applicator that was dipped in liquid nitrogen that was placed in a polystyrene cup) so as to frost lightly the lesion's surface, thereby resulting in brief whitening of the lesion's surface. This brief whitening resulting from light frosting of the lesion's surface makes horn pseudocyst holes that are present on the lesion's surface more easily visualized. One must be very careful in the handling and use of liquid nitrogen because contact with it can cause severe frostbite at the site of contact – this is due to the extremely low temperature of liquid nitrogen. Also, liquid nitrogen should be placed only in containers made of appropriate material (e.g. Styrofoam cups) or in containers with linings made of appropriate material (e.g. special, Thermos®-like, lined vessels), and liquid nitrogen should never be kept in a closed container without appropriate venting (otherwise, pressure can build up in the container to the point where a pressure explosion occurs). In addition, the cotton-tipped applicator should have a solid wooden handle, because liquid nitrogen spurts from the hollow channel in cotton-tipped applicators with hollow plastic handles and because the plastic of cotton-tipped applicators with plastic handles can crack when such cotton-tipped applicators are placed in liquid nitrogen.

The sign of Leser–Trélat

Mention should be made of the sign of Leser–Trélat, which is the eruptive appearance of multiple seborrheic keratoses. This sign has been associated with multiple types of internal malignancies, but it is not clear whether or not this indeed is a paraneoplastic sign.

Treatment of seborrheic keratoses

If treatment of seborrheic keratoses is desired, they can be treated via liquid nitrogen (see Chapter 22) or other methods.

ACROCHORDONS

Overview

Acrochordons are typically flesh-colored or brown, digitate, pedunculated papules that commonly involve the neck, axillae and/or upper inner thighs. Acrochordons are also known as skin tags, soft fibromas and fibro-epithelial polyps. 'Digitate' means that the lesion sticks up like a finger. 'Pedunculated' means that the lesion is attached to the skin via a pedicle or stalk. 'Papules' are bumps. It should be noted that melanocytic nevi can resemble acrochordons.

Treatment of acrochordons

If treatment is desired, acrochordons can be treated via liquid nitrogen (see Chapter 22) if there is no suspicion regarding the possibility that the lesions might be melanocytic nevi (see Chapter 24) rather than acrochordons, or they can be treated via other methods. Sometimes, melanocytic nevi can be pedunculated or digitate and resemble acrochordons. Melanocytic nevi should never be treated via liquid nitrogen or other forms of destruction lacking histological evaluation (see Chapters 22 and 24).

VERRUCAE

Overview

Verrucae are commonly known as warts and are growths due to the human papilloma virus. It should be mentioned that verrucae can spontaneously resolve without sequelae. (Two-thirds of verrucae in children spontaneously resolve within 2 years, and the remaining verrucae will continue to resolve at this rate.) However, since the spontaneous resolution of verrucae cannot be counted on and may take a long time if it does occur, since new verrucae can appear while others are resolving and verrucae can spread as a result of their being caused by cutaneous infection with the human papilloma virus, I feel that destruction of verrucae is indicated with few exceptions. One such exception might be a typical, asymptomatic verruca (without any features that evoke suspicion) on the sole (i.e. a typical verruca plantaris or plantar wart, which is discussed below) in a patient with diabetes mellitus and/or peripheral vascular disease in whom an attempt to destroy the wart may result in a non-healing ulcer. In such a case very careful, non-aggressive periodic paring (if needed to relieve the typical pebble-in-the-shoe type of tenderness when the patient walks) and observation (proceeding accordingly if there is evidence of enlargement or if atypical features develop) may be more advisable than destruction would be.

Verrucae vulgares

Overview

Verrucae can present in a variety of forms. Verrucae vulgares are also called common warts and are typically flesh-colored, keratotic papules that have a rough, cauliflower-like appearance on their surfaces and may have short, digitate projections extending from their surfaces. Verrucae vulgares can occur almost anywhere on the integument.

Treatment of verrucae vulgares

Overview   Verrucae vulgares can be treated by various methods.

Salicylic acid treatment of verrucae vulgares   One very common method of treatment of verrucae vulgares involves the use of topically applied salicylic acid. The salicylic acid product that in my experience provides the best over-all results in comparison to other salicylic acid products is Occlusal-HP® (17% salicylic acid in a polyacrylic vehicle), which is available over the counter. It should not be used to treat verrucae on the face, anogenital region, or mucous membranes. Because of the potential for development of non-healing ulceration, it should also not be used anywhere there is impaired circulation and/or sensation, which occurs in patients with such conditions as peripheral vascular disease and diabetes mellitus.

When Occlusal-HP is used, the patient should first soak the verruca vulgaris in warm water for 5 min. Loose, dead tissue should be removed by scraping with an emery board, nail file, or pumice stone. The verruca vulgaris is then patted dry, and Occlusal HP is applied to the verruca vulgaris itself. The patient should be advised to take care that the medication does not get onto the normal surrounding skin. (If the applicator that comes with the medication is too large for the verruca vulgaris being treated, the Occlusal-HP can be applied to the verruca vulgaris very precisely with the use of a toothpick.) The area is allowed to air dry. This sequence is performed once or twice daily until the verruca vulgaris resolves. The patient should be informed that, if irritation develops with this treatment, the treatment should be stopped, the medication should be washed off, and the patient's health-care provider should be contacted; once the irritation has subsided, the treatment can be cautiously resumed.

It should be noted that when and where a verruca is present, the normal skin lines (e.g. 'finger print' lines) are disrupted by the verruca, and when the verruca resolves, the skin lines go through, in a normal fashion, the area where the verruca was. This is a useful aid in determining whether or not a verruca is still present and in determining where the verruca is if it is still present. (In other words, if the skin lines are disrupted, the verruca is still present, and the location of the verruca is where the skin lines are disrupted; if the skin lines are no longer disrupted, the verruca has resolved.) Discussing this information with the patient will aid the patient in his or her Occlusal-HP treatment of the verruca.

Liquid nitrogen treatment of verrucae vulgares   The health-care provider can also very effectively treat verrucae vulgares via the use of liquid nitrogen (as discussed in Chapter 22).

Laser treatment and electrodesiccation treatment of verrucae vulgares   Laser treatment and electrodesiccation treatment (for which the patient can be referred to a dermatologist) are other commonly used methods of treatment for verrucae vulgares.

Verrucae filiformes

Overview and treatment

Verrucae filiformes or filiform warts or digitate warts are basically common warts that are filiform or digitate in shape. ('Filiform' means filamentous, and 'digitate' means that the lesion sticks up like a finger.) Verrucae filiformes are treated with liquid nitrogen or Occlusal-HP in the same way that is described above for verrucae vulgares. However, because of its digitate shape, a verruca filiformis is much more amenable to liquid nitrogen therapy (which is my treatment of choice for such verrucae) than it is to Occlusal-HP therapy.

Verrucae plantares

Overview

Verrucae plantares, or plantar warts, are verrucae that are located on the sole. These are typically thick, endophytic, hyperkeratotic lesions that are frequently tender when the patient walks. ('Endophytic' means that the lesion is growing inward. 'Hyperkeratotic' refers to a thickened stratum corneum, which is the dead, horny, outermost layer of the epidermis and is composed of the protein keratin. The epidermis is the cutaneous layer that is located immediately above the dermis.) The above-described tenderness that can be associated with a verruca plantaris when the patient walks can be thought of as being analogous to discomfort resulting from walking with a pebble in a shoe.

Treatment of verrucae plantares

Occlusal-HP treatment and liquid nitrogen treatment of verrucae plantares
Verrucae plantares can be treated via the use of Occlusal-HP or liquid nitrogen as described above for verrucae vulgares. However, because of the

potential for development of non-healing ulceration neither Occlusal-HP nor liquid nitrogen should be used to treat verrucae plantares in patients with impaired circulation and/or sensation, which occurs in conditions such as diabetes mellitus and/or peripheral vascular disease.

If liquid nitrogen is used to treat a verruca plantaris, it is important to remember that, for a period of time after the liquid nitrogen treatment is performed, the liquid nitrogen treatment site will be inflamed and as a result will probably be tender when the patient walks. It is also important to remember that aggressive or excessive liquid nitrogen treatment can result in scar formation, and in treating verrucae plantares it is important to be particularly careful not to produce a scar that might be tender when the patient walks, because if this problem occurs, it could end up being a permanent sequela resulting from treatment of a benign lesion that might otherwise have spontaneously resolved without sequelae.

In general, Occlusal-HP treatment of verrucae plantares is preferable to liquid nitrogen treatment of such lesions because Occlusal-HP treatment of such lesions is generally not associated with tenderness and scar problems, unlike liquid nitrogen treatment of such lesions (see above).

Paring of verrucae plantares   Prior to initiation of either Occlusal-HP treatment or liquid nitrogen treatment of a verruca plantaris, the health-care provider can carefully pare away, using a no. 15 scalpel, the hyperkeratotic layer on the surface of the lesion in order to enhance the effectiveness of Occlusal-HP treatment or liquid nitrogen treatment. Such paring can also be done to ameliorate any pebble-in-the-shoe type of tenderness (see above). Because of the associated risk of development of non-healing ulceration resulting from improper paring (e.g. paring that is too aggressive) of verrucae plantares in patients with impaired circulation and/or sensation, paring of such lesions in such patients should be performed by a dermatologist or podiatrist if the primary health-care provider is not experienced in paring such lesions in such patients.

Paring is performed by placing the no. 15 scalpel blade parallel to or, if necessary, at a slight angle in relation to the verruca plantaris's surface and then successively paring thin slices of the dead tissue, during which time the lesional skin can be pulled or stretched tautly with a finger or fingers of the free hand, if necessary. The goal is to stop the paring at a level that is estimated to be immediately above the level at which punctate bleeding would occur. In general, I stop paring when the patient reports that he or she is beginning to feel the cutting of the scalpel blade. This should be distinguished from tenderness due to pressure being applied during the paring process – such pressure tenderness is not an indication to stop paring. In order to distinguish the two types of discomfort, I ask the patient whether the pain he or she is feeling is a sharp pain due to the cutting or more of a dull pain due to pressure. If the patient reports that it is a sharp pain due to the cutting, I stop the paring, and if the patient reports that it is a dull pain due to pressure, I continue the paring.

Paring of verrucae plantares may reveal the presence of punctate black dots, which represent thrombosed capillaries seen in verrucae plantares.

The health-care provider can see the patient about every 6 weeks, at which time paring can be repeated as needed.

Treatment of recalcitrant verrucae plantares   For recalcitrant verrucae plantares, the health-care provider can pare such lesions and then treat them with liquid nitrogen, and once the inflammation from the liquid nitrogen treatment has resolved and if the verruca plantaris is still present, the patient can initiate treatment with Occlusal-HP as described above and should return to see the health-care provider in about 6 weeks, at which time the health-care provider can evaluate the patient and repeat the treatment process if the verruca plantaris is still present. Obviously, such treatment of verrucae plantares should not be performed in patients with impaired circulation and/or sensation, because of the associated risk of development of non-healing ulceration in such patients.

If the lesion still persists following such treatment, the patient should be referred to a dermatologist.

Laser treatment and electrodesiccation treatment of verrucae plantares   Laser treatment and electrodesiccation treatment are other therapeutic modalities (for which the patient can be referred to a dermatologist) that have been used to treat verrucae plantares. However, it is important to be aware that laser treatment and electrodesiccation treatment of verrucae plantares can be associated with scar and tenderness problems as described above for liquid nitrogen treatment of verrucae plantares. Also, these treatment modalities should not be used to treat verrucae plantares in patients with impaired circulation and/or sensation, because of the associated risk of development of non-healing ulceration in such patients.

Epithelioma cuniculatum

Mention should be made of epithelioma cuniculatum. This is a rare type of verrucous carcinoma, involves the sole, is felt to arise from verruca plantaris lesions, may look like a verruca plantaris initially, and is typically a large, slowly enlarging, cauliflower-like mass that is unresponsive to standard verruca plantaris therapy. Verrucous carcinoma can be considered to be a type of low-grade, locally invasive squamous cell carcinoma that is probably due to human papilloma viruses. See Chapter 26 for discussion of squamous cell carcinoma and verrucous carcinoma. If an epithelioma cuniculatum is suspected, the patient should be referred to a dermatologist.

Verrucae planae

Overview

Verrucae planae are plane warts or flat warts. Verrucae planae generally present as numerous, typically flesh-colored, smooth-surfaced, small, slightly raised lesions that are closely grouped together.

Treatment of verrucae planae

Liquid nitrogen treatment of verrucae planae   Verrucae planae can be treated via light liquid nitrogen treatment, but liquid nitrogen treatment of verrucae planae is frequently not feasible because of the large number of lesions that are usually present. (Liquid nitrogen treatment is described in Chapter 22.)

Retin-A® treatment of verrucae planae   Verrucae planae can be treated using Retin-A (tretinoin), which is indicated for the treatment of acne, although treatment of verrucae planae is not a package insert indication for this medication. When Retin-A is used to treat verrucae planae, it is applied to the lesions nightly at bed time. (Hands should be washed after the medication is applied.) If using the Retin-A every night is too drying and/or irritating, the patient can use it less often (e.g. every other or every third night) and can then try to increase the frequency of application in step-wise fashion up to every night, as tolerated. I start out having the patient use Retin-A cream 0.025%, and I gradually try to increase the strength, as tolerated, to 0.05% and, if possible, to 0.1%.

Retin-A can make the skin more sensitive to sunlight (and sunlamps), so when I prescribe it, I warn the patient about this, and I have the patient avoid sun (and sunlamp) exposure; keep the areas being treated covered, if possible; and use a sunscreen with SPF-15 or greater when outdoors during daytime. If treatment is on the face or bald scalp, I have the patient also wear a broad-brimmed hat when outdoors during daytime. Patients with sunburn should not use Retin-A until they are fully recovered. Also, it has been recommended that wax epilation should not be performed on skin treated with Retin-A because of the potential for the development of erosions (although wax epilation should not otherwise be performed on skin containing verrucae planae), and Retin-A should not be used on irritated or eczematous skin.

I do not use Retin-A in pregnant or breast-feeding patients.

Topical 5-fluorouracil treatment of verrucae planae   Verrrucae planae can be treated using topical 5-fluorouracil (Fluoroplex® cream 1% or Efudex® cream 5%), which is indicated for the treatment of the pre-cancers actinic (solar) keratoses (see Chapter 25), although treatment of verrucae planae is not a package insert indication for this medication.

When I use topical 5-fluorouracil for the treatment of verrucae planae, I have the patient start out with Fluoroplex cream 1%, which is applied twice daily to the lesions. (Hands should be washed after the medication is applied.) If this is tolerated well, but no response is seen, I have the patient switch to Efudex cream 5%.

Topical 5-fluorouracil can make the skin more sensitive to sunlight (and sunlamps), so when I prescribe it, I warn the patient about this, and I have the patient avoid sun (and sunlamp) exposure; keep the areas being treated covered, if possible; and use a sunscreen with an SPF-15 or greater when outdoors during daytime. If treatment is on the face or bald scalp, I have the patient also wear a broad-brimmed hat when outdoors during daytime.

Topical 5-fluorouracil is contraindicated in women who are or may become pregnant during therapy and should not be used in breast-feeding patients. Safety and effectiveness of topical 5-fluorouracil in children have not been established.

Aldara® treatment of verrucae planae   Aldara (imiquimod) cream is an immune response modifier that is indicated for the treatment in adults of external genital and perianal warts that do not involve mucosal surfaces. (Anogenital warts are called condylomata acuminata, which are discussed later in this chapter. Aldara is not recommended for the treatment of condylomata acuminata involving mucosal surfaces.) Although treatment of verrucae planae is not a package insert indication for Aldara cream, some dermatologists use Aldara cream for such treatment.

In treating verrucae planae with Aldara cream, the cream is applied to the lesions three times per week prior to normal sleeping hours, and 6–10 h later, the cream is washed off with mild soap and water. (Hands should be washed after the medication is applied.) The treatment with

Aldara cream should continue until there is total clearance of the verrucae planae or for a maximum of 16 weeks. If irritation from the Aldara treatment develops, the Aldara should be washed off with mild soap and water and should be discontinued until the inflammation subsides, after which treatment with Aldara can be resumed.

Safety and efficacy of Aldara cream in patients below the age of 18 years have not been established.

Condylomata acuminata

Overview

Condylomata acuminata are anogenital warts.

Clinically, these are raised lesions that can be small or large and can be smooth-surfaced or cauliflower-like on the surface. Subclinical lesions can be detected by the application for 5–10 min of gauze soaked in 5% acetic acid (white vinegar), which turns the lesions white (this is called aceto-whitening), but be aware that false-positive results can occur.

Evaluation for other sexually transmitted diseases should be performed in all patients with condylomata acuminata, and this evaluation should include, but is not limited to, obtaining a rapid plasma reagin (RPR) or Venereal Disease Research Laboratories (VDRL) and HIV test.

Patients with perianal condylomata acuminata should be checked proctoscopically for the presence of intra-anal/rectal involvement.

All women with condylomata acuminata should be checked by a gynecologist, because condylomata acuminata can be present internally within the vagina and can predispose women to such malignancies as cervical cancer.

All sexual partners of patients with condylomata acuminata should be evaluated regarding condylomata acuminata, and female sexual partners of patients with condylomata acuminata should be checked by a gynecologist for the reasons described above.

It is mandatory that child abuse be considered in all children with condylomata acuminata, but it should be noted that the presence of condylomata acuminata in a child is not of itself proof of child abuse.

Treatment of condylomata acuminata

Liquid nitrogen treatment of condylomata acuminata   Condylomata acuminata can be treated using liquid nitrogen as described in Chapter 22.

Aldara treatment of condylomata acuminata   Aldara cream has not been evaluated for the treatment of urethral, intra-vaginal, cervical, rectal, or intra-anal condylomata acuminata and is not recommended for the treatment of such lesions. Since Aldara cream can weaken condoms and vaginal diaphragms, concurrent use of Aldara cream with such devices is not recommended. Sexual (genital, oral and anal) contact should be avoided while Aldara cream is on the skin. Uncircumcised males treating condylomata acuminata under the foreskin should retract the foreskin and clean the area daily. Aldara cream is otherwise used for the treatment of condylomata acuminata as described above for the treatment of flat warts.

Podophyllin treatment of condylomata acuminata   When I use podophyllin to treat condylomata acuminata, I use 25% podophyllin in tincture of benzoin, which I apply to the lesions. Care is taken not to get the medication on the normal, surrounding skin. For large lesions I use a cotton-tipped applicator to apply the medication, and for small lesions I put the pads of my thumbs on the middle of the wooden handle of a cotton-tipped applicator and bend the handle so that it breaks where my thumbs are placed, thereby leaving a pointed tip, which I use to apply the medication to small lesions. Treatment of large areas or numerous warts can result in excessive irritation and absorption and should therefore not be done. (It has been recommended that no more than 2 cm^2 should be treated at one time.) After the medication is applied, it is allowed to air dry, after which talcum powder is applied to the treatment area so that the medication does not spread to normal skin. I have the patient wash off the medication and talcum powder 4–6 h later, or sooner if there is discomfort. This treatment is repeated weekly, until the condition clears.

The use of podophyllin is contraindicated during pregnancy and in breast-feeding patients.

It is important to note that treatment with podophyllin can cause histopathological changes (i.e. changes on biopsy) that mimic malignancy, but these changes disappear within a few days to a week after podophyllin therapy is discontinued.

Condylox® treatment of condylomata acuminata   Condylox (podofilox or podophyllotoxin, which is a component of podophyllin) gel can be used by the patient for the treatment of condylomata acuminata that do not involve mucous membranes. When using Condylox gel, the patient uses the tube's applicator tip or his or her finger to apply the medication to the lesions twice daily for 3 consecutive days followed by 4 consecutive days during which the medication is not used, with this cycle being repeated up to a minimum of four cycles as needed. Application of the medication to the surrounding normal tissue should be minimized, and treatment should be limited to 10 cm^2 or less of wart tissue and to no more than 0.5 g of the gel per day. Following each application of the medication, the gel should be allowed to air dry before the opposing skin surfaces are allowed to return to their normal positions, and the patient should wash his or her hands before and after each application of the medication.

I do not use Condylox in pregnant or breast-feeding patients, and the safety and effectiveness of Condylox in pediatric patients have not been established.

Laser treatment and electrodesiccation treatment of condylomata acuminata Condylomata acuminata can also be treated via laser treatment or electrodesiccation treatment, for which the patient can be referred to a dermatologist.

Giant condyloma acuminatum (Buschke–Lowenstein tumor) and bowenoid papulosis

Giant condyloma acuminatum (Buschke–Lowenstein tumor)   Giant condyloma acuminatum (Buschke–Lowenstein tumor) is a type of verrucous carcinoma and involves the anogenital region. Verrucous carcinoma can be considered to be a type of low-grade, locally invasive squamous cell carcinoma that is probably due to human papilloma virus. See Chapter 26 for discussion of squamous cell carcinoma and verrucous carcinoma.

Typically, giant condyloma acuminatum is large (although it can be small), cauliflower-like and unresponsive to standard condyloma acuminatum therapy. If such a lesion is suspected, the patient should be referred to a dermatologist.

Bowenoid papulosis   Bowenoid papulosis is manifested by often multiple papules and/or plaques involving the external genitalia and containing human papilloma virus. (Papules are bumps. Plaques are broad raised lesions.) The lesions may be reddish brown or violaceous in color, may be verrucous (warty) in appearance and usually resemble condylomata acuminata.

On histopathological examination (i.e. on biopsy), the lesions resemble Bowen's disease, which is squamous cell carcinoma *in situ* (see Chapter 26).

Sometimes lesions of bowenoid papulosis resolve spontaneously. In other cases, the lesions can persist for years, and in some cases there is a possible increased risk for lesions to become Bowen's disease (squamous cell carcinoma *in situ*) and invasive squamous cell carcinoma (see Chapter 26).

Female patients with bowenoid papulosis and the female sexual partners of male patients with bowenoid papulosis may be at high risk for cervical and vulvar neoplasia.

When bowenoid papulosis is suspected, the patient should be referred to a dermatologist, and female patients and the female sexual partners of male patients should be referred to a gynecologist.

Verrucous carcinoma

In addition to the sole (epithelioma cuniculatum, which is discussed above) and anogenital region (giant condyloma acuminatum or Buschke–Lowenstein tumor, which is discussed above), verrucous carcinoma may involve other sites (e.g. the trunk, buttocks, hands, fingers, face, mouth); can be considered to be a type of low-grade, locally invasive squamous cell carcinoma that is probably due to human papilloma viruses; is warty; grows slowly; and is more likely to invade adjacent tissue (it is locally aggressive) than it is to metastasize (it only rarely metastasizes). Verrucous carcinoma and squamous cell carcinoma are discussed in Chapter 26.

Because some types of human papilloma virus have oncogenic potential and because squamous cell carcinoma can be verrucous (i.e. wart-like), any patient with any verruca that has any atypical characteristics or any patient with any verruca that is recalcitrant to treatment should be referred to a dermatologist.

MOLLUSCA CONTAGIOSA

Overview

Mollusca contagiosa are growths that are caused by molluscum contagiosum virus, which is a poxvirus.

Molluscum contagiosum lesions are typically multiple and asymptomatic (although they can be pruritic) and consist of usually small, pearly or flesh-colored papules that frequently have a central umbilication and contain a white core (or 'molluscum body'). (Papules are bumps. An umbilication is a round depression.)

The central umbilication, when present, is a molluscum contagiosum characteristic that is useful in diagnosing a lesion as a molluscum contagiosum lesion. This umbilication, when present, can be more easily visualized with the use of a magnifying hand lens, or, as discussed in more detail for seborrheic keratoses previously in this chapter, the umbilication can be more easily visualized by briefly, lightly touching the surface of the lesion with a liquid nitrogen-soaked cotton-tipped applicator so as to frost lightly the lesion's surface, thereby resulting in brief whitening of the lesion's surface. This brief whitening resulting from light frosting of the lesion's surface makes an umbilication that is present on the lesion's surface more easily visualized, in which case the umbilication, if present, is seen as a round hole on the lesion's surface.

Molluscum contagiosum lesions can be located anywhere on the skin surface or mucous membranes and generally affect children but can affect adults, in whom the lesions may be sexually acquired.

Patients with AIDS, particularly uncontrolled AIDS, are at increased risk of having molluscum contagiosum lesions (in which case the involvement can be extensive), as are patients with immunodeficiency due to other causes. I consider the possibility of associated AIDS or other immuno-deficiency when adult patients have molluscum contagiosum lesions.

Patients with sexually acquired mollusca contagiosa should be evaluated for other sexually transmitted diseases, and this evaluation should include, but is not limited to, an RPR or VDRL and HIV test. Also, the sexual part-ners of such patients should be evaluated regarding sexually transmitted mollusca contagiosa.

Except for patients with immunodeficiency (in whom mollusca conta-giosa can persist for years), individual molluscum contagiosum lesions can spontaneously resolve in 2–4 months, during which time new lesions can develop, and the condition itself frequently resolves spontaneously in 6–9 months.

Treatment of mollusca contagiosa

Because in cases other than those with associated immunodeficiency mollusca contagiosa can be self-limited (i.e. the problem can resolve spon-taneously) treatment of the condition may not be necessary in all cases.

Although mollusca contagiosa can be resistant to treatment in patients with associated immunodeficiency, effective treatment of the HIV infection in patients with uncontrolled AIDS can result in improvement of a mollus-cum contagiosum problem in these patients.

Molluscum contagiosum lesions can sometimes become secondarily infected with bacteria. (When such secondary bacterial infection occurs, it usually results from the patient's scratching of itchy lesions.) Possible secondary bacterial infection can be approached as described for possible secondarily infected non-specific dermatitis in Chapter 2, although it should be noted that rupture of a molluscum contagiosum lesion's core (molluscum body) into the dermis adjacent to the lesion can result in a sterile foreign body-type inflammatory reaction that can mimic secondary bacterial infection. (The dermis is the cutaneous layer that is located immediately below the epidermis, which is the superficial cutaneous layer.)

Molluscum contagiosum lesions can be treated with light liquid nitrogen treatment or by incision and expression of the molluscum contagiosum lesion's core (molluscum body) using a no. 11 scalpel or 20-gauge needle and a comedo expresser as described for incision and expression of comedones in Chapter 9. (See Chapter 22 for discussion of liquid nitrogen treatment. Some dermatologists feel that simple pricking of the molluscum contagiosum lesion with a sterile needle without expression of the lesion's core will result in effective treatment of the molluscum contagiosum lesion.) Molluscum contagiosum lesions can also be treated with Occlusal-HP as described for verrucae vulgares previously in this chapter. However, unlike the Occlusal-HP treatment of verrucae vulgares, molluscum contagiosum lesions being treated with Occlusal-HP should not be pre-soaked in water; loose, dead tissue should not be removed by scraping with an emery board, nail file, or pumice stone; and the Occlusal-HP should be washed off 4–6 h after application, or sooner if the lesion is very painful. (Treatment of molluscum contagiosum lesions is not a package insert indication for Occlusal-HP.) Topical podophyllotoxin has been effectively used to treat molluscum contagiosum lesions, for which I would have the patient use Condylox (podophyllotoxin or podofilox) gel as described for condylomata acuminata previously in this chapter. (Treatment of molluscum contagiosum lesions is not a package insert indication for podophyllotoxin or podofilox.) There are some dermatologists who believe that simple painting of molluscum contagiosum lesions with iodine solution is helpful. Retin-A (tretinoin) as described for verrucae planae previously in this chapter, topical 5-fluorouracil (Fluoroplex cream 1% or Efudix cream 5%) as described for verrucae planae previously in this chapter, or Aldara (imiquimod) cream as described for verrucae planae previously in this chapter can be tried. (Treatment of molluscum contagiosum lesions is not a package insert indication for Retin-A, topical 5-fluorouracil and Aldara.)

It should be noted that some dermatologists feel that not every molluscum contagiosum lesion needs to be treated, because they feel that minimal trauma to a limited number of the molluscum contagiosum lesions may provoke an overall immune response that will cause regression of the non-traumatized molluscum contagiosum lesions.

EPIDERMAL CYSTS AND TRICHILEMMAL CYSTS

Overview

Lesions that in the past were called epidermal inclusion cysts – now more precisely called epidermal cysts, epidermoid cysts, or infundibular-type pilar cysts – and lesions that in the past were called pilar cysts – now more precisely called trichilemmal cysts or isthmus-catagen-type pilar cysts – typically present as firm, smooth, spherical, dermal lesions that are usually seen as dome-shaped skin protuberances that are freely moveable over underlying structures. (The dermal layer is the cutaneous layer that is located immediately below the epidermis, which is the superficial layer of the skin.)

Epidermal cysts

An epidermal cyst is a cavity lined by epithelium that resembles the epidermis; is filled with keratin; is frequently attached to the epidermis; and frequently has a punctum, which is usually located centrally but can be located eccentrically on the lesion's surface and which represents the surface opening of an epithelium-lined channel that leads to the cyst's cavity. The epidermis is the superficial cutaneous layer that is located immediately above the dermis. The keratin that fills the cyst cavity as described above is clinically a typically whitish, cheesy material and is the protein of which the stratum corneum is composed. The stratum corneum is the dead, horny, outermost layer of the epidermis. The punctum, when present, can be accentuated and more easily visualized by pinching the surface skin overlying the cyst between the thumb and index finger – if a punctum is present, the overlying, pinched skin will pucker inward at the site of the punctum, thereby making the punctum, if present, more easily visualized.

Frequently, some of the typically whitish cheesy material (keratin) in the epidermal cyst's cavity can be expressed from the cyst's punctum, when a punctum is present.

Epidermal cysts can be seen almost anywhere on the skin's surface.

An epidermal cyst can become sterilely inflamed (i.e. can become inflamed without there being infection) as the result of the cyst's epithelium-lined cavity rupturing, resulting in keratin moving from the cyst's epithelium-lined cavity into the adjacent dermis, thereby provoking a sterile foreign body-type inflammatory reaction to the keratin in the dermis. Also, an epidermal cyst can become clinically inflamed as a result of bacterial infection.

It has been said that basal cell carcinoma, Bowen's disease (squamous cell carcinoma *in situ*) and invasive squamous cell carcinoma (see Chapter 26) have on rare occasions developed within epidermal cysts, but in actuality some of these cases may have been cases of pseudo-epitheliomatous hyperplasia (which is benign epithelial proliferation that histologically looks like carcinoma) or cases of a proliferating trichilemmal cyst, also known as proliferating trichilemmal tumor (see below in this chapter). Proliferating trichilemmal cyst (proliferating trichilemmal tumor) may develop from an ordinary trichilemmal cyst (see below in this chapter); is clinically a lobulated mass that is progressively enlarging, may ulcerate and may resemble squamous cell carcinoma (see Chapter 26); and has been considered to be a biologically benign lesion that can be locally aggressive and can very rarely undergo malignant transformation, which is seen as rapid enlargement of a nodule, to a malignant proliferating trichilemmal cyst (see below in this chapter).

Trichilemmal cysts

Overview

A trichilemmal cyst is a cavity lined by epithelium that resembles the outer root sheath located around the lower portion of the hair follicle. It is filled with the protein keratin, is usually not attached to the epidermis and generally does not have a punctum.

Trichilemmal cysts are usually multiple and are usually seen on the scalp, although they can be seen elsewhere on the skin's surface.

Similar to the situation with epidermal cysts as described above, trichilemmal cysts in my experience can rarely become sterilely inflamed as a result of rupturing or can rarely become inflamed as a result of bacterial infection.

*Proliferating trichilemmal cysts and malignant
proliferating trichilemmal cysts*

Proliferating trichilemmal cyst (proliferating trichilemmal tumor) may develop from an ordinary trichilemmal cyst. It is clinically a lobulated mass that is progressively enlarging, may ulcerate and may resemble squamous cell carcinoma (see Chapter 26). It has been considered to be a biologically benign lesion that can be locally aggressive and can very rarely undergo malignant transformation, which is seen as rapid enlargement of a nodule, to a malignant proliferating trichilemmal cyst.

Treatment of epidermal and trichilemmal cysts

Overview

Lesions that clinically are clearly non-inflamed, non-infected, asymptomatic, smooth, spherical, non-changing, freely moveable (e.g. not attached to underlying structures) epidermal or trichilemmal cysts need not be treated (excised).

If the patient desires excision of the lesion, if the lesion is changing, if the lesion is symptomatic or causes problems for the patient (e.g. as a result of its location), if it is desired to prevent the lesion from becoming infected or sterilely inflamed, or if there is any doubt as to the diagnosis or benignity of the lesion, the lesion should be excised. I send all lesions that are excised for histopathological evaluation (i.e. biopsy).

Epidermal cysts and trichilemmal cysts should not be merely incised and drained but should be removed (excised) so that the entire cyst sac (i.e. the cyst's epithelial lining) is removed. Otherwise, the cyst will be likely to recur with scarring and then will be more difficult to remove properly. In general, for cysts that have never been inflamed, it is much easier to dissect out and remove the entire cyst sac than it is for cysts that have been inflamed in the past and are therefore associated with scar tissue. Such previously inflamed, scarred cysts generally require careful dissection and removal of the cyst sac from the associated scar tissue, which can encase the cyst sac, thereby making the cyst sac difficult to dissect out. Sometimes, this encasing of the cyst sac by scar tissue can be so significant that it can be very difficult to distinguish the cyst sac from the associated scar tissue, and therefore excision around the entire clinically apparent cyst itself needs to be done because trying to dissect out the cyst sac from the associated scar tissue can be too difficult to perform. Therefore, unless the health-care provider is surgically skilled for such cyst removal, the patient should be referred to a dermatologist.

Treatment of sterilely inflamed, non-infected epidermal and trichilemmal cysts

An epidermal or trichilemmal cyst that is sterilely inflamed and not infected can be treated by intralesional injection (billed as 'intralesional injection') of injectable Kenalog® (triamcinolone) suspension 2.5 mg/ml as described for intralesional injection of inflammatory acne cysts in Chapter 9. It is generally preferable to remove the cyst after the inflammation has resolved.

Treatment of infected epidermal and trichilemmal cysts

An epidermal or trichilemmal cyst that is fluctuant and probably infected should be incised and drained (before incision and drainage are performed in any patient with a heart murmur and/or artificial implant, the American Heart Association guidelines regarding incision and drainage of infected tissue in such patients should be consulted and followed accordingly to prevent bacterial seeding of the heart or artificial implant), with a bacterial culture and sensitivities (C&S) of the drained material being obtained, as described for cutaneous abscesses in Chapter 17, at which time the patient should be empirically started on a course of an oral antibiotic that covers *Staphylococcus aureus*, such as cephalexin (Keflex®) 250–500 mg every 6 h for adults if not otherwise unadvisable or, if the patient is allergic to cephalosporins or penicillins (there is evidence of partial cross-allergenicity of the cephalosporins and the penicillins), erythromycin 250–500 mg every 6 h for adults if not otherwise unadvisable. Pediatric dosage is as described in the package inserts. The oral antibiotic therapy should be subsequently modified according to the patient's response and the bacterial C&S results.

It is generally preferable to remove the cyst after the inflammation and infection have resolved.

Treatment of proliferating trichilemmal cysts and malignant proliferating trichilemmal cysts

A lesion that is suspected of being a proliferating trichilemmal cyst (proliferating trichilemmal tumor) or a malignant proliferating trichilemmal cyst should be referred to a dermatologist. A proliferating trichilemmal cyst (proliferating trichilemmal tumor) is generally seen clinically as a lobulated mass that is progressively enlarging, may ulcerate and may resemble squamous cell carcinoma (see Chapter 26). A malignant proliferating trichilemmal cyst is generally seen clinically as a rapid enlargement of a nodule.

Clinical mimickers of epidermal and trichilemmal cysts: pilomatrixomas and pilomatrix carcinomas

Pilomatrixoma (also known as pilomatricoma and calcifying epithelioma of Malherbe) is a benign lesion that can clinically resemble an epidermal or a trichilemmal cyst. The diagnosis of pilomatrixoma is most often made on histopathological examination.

Clinically, a pilomatrixoma presents as a deep dermal or subcutaneous nodule, which can be hard. The color of a pilomatrixoma can be erythematous, flesh-colored, or blue-black. Unlike epidermal cysts but like trichilemmal cysts, pilomatrixomas do not have puncta. It is not uncommon for pilomatrixomas to develop in children. Treatment of pilomatrixomas consists of complete excision.

Pilomatrix carcinoma is a rare pilomatrixoma variant that is locally aggressive and has the potential for metastasis. It is not known whether pilomatrix carcinoma develops *de novo* or develops within a pre-existing benign pilomatrixoma. Pilomatrix carcinoma cannot be reliably distinguished from pilomatrixoma clinically, and the diagnosis is most often made on histopathological examination. Treatment of pilomatrix carcinoma consists of complete local excision.

Gardner's syndrome, epidermal cysts and pilomatrixoma

The most important feature of Gardner's syndrome consists of the presence of intestinal (usually colonic) polyposis that has a high likelihood for malignant transformation. One of the other features of Gardner's syndrome is the presence of multiple epidermal cysts that are located particularly on the head and trunk. On histopathological examination, these epidermal cysts may show areas of pilomatrixoma.

MILIA

Milia are small, superficial epidermal cysts that are clinically seen as small (generally 1–2 mm in diameter), off-white papules from which whitish, cheesy material (keratin – see above) can be expressed via incision and expression using a no. 11 scalpel or 20-gauge needle and a comedo expresser as described for incision and expression of comedones in Chapter 9.

DERMATOFIBROMAS

Dermatofibromas are benign, firm, flat or raised, typically brown or reddish lesions that are typically composed of an increased number of cells of unclear histogenic origin in the dermis. (The dermis is the cutaneous layer that is located immediately below the epidermis, which is the superficial cutaneous layer.)

When the normal skin around a dermatofibroma is pinched between the thumb and index finger, a dimple-like depression frequently occurs, and this is a dermatofibroma characteristic that is a useful aid in making the diagnosis of dermatofibroma clinically.

Dermatofibromas frequently occur on the legs and are felt to result from cutaneous trauma (e.g. from arthropod bites, cutaneous nicks resulting from leg shaving, etc.).

Dermatofibromas need not be treated. If treatment is elected, excision is the treatment of choice.

24

Common benign melanocytic skin lesions

OVERVIEW

Benign melanocytic skin lesions are skin lesions that are made up of melanocytes, which are the normal, pigment-producing cells in the skin. (The pigment that is produced by melanocytes is called melanin.) The common benign melanocytic skin lesions that will be discussed in this chapter are lentigo simplex; common acquired melanocytic nevus, the types of which include common acquired junctional melanocytic nevus, common acquired compound melanocytic nevus and common acquired intradermal melanocytic nevus; Spitz nevus; acquired dysplastic melanocytic nevus, the types of which include acquired junctional dysplastic melanocytic nevus and acquired compound dysplastic melanocytic nevus; congenital melanocytic nevus; halo melanocytic nevus; blue nevus, the two main types of which include common blue nevus and cellular blue nevus; and solar lentigo.

LENTIGO SIMPLEX

A lentigo simplex is typically a small, uniform, brown, well-demarcated and well-circumscribed, symmetrical macule with regular borders. ('Uniform' indicates that the color of the lesion is the same throught the lesion. 'Well-demarcated and well-circumscribed' mean that the pigment of the lesion stops abruptly and sharply at the surrounding normal skin and does not trail off, fade, or leach into the surrounding normal skin. A macule is a non-raised, non-palpable discoloration of the skin. 'Regular boarders' indicates that the edge of the lesion is smooth and not irregular, notched or scalloped.) Histologically (i.e. on biopsy) there is an increased number of single (i.e. not nested or grouped) melanocytes in the basal layer of the epidermis in a lentigo simplex lesion in comparison to the number of melanocytes in the basal layer of the epidermis in normal skin. (The epidermis is the superficial cutaneous layer that is located immediately above the dermis.)

COMMON ACQUIRED MELANOCYTIC NEVI

Common acquired junctional melanocytic nevi

It has been suggested that common acquired junctional melanocytic nevi can evolve from lentigo simplex lesions.

Common acquired junctional melanocytic nevi typically look basically the same clinically as lentigo simplex lesions, except that common acquired junctional melanocytic nevi may sometimes be slightly larger than lentigo simplex lesions.

Histologically, there are nests (i.e. groups) of melanocytes at the junction of the epidermis and dermis (i.e. at the so-called dermoepidermal junction) in common acquired junctional melanocytic nevi.

Common acquired compound melanocytic nevi

It has been suggested that common acquired compound melanocytic nevi evolve from common acquired junctional melanocytic nevi.

Common acquired compound melanocytic nevi typically look the same clinically as common acquired junctional melanocytic nevi except that common acquired compound melanocytic nevi are generally palpable; may be raised; can be dome-shaped, flat-topped, or pedunculated; and in my experience are usually brown but can be flesh-colored or pink. ('Pedunculated' means that the lesion is on a pedicle or stalk, like an acrochordon (see Chapter 23)).

Histologically, there are nests of melanocytes in the dermis as well as at the dermoepidermal junction in common acquired compound melanocytic nevi.

Common acquired intradermal melanocytic nevi

It has been suggested that common acquired intradermal melanocytic nevi evolve from common acquired compound melanocytic nevi.

Common acquired intradermal melanocytic nevi typically look the same clinically as common acquired compound melanocytic nevi, but in my experience common acquired intradermal melanocytic nevi are usually flesh-colored but can be pink or brown.

Histologically, there are nests of melanocytes only in the dermis in common acquired intradermal melanocytic nevi.

Relationship of malignant melanoma to common acquired melanocytic nevi

Malignant melanoma (see Chapter 26) can develop within common acquired melanocytic nevi, and it has been considered that common acquired melanocytic nevi have a slightly greater risk of malignant melanoma developing within them than does normal skin. However, it can be thought that the majority of malignant melanomas arise on normal skin and not within common acquired melanocytic nevi. This can be accounted for by the idea that the risk of malignant melanoma developing within a given area of a common acquired melanocytic nevus is slightly greater than is the risk of malignant melanoma developing within the same-size area of normal skin, but because the total surface area of normal skin is greater than the total amount of skin area occupied by common acquired melanocytic nevi, it can be concluded that it would be more likely overall for malignant melanoma to develop on normal skin.

EVALUATION OF LENTIGO SIMPLEX LESIONS AND COMMON ACQUIRED MELANOCYTIC NEVI

Overview

Lentigo simplex lesions and common acquired melanocytic nevi without change and without features (as described below) suggestive of malignant melanoma are not prophylactically excised but are watched. However, if change or features suggestive of malignant melanoma are present or develop, complete excisional biopsy of the lesion is performed (as discussed below).

Clinical features suggestive of malignant melanoma

Features that are suggestive of malignant melanoma can be remembered by thinking of 'A, B, C and D'.

'A' stands for asymmetry – malignant melanomas tend to be asymmetrical (meaning that the lesion does not look the same on both sides of imaginary lines that are located through the center of the lesion).

'B' stands for border – malignant melanomas tend to have borders that are irregular and/or poorly demarcated or poorly circumscribed. (Irregular borders are borders that are jagged, scalloped and/or notched. Poorly demarcated or poorly circumscribed borders are borders at which the pigment of the lesion trails off, fades, or leaches into the surrounding normal skin instead of stopping sharply and abruptly at the surrounding normal skin.)

'C' stands for color – malignant melanomas tend to have irregular pigmentation and may have within them red, white, blue and/or gray coloration. (Irregular pigmentation refers to pigmentation that is characterized by different tan and/or brown shades that are present irregularly or haphazardly within the lesion. Red coloration can be a manifestation of inflammation, which can occur in malignant melanomas. White coloration can be a manifestation of lesional regression, which can occur in malignant melanomas and is considered to be a sign of poorer prognosis when seen in malignant melanomas. With regard to blue coloration, melanin, which is brown in color, can be located deeply in the dermis in malignant melanomas (this can also occur in some benign lesions), and when such deeply located melanin is seen through the dermis overlying it, it is seen as blue in color as the result of an optical effect.) Mention should be made of amelanotic malignant melanoma, which is uncommon. This presents without tan, brown, blue, gray and black pigmentation (i.e. it is amelanotic) and is generally reddish in color.

'D' stands for diameter – when combined with other clinical features of malignant melanoma, a lesional size ≥ 5 mm (roughly the size of a pencil's eraser head) is suggestive of malignant melanoma. (This characteristic can be considered to reflect the size of malignant melanomas at the time of diagnosis, and one must be aware that malignant melanoma starts out tiny and grows from there.)

'D' can also stand for dark – the presence of very dark brown or black coloration can be suggestive of malignant melanoma. [Very dark brown and black are unusual colors for common acquired melanocytic nevi in individuals who have lightly pigmented skin, although dark pigmentation is not unusual for common acquired melanocytic nevi in individuals with darkly pigmented skin. However, regardless of an individual's skin color, one should be suspicious of very dark brown or black in lesions that are located on peripheral sites (e.g. hands or feet) or on mucous membranes.]

Common acquired melanocytic nevi normally tend to grow in accordance with the growth of their anatomic location, and all melanocytic nevi within the area of anatomic growth should be growing similarly. The growth of a lesion without the associated similar growth of other melanocytic nevi in the area should make one suspicious of the differently growing lesion.

Any change in color, shape, border, etc. of an individual pre-existing lesion should make one suspicious of the changing lesion.

SPECIAL CONSIDERATIONS REGARDING LENTIGO SIMPLEX LESIONS AND BENIGN MELANOCYTIC NEVI

It is important to remember that lentigo simplex lesions and benign melanocytic nevi can involve mucous membranes and nail beds.

PIGMENTED NAIL STREAKS

Lentigo simplex lesions and benign melanocytic nevi can be present in the nail matrix and as a result can produce pigmented nail streaks, which are typically brown streaks that are oriented longitudinally in the nail plate and extend from the proximal nail fold to the distal edge of the nail (see Chapter 20). The nail matrix is located under the proximal nail fold and produces the nail plate. The proximal nail fold is the skin fold that is located at the proximal edge of the nail plate.

Pigmented nail streaks can also be caused by malignant melanoma (see Chapter 26) in the nail matrix or by drugs, e.g. minocycline (Minocin®). They can be solitary or multiple, and can involve a single nail or multiple nails.

Benign pigmented nail streaks are seen not uncommonly in Black individuals, who nonetheless can have pigmented nail streaks due to malignant melanoma in the nail matrix.

Patients with pigmented nail streaks, especially patients with pigmented nail streaks that have features that make one suspect the presence of malignant melanoma in the nail matrix, should be referred to a dermatologist for evaluation and consideration of performing a nail matrix biopsy to rule out the presence of malignant melanoma in the nail matrix. (Nail matrix biopsy is discussed below in this chapter.) Pigmented nail streak features that make one suspect the presence of malignant melanoma in the nail matrix include a solitary streak (if there are multiple streaks, they are not likely to be due to malignant melanoma, because it is not likely for a patient to have multiple malignant melanomas in multiple nail matrices at one time); a streak in a White patient; a streak that is irregular in any patient (e.g. a streak that has different shades of color and/or has edges that are not sharply demarcated in that the pigment trails off, fades, or leaches into the adjacent normal nail and does not stop sharply and abruptly at the juncture with the adjacent normal nail); a streak that is changing in any patient; a streak that is very dark in any patient; a streak that is very wide in any patient; or a streak that is associated with pigment involving the skin of the proximal nail fold in any patient (this is called Hutchinson's sign and is a late finding of malignant melanoma involving the nail matrix).

If there is any uncertainty at all as to the cause of a pigmented nail streak, the patient should be referred to a dermatologist.

BIOPSY OF SUSPECT MELANOCYTIC LESIONS

Overview

If a patient has a lesion that has features (as described above) that make one suspect the possibility of malignant melanoma, the lesion optimally needs complete excisional biopsy, because if there is malignant melanoma present within the lesion, the entire lesion needs to be present in the biopsy specimen so that the maximum depth and thickness of the malignant melanoma can be determined histologically (i.e. microscopically) on the initial biopsy for staging purposes that determine prognosis and optimal treatment. In addition, complete excisional biopsy should be performed because the entire lesion should be present in the biopsy specimen so that the overall architecture of the entire lesion can be assessed histologically (e.g. to see whether the lesion is symmetrical histologically) and because a narrow rim of normal skin surrounding the lesion should be present in the biopsy specimen so that the peripheral margins of the lesion can be assessed histologically (e.g. to see whether the peripheral margins of the lesion are well-demarcated histologically). In difficult cases such assessments can be important in determining whether the lesion is a malignant melanoma or a benign melanocytic lesion. Complete excisional biopsy is also optimal because there is no risk of missing malignant melanoma developing within a melanocytic nevus, as a result of sampling error, which can occur if only a portion of the lesion is removed for biopsy. Therefore, unless one is skilled in performing the necessary complete excisional biopsy, the patient should be referred to a dermatologist. When doing a biopsy of a lesion on a mucous membrane, appropriate systemic antibiotic prophylaxis (e.g as recommended in the American Heart Association's guidelines) should be administered to patients with heart murmurs and/or artificial implants to prevent bacterial seeding of the heart or artificial implant.

If the lesion is too large for a complete excisional biopsy to be feasible, a dermatologist would be the optimal physician for determining the best way to biopsy a portion of the lesion so as to obtain the best specimen possible for obtaining the best histological information possible, short of complete excisional biopsy.

Biopsy regarding pigmented nail streaks

If a patient has a pigmented nail streak that has features (see above) that make one suspect the presence of malignant melanoma involving the nail matrix, the patient should be referred to a dermatologist for evaluation and consideration of performing a nail matrix biopsy to rule out the presence of malignant melanoma in the nail matrix. (Biopsy of the nail matrix involves temporarily reflecting back the proximal nail fold as a flap in order to gain access to the underlying nail matrix so that biopsy of the lesion in the nail matrix can be performed.)

If there is any uncertainty at all as to the cause of a pigmented nail streak, the patient should be referred to a dermatologist.

SPITZ NEVI

Clinically, Spitz nevi typically present as papules that can be pink, reddish, tan, darkly pigmented, bluish, or somewhat orange or yellowish, although there are other ways in which Spitz nevi can present clinically.

Histologically, melanocytic cells are present at the dermoepidermal junction and/or in the dermis in Spitz nevi. Of significance is the fact that Spitz nevi have histological features that resemble malignant melanoma, but they typically also have other histological features that distinguish them from malignant melanoma and establish them as Spitz nevi rather than malignant melanoma.

Spitz nevi are generally considered to be benign melanocytic nevi, but there has been a concern that some Spitz nevi may become malignant melanoma or are malignant melanoma from the beginning, and there are cases in which malignant melanoma looked histologically like a Spitz nevus. However, in support of those who believe that Spitz nevi are truly benign lesions, it is suggested that lesions that did not follow a benign course were in fact malignant melanomas (which may have been misdiagnosed) and not Spitz nevi.

In any case, any patient with a suspected or histologically confirmed Spitz nevus should be seen in conjunction with a dermatologist.

ACQUIRED DYSPLASTIC MELANOCYTIC NEVI

Overview

The two types of acquired dysplastic melanocytic nevi are acquired junctional dysplastic melanocytic nevi (in which there are nests or groups of melanocytes at the dermoepidermal junction, along with other histological features, including what has been called 'architectural disorder') and acquired compound dysplastic melanocytic nevi (in which there are nests or groups of melanocytes in the dermis as well as at the dermoepidermal junction, along with other histological features, including what has been called 'architectural disorder').

Acquired dysplastic melanocytic nevi have been said to have clinical and histological features that tend to be somewhat intermediate between those of a common acquired melanocytic nevus and those of malignant melanoma.

Relationship of acquired dysplastic melanocytic nevi to malignant melanoma

Overview

There is disagreement among dermatologists regarding the extent to which dysplastic melanocytic nevi are precursor lesions for malignant melanoma (i.e. the extent to which there is an increased risk for the development of malignant melanoma within dysplastic melanocytic nevi) and the extent to which dysplastic melanocytic nevi are marker lesions for malignant melanoma (i.e. the extent to which the presence of dysplastic melanocytic nevi is a risk factor for the development of malignant melanoma at sites that are not necessarily within dysplastic melanocytic nevi).

Some dermatologists, who can be said to be in agreement with what one may call Dr Wallace H. Clark Jr's school of thought, feel that dysplastic melanocytic nevi are precursor and marker lesions for malignant melanoma to a greater extent than are common melanocytic nevi and *per se* significantly increase an individual's risk for malignant melanoma. However, other dermatologists, who can be said to be in agreement with what one may call Dr A. Bernard Ackerman's school of thought, feel that so-called dysplastic melanocytic nevi are no different from so-called common melanocytic nevi with regard to being precursor and marker lesions for malignant melanoma and therefore are no more significant with regard to malignant melanoma risk than are so-called common melanocytic nevi. It should be noted that members of neither school of thought advocate prophylactic excision in general of so-called dysplastic melanocytic nevi that are without change and without features (as described above) suggestive of malignant melanoma; such lesions are in general watched instead of being prophylactically excised, and if change or if features or lesions suggestive of malignant melanoma develop, complete excisional biopsy is performed, as described above.

This disagreement may be reflected in the fact that it has been variously recommended that so-called dysplastic melanocytic nevi be called 'atypical melanocytic nevi', 'Clark's nevi', and 'melanocytic nevi with architectural disorder' (the latter more specifically being a histopathological term). In fact, Ackerman seems to prefer not to use the terms 'common' melanocytic nevi and 'dysplastic' melanocytic nevi but instead classifies melanocytic nevi as Clark's nevi, Miescher's nevi, Unna's nevi, Spitz's nevi, congenital nevi, blue nevi, etc. (the details of this classification are beyond the scope of this guide). Since it seems that the terms dysplastic melanocytic nevus and common melanocytic nevus are somewhat more universally recognized by all physicians of all specialties, I tend to use these terms, which I use throughout this discussion.

Recommendation regarding dysplastic melanocytic nevi

I feel that patients with what is clinically felt to be a dysplastic melanocytic nevus should be seen in conjunction with a dermatologist because a health-care provider with an untrained eye might mistakenly clinically diagnose what is in actuality a malignant melanoma as a dysplastic melanocytic nevus, and also because there are dermatologists who feel that dysplastic melanocytic nevi are precursor and marker lesions for malignant melanoma and *per se* increase an individual's risk for malignant melanoma (although, as discussed above, there is disagreement among dermatologists regarding this).

Also, patients with a histologically confirmed (i.e. biopsy-proven) dysplastic melanocytic nevus should also be seen in conjunction with a dermatologist, again because there are dermatologists who feel that dysplastic melanocytic nevi *per se* increase an individual's risk for malignant melanoma as discussed above (although, again, as discussed above, there is disagreement among dermatologists regarding this).

CONGENITAL MELANOCYTIC NEVI

Overview

A congenital melanocytic nevus is a melanocytic nevus that is present at birth or during the first year of life.

Clinically, they can look like any kind of melanocytic nevus discussed in this chapter, and they can range in size from small (less than 1.5 cm in diameter) to large (≥ 20 cm in diameter – some congenital melanocytic nevi are so large as to cover a significant area of a major anatomic site).

Problems associated with congenital melanocytic nevi

There is an association between giant congenital melanocytic nevi and neurofibromatosis.

Also, large congenital melanocytic nevi involving the head or neck or overlying the spinal area may be associated with underlying melanocytosis involving the cranial or spinal leptomeninges; such central nervous system (CNS) melanocytosis can be asymptomatic or can be associated with significant CNS problems, including CNS malignant melanoma.

Relationship of malignant melanoma to congenital melanocytic nevi

It is not entirely clear as to the exact risk regarding small versus large congenital melanocytic nevi developing malignant melanoma within them, but it is reasonable to say that congenital melanocytic nevi, especially large ones, have a risk of malignant melanoma developing within them (even deeply within them, in which case early detection may not be possible) that is greater than is the risk of malignant melanoma developing within common acquired melanocytic nevi, and prophylactic excision versus observation of congenital melanocytic nevi is performed accordingly.

Therefore, all patients with a congenital melanocytic nevus should be seen in conjunction with a dermatologist.

HALO MELANOCYTIC NEVI

Overview

A halo melanocytic nevus (or halo nevus) occurs when a melanocytic nevus becomes surrounded by a depigmented ring (or halo) of normal skin, after which the central melanocytic nevus may or may not regress. This phenomenon is not entirely understood, but it appears to represent an immunological reaction.

A patient may have one or more halo nevi.

Problems associated with halo nevi and relationship of malignant melanoma to halo nevi

Halo nevi may be associated with vitiligo (see Chapter 7); a personal or family history of cutaneous malignant melanoma (see Chapter 26) and/or dysplastic melanocytic nevi (see above in this chapter); ocular malignant melanoma; and pernicious anemia.

Evaluation of halo nevi

If the nevus component of a patient's halo nevus is benign-appearing (i.e. there are no features that are suggestive of malignant melanoma – features that are suggestive of malignant melanoma are discussed previously in this chapter) and is positioned centrally within a depigmented halo component that is symmetrical, the lesion need not be removed for biopsy but should be watched. If features that are suggestive of malignant melanoma develop in the nevus component, if asymmetry regarding the depigmented halo component develops, or if the nevus component becomes no longer centrally positioned within the depigmented halo component, complete excisional biopsy (as discussed previously in this chapter) should be performed.

On the other hand, if the patient first presents with a halo nevus in which the nevus component is not benign-appearing or is not positioned centrally within a depigmented halo component that is symmetrical, complete excisional biopsy should be performed at the time of the patient's first presentation.

As noted above, halo nevi may be associated with a personal or family history of cutaneous malignant melanoma and/or dysplastic melanocytic nevi. Therefore, if a patient has a halo nevus or halo nevi, it is advisable to find out whether he or she has a personal or family history of malignant melanoma or dysplastic melanocytic nevi. Personal history of malignant melanoma is a risk factor for developing additional, new primary malignant melanomas. Family history of malignant melanoma (particularly in first-degree relatives, i.e. parents, siblings, children) is considered to be a risk factor for malignant melanoma. Dysplastic melanocytic nevi are felt to be risk factors for malignant melanoma, although there is disagreement among dermatologists regarding this, as discussed previously in this chapter.

Lastly, since halo nevi may be associated with cutaneous malignant melanoma, dysplastic nevi and vitiligo, I perform total body examination in which I check for these conditions in patients with halo nevi.

BLUE NEVI

Overview

The two main types of blue nevus are common blue nevus and cellular blue nevus, both of which contain melanocytic cells in the dermis, but each of these two types of blue nevus have other histological features and clinical features by which they can be distinguished.

The blue color of these lesions results from melanin located deeply in the dermis. When such deeply located melanin, which is brown in color, is seen through the dermis overlying it, it is seen as blue in color as the result of an optical effect.

Common blue nevi and relationship to malignant blue nevus

Clinically, a common blue nevus is typically seen as a blue, blue-gray, or blue-black papule (small bump). Common blue nevi are usually less than 1 cm in diameter and have not been associated with the development of malignant melanoma (e.g. malignant blue nevus, which may be a variant of malignant melanoma rather than a distinct entity).

Cellular blue nevi and relationship to malignant blue nevus

Clinically, a cellular blue nevus is typically seen as a blue-gray or blue-brown nodule (large bump) or plaque (a broad, raised lesion), the surface of which is usually smooth but is sometimes irregular. In contrast to common blue nevi, which are usually less than 1 cm in diameter, cellular blue nevi are usually 1–3 cm or greater in diameter.

Malignant blue nevus (which may be a variant of malignant melanoma rather than a distinct entity) can develop in a cellular blue nevus, unlike the situation with common blue nevus. (Malignant blue nevus can also develop *de novo*, i.e. unassociated with a preceding lesion.) Malignant blue nevus is typically seen as an enlarging blue nodule in which there may or may not be ulceration.

Evaluation of blue nevi

A common blue nevus that is less than a centimeter in size and has been unchanging for many years in an adult can generally be observed. However, if the lesion is a blue nodule that has suddenly appeared, if a pre-existing blue nodule is enlarging, if a blue nodule is congenital, or if a blue nodule or plaque is greater than 1 cm in diameter, complete excisional biopsy of the lesion should be performed, as discussed previously in this chapter.

I feel that cellular blue nevi should be excised prophylactically because of the potential for malignant blue nevus to develop within them.

SPECIAL CONSIDERATIONS REGARDING MELANOCYTIC NEVI

Destruction of melanocytic nevi

A melanocytic nevus of any type should never be destroyed (i.e. treated without histological examination (biopsy)) because malignant melanoma can be associated with melanocytic nevi. Therefore, removal of melanocytic nevi should always be performed in such a way that the specimen can be sent for histological examination. Also, partially removed or partially destroyed melanocytic nevi can recur and clinically and histologically look like malignant melanoma but not be malignant melanoma (this condition can be called 'pseudomelanoma'). This can be confusing and cause problems in patients for whom no prior biopsy to confirm the benignity of the original lesion was performed.

Significance of number of melanocytic nevi

It should also be noted that patients with a large number of melanocytic nevi are considered to have an increased risk for developing malignant melanoma (see Chapter 26). Therefore, patients with more than the average number of melanocytic nevi can be considered, with regard to this risk factor, to be at increased risk, relative to the average person in the population for which the average number of melanocytic nevi was determined, for the development of malignant melanoma. Regarding the average number of melanocytic nevi, consider the following. According to Dr Arthur R. Rhodes, referring to studies involving Europeans and Australians, in *Fitzpatrick's Dermatology in General Medicine*, 5th edn., 'In 432 European whites between the ages of 4 days and 96 years, nevi that were 3 mm in diameter or larger were detected in females and males, respectively, at a median number of 0 and 2 in the first decade, 16 and 10 in the second decade, 24 and 16 in the third decade, 19 and 10 in the fourth decade, 12 and 15 in the fifth decade, 12 and 4 in the sixth decade, and 3.5 and 2 from the seventh through the ninth decades. In a series of Australian whites, the average number of nevi per person peaked at 43 for males and 27 for females during the second and third decades, respectively, and decreased to very few in the sixth and seventh decades.'

Also, it has been said that patients with 50–99 small, non-dysplastic melanocytic nevi or more than ten large, non-dysplastic melanocytic nevi have a risk for the development of malignant melanoma that is twice the ordinary risk. As noted previously in this chapter, there is disagreement among dermatologists regarding malignant melanoma risk associated with dysplastic melanocytic nevi, but it is safe to say that the risks regarding dysplastic melanocytic nevi are at least as great as those regarding non-dysplastic melanocytic nevi.

SOLAR LENTIGO

A solar lentigo typically is a uniform tan or brown, symmetrical, well-demarcated, well-circumscribed macule with smooth, regular borders (although the borders in some solar lentigines can be irregular). (A macule is a non-raised, non-palpable discoloration of the skin.) Solar lentigines are usually multiple, are due to chronic sun exposure, are located on sun–exposed areas of the skin and are typically seen in older adults.

Unlike melanocytic nevi, solar lentigines can be treated with light liquid nitrogen therapy using the cotton-tipped applicator technique (see Chapter 22), if desired for cosmetic purposes.

QUANTITATIVE ASSESSMENT OF MALIGNANT MELANOMA RISK ASSOCIATED WITH BENIGN MELANOCYTIC LESIONS

According to Dr. Arthur R. Rhodes in *Fitzpatrick's Dermatology in General Medicine*, 5th edn., individuals who have a new melanocytic nevus or a melanocytic nevus that has changed or is changing have a very high relative risk regarding the development of cutaneous malignant melanoma (where relative risk represents the degree of estimated increased risk for individuals who have the risk factor compared to individuals who do not have the risk factor and where a relative risk of 1 implies no increased risk). Individuals who have a congenital melanocytic nevus have a relative risk of 2–21 regarding the development of cutaneous malignant melanoma. Individuals who have 50 melanocytic nevi that are ≥ 2 mm in diameter have a relative risk of 4–54 regarding the development of cutaneous malignant melanoma. Individuals who have 12 melanocytic nevi that are ≥ 5 mm in diameter have a relative risk of 41 regarding the development of cutaneous malignant melanoma. Individuals who have five melanocytic nevi that are ≥ 5 mm in diameter have a relative risk of 7–10 regarding the development of cutaneous malignant melanoma. Individuals who have marked sun-induced freckles have a relative risk of 4 regarding the development of cutaneous malignant melanoma. Individuals who have a dysplastic melanocytic nevus or dysplastic melanocytic nevi in addition to having a personal history of malignant melanoma and being in a familial melanoma family have a relative risk of 500 regarding the development of cutaneous malignant melanoma. Individuals who have a dysplastic melanocytic nevus or dysplastic melanocytic nevi in addition to being in a familial melanoma family but who do not have a personal history of malignant melanoma have a relative risk of 148 regarding the development of cutaneous malignant melanoma. Individuals who have a dysplastic melanocytic nevus or dysplastic melanocytic nevi, have no personal history of malignant melanoma, and are not in a familial melanoma family have a relative risk of 7–27 regarding the development of cutaneous malignant melanoma. As noted previously, there is disagreement among dermatologists regarding malignant melanoma risk associated with dysplastic melanocytic nevi. Also, it should be noted that some dermatologists feel that the number of families with true familial melanoma is very small (see Chapter 26).

CONCLUDING CAVEAT

In conclusion, if there is any suspicion, doubt, or concern regarding a melanocytic nevus or other pigmented lesion, complete excisional biopsy as discussed previously in this chapter or referral to a dermatologist should be done, because of the association of malignant melanoma with melanocytic lesions.

25

Actinic (solar) keratoses

OVERVIEW

Actinic (solar) keratoses are generally seen clinically as flat, rough, scaly or keratotic, sometimes erythematous lesions that can sometimes be pigmented with shades of brown. (Keratotic lesions are made up of keratinocytes and contain the protein keratin. Keratinocytes make up the bulk of the epidermis and produce keratin. The epidermis is the superficial cutaneous layer that is located immediately above the dermis. Keratin is the substance of which hair, nails and the stratum corneum are composed. The stratum corneum is the dead, horny, most superficial layer of the epidermis.) Actinic keratoses are sometimes more easily palpated (e.g. as roughness) than they are visualized, particularly when the lesions are not erythematous or pigmented. When present, actinic keratoses are generally multiple.

Histologically (i.e. on biopsy), an actinic keratosis is noted to have atypical keratinocytes involving the lower portion of the epidermis.

RELATIONSHIP OF ACTINIC KERATOSES TO SUN EXPOSURE

Actinic keratoses are caused by chronic, long-term, cumulative sun exposure and therefore occur on skin surfaces that have been exposed to the sun.

Since sun exposure is an etiological/risk factor regarding actinic keratoses, it follows that patients who have deficient melanin pigmentation – e.g. fair-skinned patients and patients with vitiligo (see Chapter 7) – have a greater risk for the development of actinic keratoses than do patients who do not have deficient melanin pigmentation.

RELATIONSHIP OF ACTINIC KERATOSES TO SQUAMOUS CELL CARCINOMA AND OTHER SKIN CANCERS

An actinic keratosis is a precancer in that it is a precursor lesion to squamous cell carcinoma (see Chapter 26). An individual actinic keratosis has a

1 in 1000 chance of progressing to squamous cell carcinoma, but 12–25% of patients with actinic keratoses develop squamous cell carcinoma within 10 years.

It has been felt that invasive squamous cell carcinomas that develop within actinic keratoses and squamous cell carcinomas that develop on sun-damaged sun-or exposed skin tend to be less aggressive/likely to metastasize than are squamous cell carcinomas that develop *de novo* (i.e. without a preceding actinic keratosis) and squamous cell carcinomas that develop on skin that is not sun-damaged or sun-exposed, respectively. However, there is some dispute regarding this. For example, it can be difficult to determine with certainty whether a squamous cell carcinoma developed within a preceding actinic keratosis or developed *de novo*, because the squamous cell carcinoma can destroy any preceding actinic keratosis by the time that the patient seeks medical attention for the squamous cell carcinoma. Other factors (see Chapter 26) are undoubtedly more important in terms of determining the degree of such aggressiveness of squamous cell carcinomas. The degree to which such factors are involved in the squamous cell carcinoma cases that comprise any given study can skew the results of that study accordingly if those factors were not properly taken into account. Study conclusions can also be skewed by such factors as hypertrophic actinic keratoses (see below) being interpreted as squamous cell carcinomas and being included in studies dealing with squamous cell carcinoma.

Actinic keratoses are also markers for an increased risk for the development of skin cancer in general, because actinic keratoses are indicative of a patient who has had long-term, chronic, cumulative sun exposure, which is a risk factor for the development of skin cancer in general.

TREATMENT OF ACTINIC KERATOSES

Liquid nitrogen treatment of actinic keratoses

Actinic keratoses can be treated with liquid nitrogen as described in Chapter 22.

Topical 5-fluorouracil treatment of actinic keratoses

Actinic keratoses can also be treated by patient-applied topical 5-fluorouracil (Efudex® cream 5%, Efudex solution 2%, Efudex solution 5%, Fluoroplex® cream 1%, and Fluoroplex solution 1%), which is a particularly good treatment modality for areas of the skin where there are numerous, confluent actinic keratoses.

Topical 5-fluorouracil is a specific treatment in that its application causes inflammation and destruction of actinic keratoses but has no effect on normal skin (assuming the patient is not allergic to topical 5-fluorouracil) and treats subclinical, microscopic actinic keratoses that are not visible to the naked eye.

Since topical 5-fluorouracil can make the patient's skin more sensitive to sunlight (and sunlamps), I accordingly have the patient avoid sun (and sun-lamp) exposure, and keep the areas being treated covered, if possible, when outdoors during the daytime. I have the patient wear a broad-brimmed hat if the areas being treated are on the bald scalp or face, and have the patient use a sunscreen with SPF-15 or greater when the patient is outdoors during the daytime.

When I use topical 5-fluorouracil to treat actinic keratoses, I use Efudex cream 5% and have the patient apply it to the skin area to be treated twice daily. When this is done, actinic keratosis lesions that are present will develop erythema usually followed by vesiculation (blister formation), desquamation, erosion and re-epithelialization. I have the patient discontinue the Efudex when the inflammatory reaction reaches the erosion stage, which usually takes 2–4 weeks of treatment. Complete healing may not occur until 1–2 months after the Efudex treatment is discontinued.

Since the expected inflammatory reaction to Efudex can be severe and sometimes uncomfortable, I warn the patient regarding this, and generally I have the patient treat a small section of skin at first, after which the size of the areas treated can be increased if the patient wishes to do so, once the patient has experienced the Efudex reaction.

If the reaction is severe and uncomfortable, the patient can use cool, plain water open wet compresses (as described for non-specific dermatitis in Chapter 2), which are soothing and do not decrease the effectiveness of the inflammatory reaction produced by the Efudex.

If the reaction is very severe and bothersome to the patient, a topical steroid can be used (as described for non-specific dermatitis in Chapter 2), but one should be aware that such topical steroid use can decrease the inflammatory reaction produced by the Efudex and may therefore decrease the effectiveness of the Efudex treatment.

Topical 5-fluorouracil is contraindicated in women who are or may become pregnant during therapy and should not be used in breast-feeding patients.

HYPERTROPHIC ACTINIC KERATOSES

Overview

Mention should be made of hypertrophic actinic keratoses, which can be considered to be lesions that are at an intermediate stage between ordinary actinic keratoses and squamous cell carcinomas.

Hypertrophic actinic keratoses are generally thicker than are ordinary actinic keratoses. A hypertrophic actinic keratosis should be distinguished from a hyperkeratotic actinic keratosis. In a hyperkeratotic actinic keratosis, the dead, outer, horny layer (which is made of keratin) of the lesion is thickened, but the actinic keratosis itself is not thickened and therefore biologically acts the way that an ordinary actinic keratosis biologically acts. In a hypertrophic actinic keratosis, the lesion itself (and not its dead, outer, horny layer) is thickened, so that the hypertrophic actinic keratosis can be considered to be at an intermediate stage between an ordinary actinic keratosis and a squamous cell carcinoma.

Treatment of hypertrophic actinic keratoses

Hypertrophic actinic keratoses can be treated with more aggressive liquid nitrogen treatment than would be used for an ordinary actinic keratosis (see Chapter 22 for discussion of liquid nitrogen treatment). For example, the liquid nitrogen-soaked cotton-tipped applicator can be applied with greater pressure to the lesion and/or the lesion can be kept frozen (during the time that an area is frozen, it is white) for a longer period of time when a hypertrophic actinic keratosis is being treated than when an ordinary actinic keratosis is being treated. Also, when a hypertrophic actinic keratosis is being treated, it can be treated (i.e. frozen) a second time after the first treatment thaws.

When a hypertrophic actinic keratosis is treated, the patient should be watched for non-resolution or recurrence of the lesion even more closely than following treatment of an ordinary actinic keratosis.

Alternatively, a patient with a hypertrophic actinic keratosis can be referred to a dermatologist for such treatment as curettage and electrodesiccation (which consists of scraping with a curette followed by burning with an electrodesiccator).

FOLLOW-UP REGARDING ACTINIC KERATOSES
AND HYPERTROPHIC ACTINIC KERATOSES

Following treatment of actinic keratoses or hypertrophic actinic keratoses, the patient should be followed to ensure that the lesions resolve and do not recur. If a lesion does not resolve as expected or recurs unexpectedly, the lesion should be biopsied (see the discussion of shave biopsy in Chapter 26), or the patient should be referred to a dermatologist.

Since a history of actinic keratoses and/or hypertrophic actinic keratoses is indicative of chronic, long-term, cumulative sun exposure (which is a risk factor for the development of actinic keratoses, hypertrophic actinic keratoses and skin cancer in general), patients with a history of actinic keratoses and/or hypertrophic actinic keratoses are in general at increased risk for the presence and development of additional actinic keratoses and hypertrophic actinic keratoses and of skin cancer (see Chapter 26) in general (as well as squamous cell carcinoma in particular) and should therefore be evaluated and followed accordingly in this regard as well as followed regarding adequacy of treatment regarding treated lesions. Also, patients should be told to avoid sun exposure, keep covered, wear a broad-brimmed hat, and use a sunscreen with an SPF of 15 or greater when outdoors during the daytime.

26

Common skin cancers

OVERVIEW

The skin cancers that will be discussed in this chapter are basal cell carcinoma, squamous cell carcinoma (and its variants, including verrucous carcinoma and keratoacanthoma) and malignant melanoma.

BASAL CELL CARCINOMA

Overview

Basal cell carcinoma is the most common skin cancer, can occur as an ordinary basal cell carcinoma or as an aggressive-growth basal cell carcinoma, and can occur anywhere on the skin.

Etiological/risk factors regarding basal cell carcinoma

Sun exposure

Although it has been felt that basal cell carcinomas can be caused by long-term, chronic, cumulative sun exposure, childhood and adolescent intermittent sun exposure producing severe sunburns may be of more significance. Also, adults who have sun-induced freckles have about a two-fold to four-fold increase in the risk for non-melanoma skin cancer (i.e. basal cell carcinoma and squamous cell carcinoma).

Since sun exposure is an etiological/risk factor regarding basal cell carcinoma, it follows that patients who have deficient melanin pigmentation – i.e. fair-skinned patients and patients with vitiligo (see Chapter 7) – have a greater basal cell carcinoma risk than do patients who do not have deficient melanin pigmentation.

However, it is important to note that the issue regarding sun exposure and basal cell carcinoma is complicated by the fact that 20% of basal cell carcinomas develop on non-sun-exposed areas.

X-rays/Grenz rays/gamma rays (radiation)

Basal cell carcinomas can be due to radiation.

Heredity

Basal cell carcinomas can be part of hereditary conditions in the form of such syndromes as the nevoid basal cell carcinoma syndrome (NBCCS), in which patients begin developing multiple basal cell carcinomas at an early age (usually beginning between puberty and 35 years of age, although NBCCS patients as young as 2 years of age have developed basal cell carcinoma), develop a range of other tumors and have multiple developmental defects. NBCCS is rare. Its prevalence has been estimated to be 1 in 56 000, and in 18 years of clinical practice I have seen only a few cases of this syndrome. However, NBCCS should be considered in any young patient with multiple basal cell carcinomas.

Immunodeficiency

Patients who are immunodeficient (e.g. immunosuppressed transplant patients, AIDS patients) should be considered to have an increased risk for basal cell carcinoma.

Aggressiveness/prognosis of basal cell carcinoma

Metastasis of basal cell carcinoma

It is very rare for basal cell carcinomas to metastasize. (The rate of metastasis for basal cell carcinoma has been said to range from 0.0028% to 0.1%.) Basal cell carcinomas that metastasize tend to be lesions that are large, ulcerated, and neglected or frequently recurrent following treatment, and most cases have occurred in men. In my 18 years of clinical practice, I have not personally seen a single case in which basal cell carcinoma metastasized.

Local aggressiveness of basal cell carcinoma

Although it is very rare for basal cell carcinomas to metastasize, they are characteristically locally invasive and destructive.

A special category of basal cell carcinoma called aggressive-growth basal cell carcinoma (discussed below) has an overall cure rate that is lower than that for ordinary basal cell carcinoma (discussed below).

'High-risk' locations for basal cell carcinoma

Basal cell carcinomas involving certain locations, including those constituting embryonic fusion planes and those involving resistance planes, are more likely to extend more extensively than is clinically apparent and have a higher recurrence rate after treatment. Such locations include the nasolabial folds (i.e. the bilateral facial creases that extend from the side of the nose to the side of the mouth), the alar grooves (i.e. the bilateral facial creases that are adjacent to the sides of the nasal alae), the nose (including the nasal columella, which is the column of skin that separates the nostril openings), the periauricular regions (i.e. the areas around the ears), the ears, the area around the mouth and the areas around the eyes.

Superficial basal cell carcinoma

A superficial basal cell carcinoma typically presents clinically as a usually erythematous flat lesion that may be slightly scaly; may be slightly pearly, opalescent, translucent and/or waxy; may have a fine, rolled, thread-like, raised, pearly, opalescent, translucent and/or waxy border; may have erosions and/or crusting within it; and may have papules (small bumps) develop within it.

Histologically, a superficial basal cell carcinoma has tumor buds (made up of basaloid cells) that extend from the undersurface of the epidermis with essentially no islands of tumor present free in the dermis. (Basaloid cells are cells that histologically resemble cells that comprise the basal layer of the epidermis. The epidermis is the superficial cutaneous layer that is located immediately above the dermis.)

Nodular basal cell carcinoma

Nodular basal cell carcinomas typically are pearly, opalescent, translucent and/or waxy raised or flat lesions that may or may not be erythematous, may or may not be ulcerated and may or may not be associated with overlying telangiectases (small, superficial, cutaneous blood vessels that present as fine, red lines that may or may not blanch when pressure is applied to them).

Some nodular basal cell carcinomas are endophytic (i.e. grow inward) and present as a non-ulcerated pit or crater and can be noted by palpation to extend beyond what is clinically apparent on visual inspection.

Histologically (i.e. on biopsy), an *ordinary* nodular basal cell carcinoma is made up of relatively large islands of basaloid cells in the dermis, and the edges of these tumor islands are smooth and non-spiky.

See below for the histological appearance of *aggressive-growth* nodular basal cell carcinomas and for discussion regarding *aggressive-growth* basal cell carcinomas in comparison to *ordinary* nodular basal cell carcinomas.

Aggressive-growth basal cell carcinoma

Aggressive-growth basal cell carcinomas are more difficult to treat effectively and are associated with a lower cure rate than are ordinary nodular basal cell carcinomas, because aggressive-growth basal cell carcinomas have a greater tendency to extend beyond what is clinically apparent.

Histologically, aggressive-growth basal cell carcinomas can show a micro-nodular pattern (in which there are small groups, rather than relatively large islands, of basaloid cells in the dermis), an infiltrative pattern (in which the edges of the tumor masses in the dermis are irregular and spiky), and a sclerosing or morpheaform pattern (in which elongated strands of basaloid cells are associated with an increase in collagen deposition).

Clinically, sclerosing or morpheaform basal cell carcinomas typically present as whitish, firm, indurated flat lesions with poorly demarcated borders and may be difficult to visualize. Aggressive-growth basal cell carcinomas that are not sclerosing or morpheaform but are nonetheless histologically micronodular or infiltrative have the clinical appearance of nodular basal cell carcinomas and can therefore be called aggressive-growth nodular basal cell carcinomas.

Pigmentation of basal cell carcinoma

It should be noted that it is not uncommon, especially in dark-skinned patients, for basal cell carcinomas to be pigmented and resemble melanocytic nevi or malignant melanoma clinically.

Atypical clinical presentations of basal cell carcinoma

Basal cell carcinomas may also appear clinically as pimples, papules, cysts, scaly patches (non-raised, non-palpable lesions), or crusts. Therefore, particularly in patients with a history of or at risk for skin cancer, any persistent lesion should be biopsied (see below for discussion regarding biopsy).

Biopsy of lesions suspected of being basal cell carcinoma

The optimal type of biopsy for histological confirmation of the diagnosis for lesions clinically suspected of being basal cell carcinoma is in general the shave biopsy, which is discussed later in this chapter. However, a punch biopsy is preferable when the diagnosis is not obvious or when tumor is suspected within scar tissue. If the health-care provider is not trained in performing punch biopsies, the patient can be referred to a dermatologist for the punch biopsy.

Treatment of basal cell carcinoma

Basic treatment modalities

The basic treatment modalities that are effective for the treatment of appropriate types of basal cell carcinoma that involve appropriate sites in appropriate patients include curettage and electrodesiccation (scraping with a curette and burning with an electrodesiccator), excision with the specimen being sent for histological examination using standard sectioning techniques, and radiation therapy.

Mohs surgery

Special note should be made regarding treatment of aggressive-growth basal cell carcinomas, which can be thought of as expanding by way of narrow tumor extensions so that these tumors can involve tissue far beyond the clinically apparent involvement. These narrow tumor extensions can be missed by basic treatment modalities and by standard histological sectioning techniques for determining clearance of margins when such lesions are excised, in which case the margins would appear to be clear clinically and histologically when in actuality they are not clear. These factors would account for the higher recurrence rate and lower cure rate for aggressive-growth basal cell carcinomas treated with the above-described basic treatment modalities, including excision with standard histological sectioning for determination of clearance of margins.

Mohs surgery is a technique of micrographically controlled excision in which the histological sectioning of the excision specimens is performed differently from the standard method of specimen sectioning, and the tumor is mapped as it is excised. As a result of this, Mohs surgery provides a lower recurrence rate, a higher cure rate and greater sparing of normal tissue in comparison to the basic treatment modalities in the treatment of all types of basal cell carcinoma, including aggressive-growth basal cell carcinoma, as well as in the treatment of certain other types of skin cancer.

Although there is generally a lower recurrence rate, higher cure rate and greater sparing of normal tissue with Mohs surgery in comparison to other treatment modalities, Mohs surgery requires special training and is generally more expensive and more labor intensive than are other treatment modalities.

Therefore, treatment of basal cell carcinomas by Mohs surgery is generally reserved for recurrent basal cell carcinomas (recurrent basal cell carcinomas are generally more aggressive and more likely to recur than are primary basal cell carcinomas), basal cell carcinomas with an aggressive-growth histological pattern (as discussed above), basal cell carcinomas involving sites where there is a statistically high risk of recurrence (as discussed above), basal cell carcinomas that are greater than 2 cm in diameter (very large basal cell carcinomas can have an increased risk of recurrence, and sparing of normal tissue can be of greater importance when treating very large basal cell carcinomas), basal cell carcinomas with poorly demarcated clinical margins (clinically, it is more difficult to determine adequate margins for treatment of such lesions, and such lesions can have a high recurrence rate) and basal cell carcinomas involving locations where sparing of normal tissue is particularly important (e.g. the lips, digits, eyelids, and the tip and alae of the nose).

Follow-up regarding basal cell carcinoma

In checking for recurrence of a treated basal cell carcinoma, the treatment site should be examined on a regular basis for the presence of recurrence for at least 5 years but preferably 10 years. Recurrence of basal cell carcinoma is most likely to become apparent during the first year following treatment, so the treatment site should be examined for the presence of recurrence more frequently during this period. Subsequently, the site should be checked for recurrence once a year, or sooner if the patient notices anything at the site.

In addition, patients with a history of basal cell carcinoma are in general at increased risk for the presence and development of actinic keratoses and additional primary skin cancers and should therefore be evaluated and followed at intervals accordingly. Some statistics follow. A new skin cancer – usually a basal cell carcinoma – was found during a 1-year study period in 20% of patients treated for one basal cell carcinoma; 41% of patients treated for two or more basal cell carcinomas developed a new skin cancer during the study period; 56% of patients treated for three or more basal cell carcinomas developed a new skin cancer during the study period; 45% of patients treated for basal cell carcinoma develop another basal cell carcinoma within 5 years; and 22–38% of patients treated for skin cancer subsequently develop additional basal cell carcinomas or squamous cell carcinomas.

Also, since sun exposure has an etiological role in the development of skin cancer, patients should accordingly be told to avoid excessive sun exposure, keep covered, wear a broad-brimmed hat and use a sunscreen with a sun protection factor (SPF) of 15 or greater when outdoors during the daytime.

SQUAMOUS CELL CARCINOMA

Overview

There are various types of squamous cell carcinoma. These types include squamous cell carcinoma *in situ* involving the skin (Bowen's disease); invasive squamous cell carcinoma, which is distinguished from the entity verrucous carcinoma (see below), involving the skin; squamous cell carcinoma *in situ* involving mucous membranes (including erythroplasia, leukoplakia and erythroleukoplakia); invasive squamous cell carcinoma, which is distinguished from the entity verrucous carcinoma (see below), involving mucous membranes (including erythroplasia, leukoplakia and erythroleukoplakia); and verrucous carcinoma.

There is disagreement among dermatologists regarding the classification of keratoacanthoma (see discussion later in this chapter).

All of the above-described lesions are discussed later in this chapter, along with actinic (solar) keratosis and bowenoid papulosis.

Etiological/risk factors regarding squamous cell carcinoma

Sun exposure

Squamous cell carcinoma is most commonly due to chronic, long-term, cumulative sun exposure. Adults who have sun-induced freckles have about a two-fold to four-fold increase in the risk for non-melanoma skin cancer (i.e. squamous cell carcinoma and basal cell carcinoma).

Since sun exposure is an etiological/risk factor regarding squamous cell carcinoma, it follows that patients who have deficient melanin pigmentation – i.e. fair-skinned patients and patients with vitiligo (see Chapter 7) – have a greater squamous cell carcinoma risk than do patients who do not have deficient melanin pigmentation.

Actinic (solar) keratoses

Squamous cell carcinoma can develop in premalignant precursor lesions known as actinic (solar) keratoses (discussed in Chapter 25).

Actinic keratoses are caused by chronic, long-term, cumulative sun exposure and therefore occur on sun-exposed skin surfaces. An individual actinic keratosis has a 1 in 1000 chance of progressing to squamous cell carcinoma, but 12–25% of patients with actinic keratoses develop squamous cell carcinoma within 10 years.

As described in Chapter 25, actinic keratoses are generally seen clinically as flat, rough, scaly or keratotic, sometimes erythematous lesions that can sometimes be pigmented with shades of brown. (Keratin is the substance of which hair, nails and the stratum corneum are composed. The stratum corneum is the dead, horny, most superficial layer of the epidermis, which is the cutaneous layer immediately above the dermis). Actinic keratoses are sometimes more easily palpated (e.g. as roughness) than they are visualized, particularly when the lesions are not erythematous or pigmented. When present, actinic keratoses are generally multiple.

Histologically (i.e. on biopsy) an actinic keratosis is noted to have atypical keratinocytes involving the lower portion of the epidermis with no involvement of the dermis.

Actinic keratoses are discussed in more detail in Chapter 25.

Chronic scars and chronic inflammation

Squamous cell carcinoma can develop in chronic scars (it can take an average of about 45 years for squamous cell carcinoma to develop in acute burn scars) and at sites of chronic inflammation (e.g. chronic ulcers, chronic sinus tracts, chronic fistulas).

X-rays/Grenz rays/Gamma rays (radiation)

Squamous cell carcinoma can develop as a result of radiation (it can take an average of 25 years for the development of squamous cell carcinoma due to radiation).

Immunodeficiency

Patients who are immunodeficient (e.g. immunosuppressed transplant patients, AIDS patients) should be considered to have an increased risk for squamous cell carcinoma, which may be more aggressive in such patients.

About 7% of immunosuppressed renal transplant patients developed neoplasms, most of which were squamous cell carcinomas on sun-exposed skin, in one study. This is about 16 times the rate in the normal population. It was observed that patients showing less evidence of rejection were more likely to develop squamous cell carcinomas, presumably because these patients were more greatly immunosuppressed.

Human papilloma virus

Squamous cell carcinoma can be due to certain types of human papilloma virus, which is the virus that causes warts (see Chapter 23), causes bowenoid papulosis (see below) and probably causes verrucous carcinoma, which can be considered to be a low-grade squamous cell carcinoma and which is discussed later in this chapter.

Bowenoid papulosis

Bowenoid papulosis (see also Chapter 23) is manifested by often multiple papules and/or plaques involving the external genitalia and containing human papilloma virus. (Papules are bumps. Plaques are broad, raised lesions.) The lesions may be reddish brown or violaceous in color, may be verrucous (i.e. warty in appearance) and usually resemble condylomata acuminata (see Chapter 23).

Sometimes lesions of bowenoid papulosis resolve spontaneously. In other cases, the lesions can persist for years, and in some cases there is a possible increased risk for lesions to become Bowen's disease (squamous cell carcinoma *in situ*) and invasive squamous cell carcinoma.

Female patients with bowenoid papulosis and the female sexual partners of male patients with bowenoid papulosis may be at high risk for cervical and vulvar neoplasia.

Histologically, bowenoid papulosis lesions resemble Bowen's disease, which is squamous cell carcinoma *in situ* involving the skin (see below).

Alcohol and tobacco products

Alcohol ingestion and use of tobacco products can cause oral/aerodigestive squamous cell carcinoma.

Lack of penile circumcision

Squamous cell carcinoma of the glans penis can be seen in men who have not undergone circumcision in early childhood.

Aggressiveness/prognosis of squamous cell carcinoma

Overview

Squamous cell carcinoma can be locally aggressive and destructive and can metastasize. It is important to emphasize that, even if a squamous cell carcinoma has a low metastatic potential and does not metastasize, it can still be locally aggressive and destructive.

Squamous cell carcinomas involving certain locations, including those constituting embryonic fusion planes and those involving resistance planes, are more likely to extend more extensively than is clinically apparent, are more likely to be treated inadequately and have a higher recurrence rate after treatment. Such locations include the nasolabial folds (i.e. the bilateral facial creases that extend from the side of the nose to the side of the mouth), the alar grooves (i.e. the bilateral facial creases that are adjacent to the sides of the nasal alae), the nose (including the nasal columella, which is the column of skin that separates the nostril openings), the periauricular regions (i.e. the areas around the ears), the ears, the area around the mouth and the areas around the eyes.

The incidence of metastasis reported for patients with squamous cell carcinoma has varied from 0% to more than 50%, with differences in case selection most likely to account for this wide range. In most surveys, the incidence of metastasis ranges from 1% to 20%. (However, in my 18 years of general dermatological practice, I have seen only a couple of patients with metastatic cutaneous squamous cell carcinoma.)

In one study the 5-year survival rate for patients with squamous cell carcinoma that was metastatic to regional lymph nodes was 26%, and for patients with distant metastases it was 23%.

It has been felt that invasive squamous cell carcinomas that develop within actinic keratoses and squamous cell carcinomas that develop on sun-damaged or exposed skin tend to be less aggressive/likely to metastasize than are squamous cell carcinomas that develop *de novo* (i.e. without a preceding actinic keratosis) and squamous cell carcinomas that develop on skin that has not been sun-damaged or sun-exposed, respectively. However, there is some dispute regarding this. For example, it can be difficult to determine with certainty whether a squamous cell carcinoma developed within a preceding actinic keratosis or developed *de novo*, because the squamous cell carcinoma can destroy any preceding actinic keratosis by the time that the patient seeks medical attention for the squamous cell carcinoma. Other factors (see below) are undoubtedly more important in determining the degree of such aggressiveness of squamous cell carcinomas, and the degree to which such factors are involved in the squamous cell carcinoma cases that comprise any given study can skew the results of that study accordingly if those factors were not properly taken into account. Study conclusions can also be skewed by such factors as hypertrophic actinic keratoses (see Chapter 25) being interpreted as squamous cell carcinomas and being included in studies dealing with squamous cell carcinoma.

Cutaneous invasive squamous cell carcinomas that are large (e.g. greater than 2 cm), deeply invasive (e.g. 4 mm or greater) and/or less well differentiated are associated with a greater risk for local recurrence and for metastasis. Prognosis is also poorer for cutaneous invasive squamous cell carcinomas with perineural involvement (i.e. with involvement of the perineural space) and is poorer in immunosuppressed patients.

Invasive squamous cell carcinomas developing in lesions of Bowen's disease (squamous cell carcinoma *in situ* involving the skin), in lesions of erythroplasia of Queyrat (squamous cell carcinoma *in situ* involving the glans penis), in chronic scars/sites of chronic inflammation, due to radiation, or *de novo* (i.e. on normal skin without a precursor lesion) have been reported to be more aggressive/likely to metastasize than are invasive squamous cell carcinomas developing in actinic keratoses, but it must be remembered that study results can be skewed if certain factors are not taken into account, as discussed above.

In addition, it has been held that invasive squamous cell carcinomas developing at certain anatomic sites tend to be more aggressive/likely to metastasize in comparison to those developing at other anatomic sites, but, again, it must be remembered that study results can be skewed, as discussed above.

Also, it is held that invasive squamous cell carcinomas developing on mucous membranes tend to be more aggressive/likely to metastasize in comparison to those developing on ordinary skin, although delay in detection may be a factor (e.g. with oral squamous cell carcinomas).

Verrucous carcinoma can be considered to be a low-grade squamous cell carcinoma that is more likely to invade adjacent tissue (it is locally aggressive) than it is to metastasize (it only rarely metastasizes).

There is disagreement among dermatologists regarding the classification and aggressiveness/metastatic potential of keratoacanthomas (see discussion below).

Aggressiveness/prognosis of actinically derived
invasive squamous cell carcinoma

It has traditionally been held that the metastatic potential of actinically derived invasive squamous cell carcinomas is low and that such lesions do not commonly metastasize. Although reported metastatic rates for such lesions have ranged from 0.3% to 5%, in my 18 years of general dermatological practice I have seen only a couple of patients with metastatic cutaneous squamous cell carcinoma.

Aggressiveness/prognosis of invasive squamous cell carcinoma developing in a lesion of Bowen's disease

It has been reported that, without adequate therapy, at least one-third of patients with invasive squamous cell carcinoma that has developed in a lesion of Bowen's disease develop metastases. (However, because squamous cell carcinoma *in situ* that has truly not progressed to invasive squamous cell carcinoma is confined to the epidermis and has not gone below the basement membrane of the epidermis, squamous cell carcinoma *in situ* as such theoretically has no potential for metastasis.)

Aggressiveness/prognosis of invasive squamous cell carcinoma developing in a lesion of erythroplasia of Queyrat

It has been reported that 20% of patients with erythroplasia of Queyrat in which invasive squamous cell carcinoma developed and invaded the penile submucosa displayed metastases. (However, because squamous cell carcinoma *in situ* that has truly not progressed to invasive squamous cell carcinoma is confined to the epidermis and has not gone below the basement membrane of the epidermis, squamous cell carcinoma *in situ* as such theoretically has no potential for metastasis.)

Aggressiveness/prognosis of invasive squamous cell carcinoma developing in chronic scars/sites of chronic inflammation

Although the risk of squamous cell carcinoma developing in scars, ulcers and sinus tracts is low, it has been reported that such squamous cell carcinomas have a high potential for metastasis and are aggressive.

The reported incidence of metastasis for invasive squamous cell carcinomas developing in osteomyelitis scars and sinus tracts ranges from 11% to 37%, and patients with squamous cell carcinoma developing in scars have been reported to have a 5-year survival rate of about 55%.

Aggressiveness/prognosis of invasive squamous cell carcinoma due to X-rays/Grenz rays/Gamma rays (radiation)

It has been reported that squamous cell carcinomas due to radiation have a high potential for metastasis and are aggressive.

Reported rates of metastasis for invasive squamous cell carcinoma due to radiation have been 20–25%, and patients with radiation-induced squamous cell carcinoma have been reported to have a 5-year survival rate of 50%.

Aggressiveness/prognosis of invasive squamous cell carcinoma developing de novo

It has been held that invasive squamous cell carcinomas that develop *de novo* have a tendency to metastasize and exhibit rapid invasiveness. Although the exact metastatic rate for invasive squamous cell carcinomas that develop *de novo* is unclear, the rate has been reported to be 8%.

Aggressiveness/prognosis of invasive squamous cell carcinoma developing on mucous membranes and at certain higher-risk anatomic sites

Overview   Invasive squamous cell carcinoma involving mucous membranes and involving certain body sites (e.g. the lower lip, mouth, and genitals, as well as the temples, ears, scalp, dorsal aspects of the hands) have been reported to be more aggressive/likely to metastasize and have been reported to have a worse prognosis in comparison to non-mucosal skin and to other body sites.

Aggressiveness/prognosis of invasive squamous cell carcinoma involving the lower lip   Overall, the reported metastatic rate for lower lip squamous cell carcinoma ranges from 15% up to 40%.

It has been reported that about 75% of lip squamous cell carcinomas that were 6 mm or greater in thickness, 60% of lip squamous cell carcinomas with perineural invasion (i.e. invasion involving the perineural space) and about 90% of lip squamous cell carcinomas that had a Broders grade 4 histological pattern (i.e. extremely poorly differentiated histologically) were associated with metastasis. However, lip squamous cell carcinomas treated when they are still at an early stage can be easily cured. The prognosis is poor when there is metastasis.

Younger patients with lip squamous cell carcinoma that has metastasized tend to have a poorer prognosis than do older patients. Patients under 40 years of age with lip squamous cell carcinoma that was metastatic had a 5-year mortality rate of about 20%.

Aggressiveness/prognosis of invasive squamous cell carcinoma involving the mouth   It has been reported that at least 50% of patients with mouth squamous cell carcinoma have lymph node metastases, but when the cancer is detected at an early, asymptomatic stage, metastases are few.

Patients with squamous cell carcinoma involving the mouth have an overall 5-year survival rate of 30–40%, but mouth squamous cell carcinoma is often curable if treated early. Patients with mouth squamous cell carcinoma that was treated when the lesion was in an early asymptomatic stage had a 5-year survival rate of about 90%.

It should be noted that patients with mouth squamous cell carcinoma are at increased risk for additional oral/aerodigestive squamous cell carcinomas.

Aggressiveness/prognosis of invasive squamous cell carcinoma involving the penis   As many as 60% of patients with penile squamous cell carcinoma have been reported to have inguinal lymph node metastases at the time of presentation.

Patients with penile squamous cell carcinoma without clinical metastases have a 5-year survival rate of 60–90%, but the 5-year survival rate is about 10–30% when there has been regional lymph node metastasis.

Aggressiveness/prognosis of invasive squamous cell carcinoma involving the scrotum   A metastatic rate for scrotal squamous cell carcinoma was reported to be as high as about 70%, although delay in seeking medical attention may be a factor.

The 5-year survival rate for patients with scrotal squamous cell carcinoma has been reported to range from 8% to 70%, depending on the stage of the disease.

Aggressiveness/prognosis of invasive squamous cell carcinoma involving the vulva   In studies, 29% and 38% of cases of vulvar squamous cell carcinoma were associated with lymph node metastasis, and when the tumor thickness was greater than 4 mm, over 40% of cases of vulvar squamous cell carcinoma were associated with lymph node metastasis.

The 5-year survival rate for patients with vulvar squamous cell carcinoma is about 70% (the larger the tumor, the poorer the prognosis).

Patients with vulvar squamous cell carcinoma *in situ* have a high incidence of upper vaginal, cervical and uterine cancer. It has been reported that primary squamous cell carcinoma of the uterine cervix is present in up to 30% of patients who have squamous cell carcinoma of the vulva.

Aggressiveness/prognosis of verrucous carcinoma

Verrucous carcinoma can be considered to be a low-grade squamous cell carcinoma with a relatively low degree of aggressiveness. Although it rarely metastasizes (typically after many years), it is locally invasive and destructive.

Aggressiveness/prognosis of keratoacanthomas

There is disagreement among dermatologists regarding the classification and aggressiveness/metastatic potential of keratoacanthomas (see discussion below).

Squamous cell carcinoma *in situ* involving the skin

Invasive squamous cell carcinoma develops in at least 5% of patients with squamous cell carcinoma *in situ* involving the skin (Bowen's disease).

Common Bowen's disease typically presents clinically as a reddish, scaly, sometimes keratotic, sometimes verrucous, sometimes fissured, sometimes eroded, sometimes crusted, flat or raised, sharply demarcated lesion without hair within it. (Verrucous means warty. Sharply demarcated means that the border between the lesion and normal skin is sharply defined.) Less than 2% of lesions are pigmented. Lesions of Bowen's disease can sometimes resemble dermatitis (see Chapter 2), psoriasis (see Chapter 4), or tinea (see Chapter 18). Bowen's disease can occur just about anywhere on the skin, including the nail beds.

Histologically, squamous cell carcinoma *in situ* exhibits keratinocytic atypia throughout the full thickness of the epidermis with no involvement of the dermis. It is important to note that squamous cell carcinoma *in situ* can extend down the epithelium of hair follicles (the epithelium of hair follicles is continuous with the surface epidermis), in which case superficial treatment of the lesion would be expected to be inadequate.

Invasive squamous cell carcinoma involving the skin

This is non-*in situ* squamous cell carcinoma and typically presents clinically as a reddish or skin-colored, usually keratotic, raised or palpable lesion, which may or may not be eroded/ulcerated or crusted, and the surface may be smooth or may become verrucous. The lesions can be scaly. An erosion/ulcer can sometimes be an early manifestation of invasive squamous cell carcinoma. Sometimes lesions of invasive squamous cell carcinoma can present as flat, scaly lesions resembling dermatitis (see Chapter 2) or tinea (see Chapter 18).

Like Bowen's disease, invasive squamous cell carcinoma can occur almost anywhere on the skin, including the nail beds.

Histologically, invasive squamous cell carcinoma consists of groups of atypical keratinocytes in the dermis.

Squamous cell carcinoma *in situ* and invasive squamous cell carcinoma involving mucous membranes

Overview

Mucosal squamous cell carcinoma *in situ* and mucosal invasive squamous cell carcinoma can be difficult to distinguish from each other clinically, although granularity or roughness suggests invasive squamous cell carcinoma.

Squamous cell carcinoma *in situ* and invasive squamous cell carcinoma involving mucous membranes (such as the mouth, mucosal areas of the vulva and mucosal areas of the penis) can be red, flat or raised, and smooth, with minimal or no white components, or they can be red, raised and velvety, with or without white components. These clinical presentations are called erythroplasia.

Alternatively, rarely, such mucous membrane squamous cell carcinoma *in situ* and invasive squamous cell carcinoma lesions can be white, flat or raised, and smooth or verrucous, with or without red components. In this case, such lesions without red components can be called leukoplakia (although leukoplakia can also represent benign mucous membrane lesions); when such white lesions have red components, they can be called leukoerythroplakia and are classified as a type of erythroplasia.

In terms of the significance of the above-described red versus white mucous membrane changes, it is important to note that the association of oral squamous cell carcinoma is much greater with oral erythroplasia and leukoerythroplakia than with leukoplakia. More than 95% of oral squamous cell carcinomas begin as erythroplasia (in which there may or may not be a white component), and only about 2% of oral squamous cell carcinomas are manifested by changes that are primarily those of leukoplakia. Also, about 2–4% of oral clinical leukoplakia lesions turn out to be squamous cell carcinoma *in situ* or invasive squamous cell carcinoma. On the other hand, a high percentage of oral clinical erythroplasia lesions turn out to be squamous cell carcinoma. For high-risk oral sites (which include the floor of the mouth, the venterolateral tongue and the soft palate complex), 80% of clinical erythroplasia lesions turned out to be invasive squamous cell carcinoma.

Squamous cell carcinoma *in situ* and invasive squamous cell carcinoma involving mucous membranes can also present as a verrucous raised lesion.

Erythroplasia of Queyrat

Erythroplasia of Queyrat is squamous cell carcinoma *in situ* involving the penile mucosa. It typically presents clinically as a bright reddish, velvety, sharply demarcated plaque that may have crusting and scaling involving the glans penis, and it usually occurs in men who were not circumcised in early childhood. (A plaque is a broad, raised lesion.) Without treatment, 10% of patients with erythroplasia of Queyrat develop invasive squamous cell carcinoma. Also, 10% of patients with erythroplasia of Queyrat have invasive squamous cell carcinoma in their erythroplasia of Queyrat lesions.

Histological changes of squamous cell carcinoma in situ
and invasive squamous cell carcinoma involving mucous membranes

Histologically, squamous cell carcinoma *in situ* exhibits keratinocytic atypia throughout the full thickness of the epidermis with no involvement of the dermis, whereas invasive squamous cell carcinoma consists of groups of atypical keratinocytes in the dermis.

Verrucous carcinoma

In comparison to conventional invasive squamous cell carcinoma, verrucous carcinoma, which can be considered to be a type of low-grade, locally invasive squamous cell carcinoma that is probably due to human papilloma viruses, is warty, grows slowly and is more likely to invade adjacent tissue (it is locally aggressive) than it is to metastasize (it only rarely metastasizes). Verrucous carcinoma is also mentioned in Chapter 23.

Types of verrucous carcinoma include epithelioma cuniculatum and giant condyloma acuminatum (also called Buschke–Lowenstein tumor).

Epithelioma cuniculatum is rare, involves the sole, is felt to arise from a plantar wart (see Chapter 23), may look like a plantar wart initially and is typically a large, slowly enlarging, cauliflower-like mass that is unresponsive to standard plantar wart therapy.

Giant condyloma acuminatum contains human papilloma virus, involves the anogenital region and is typically large (although it can be small), cauliflower-like and unresponsive to standard condyloma acuminatum therapy (see Chapter 23).

Verrucous carcinoma may involve other sites (e.g. the trunk, buttocks, hands, fingers, face, mouth).

Histologically, verrucous carcinoma exhibits groups of minimally atypical keratinocytes extending from the epidermis into the dermis in a pattern similar to that seen in verrucae (warts).

Keratoacanthoma

Keratoacanthoma has been considered by some dermatologists to be a benign lesion that typically resolves spontaneously and, in the opinion of these dermatologists, never metastasizes. Persistence with significant local invasiveness and associated tissue destruction by such lesions and occurrence of distant metastasis, especially in immunocompromised patients, have been accounted for by the opinion that such lesions were in fact squamous cell carcinomas misdiagnosed as keratoacanthomas or were keratoacanthomas that underwent malignant transformation. Other dermatologists account for such behavior by considering keratoacanthomas to be well-differentiated squamous cell carcinomas that usually, but not always, spontaneously resolve. The term used by these dermatologists for keratoacanthoma is 'squamous cell carcinoma, keratoacanthoma type', which corresponds to my view regarding keratoacanthomas. In any case, in light of their potential for aggressive behavior, I feel that it is best to treat keratoacanthomas as well-differentiated squamous cell carcinomas.

Typically, keratoacanthomas develop and grow rapidly to a size of about 1–2.5 cm over a period of about 6 weeks and subsequently spontaneously resolve gradually over a period of about 2–6 months, although some lesions can take over a year to resolve. However, as noted above, some lesions have been noted to persist and to behave biologically in the way that a malignant lesion behaves.

Typically, when fully developed, a keratoacanthoma is clinically seen as a fleshy, flesh-colored or slightly erythematous, dome-shaped nodule with a central, keratin-filled crater.

Histologically, a keratoacanthoma consists of a mass of atypical keratinocytes. On high-magnification light microscopy, a keratoacanthoma can be difficult to distinguish from an ordinary higher-grade invasive squamous cell carcinoma. However, on low-magnification light microscopy, when the outline and architecture of the entire lesion (including its base) can be examined, a keratoacanthoma can generally be distinguished from an ordinary higher-grade invasive squamous cell carcinoma.

Biopsy of lesions suspected of being squamous cell carcinoma and keratoacanthoma

Biopsy of a lesion suspected of being squamous cell carcinoma

The optimal type of biopsy for histological confirmation of diagnosis for lesions clinically suspected of being squamous cell carcinoma (excluding keratoacanthoma, biopsy of which is discussed below) is in general the shave biopsy, which is discussed later in this chapter. However, a punch biopsy is preferable when the diagnosis is not obvious or when tumor is suspected within scar tissue. If the health-care provider is not trained in performing punch biopsies, the patient can be referred to a dermatologist for the punch biopsy.

When performing a biopsy of a lesion on a mucous membrane, appropriate systemic antibiotic prophylaxis (e.g. as recommended in the American Heart Association's guidelines) should be administered to patients with heart murmurs and/or artificial implants to prevent bacterial seeding of the heart or artificial implant.

Biopsy of a lesion suspected of being a keratoacanthoma

On high-magnification light microscopy, a keratoacanthoma can be difficult to distinguish from an ordinary higher-grade invasive squamous cell carcinoma. However, on low-magnification light microscopy, when the outline and architecture of the entire lesion (including its base) can be examined, a keratoacanthoma can generally be distinguished from an ordinary higher-grade invasive squamous cell carcinoma.

If the specimen for histological examination is such that the outline and architecture of the entire lesion (including its base) cannot be examined, distinguishing a keratoacanthoma from an ordinary higher-grade invasive squamous cell carcinoma can be very difficult, if not impossible (although a clinical history of rapid development and growth over a period of about 6 weeks followed by cessation of growth can be suggestive of the diagnosis of keratoacanthoma). Therefore, if a keratoacanthoma is suspected clinically, a complete excisional biopsy of the lesion (including its base) is preferable to a biopsy of a portion of the lesion, because a complete excisional biopsy, unlike a biopsy of a portion of the lesion, will provide a specimen for histological examination such that the outline and architecture of the entire lesion (including its base) can be examined, thereby making it easier to distinguish a keratoacanthoma from an ordinary higher-grade invasive squamous cell carcinoma.

Treatment of actinic keratoses, bowenoid papulosis, squamous cell carcinoma and keratoacanthomas

Treatment of actinic keratoses

Treatment of actinic keratoses is as discussed in Chapter 25.

Treatment of bowenoid papulosis

Sometimes lesions of bowenoid papulosis resolve spontaneously. In other cases, the lesions can persist for years, and in some cases there is a possible increased risk for lesions to become Bowen's disease (squamous cell carcinoma *in situ*) and invasive squamous cell carcinoma.

Female patients with bowenoid papulosis and the female sexual partners of male patients with bowenoid papulosis may be at high risk for cervical and vulvar neoplasia.

When bowenoid papulosis is suspected, the patient should be referred to a dermatologist, and female patients and the female sexual partners of male patients should be referred to a gynecologist.

Treatment of squamous cell carcinoma in situ *involving the skin*

In my opinion, squamous cell carcinoma *in situ* involving the skin (Bowen's disease) is generally best treated by complete excision, because Bowen's disease can extend down hair follicles, in which case superficial treatment modalities would not be expected to be effective.

Treatment of invasive squamous cell carcinoma *involving the skin*

Because invasive squamous cell carcinoma has the potential for metastasis, patients with this lesion should be evaluated for the presence of metastasis. Also, because of the metastatic potential of invasive squamous cell carcinoma, I feel that it is generally best treated by excision. Patients with treated invasive squamous cell carcinoma should be followed for the development of metastasis as well as for the development of recurrence of the treated lesion.

Treatment of squamous cell carcinoma in situ *involving mucous membranes*

Squamous cell carcinoma *in situ* involving mucous membranes (erythroplasia of Queyrat and other types of squamous cell carcinoma *in situ* involving mucous membranes) can be treated by topical 5-fluorouracil (which should be done under the care of a dermatologist) or by excision.

Treatment of invasive squamous cell carcinoma *involving mucous membranes*

Because invasive squamous cell carcinoma has the potential for metastasis, patients with this lesion should be evaluated for the presence of metastasis. Also, because of the metastatic potential of invasive squamous cell carcinoma, I feel that it is generally best treated by excision. Patients with treated invasive squamous cell carcinoma should be followed for the development of metastasis as well as for the development of recurrence of the treated lesion.

Treatment of verrucous carcinoma

Because verrucous carcinoma can be considered to be a low-grade squamous cell carcinoma that has a potential for metastasis (albeit low), I feel that verrucous carcinoma is generally best evaluated, treated and followed as described above for invasive squamous cell carcinoma.

Treatment of keratoacanthomas

Because I am in agreement with those who consider keratoacanthomas to be well-differentiated squamous cell carcinomas, I feel that keratoacanthomas are generally best evaluated, treated and followed as described above for invasive squamous cell carcinoma.

Other treatment modalities for squamous cell carcinoma

Other modalities that have been used to treat appropriate squamous cell carcinomas involving appropriate sites in appropriate patients include curettage and electrodesiccation (scraping with a curette and burning with an electrodesiccator) and radiation therapy (radiation therapy should not be used for the treatment of verrucous carcinoma, because it may increase the risk for early metastasis).

Mohs micrographic surgery is indicated for the treatment of squamous cell carcinomas that are high risk or are located at sites where sparing of normal tissue when the lesion is treated is essential. (Mohs surgery is discussed in detail in the discussion of the treatment of basal cell carcinomas previously in this chapter.)

Surgical treatment of lesions on mucous membranes

When doing surgical treatment of lesions on mucous membranes, appropriate systemic antibiotic prophylaxis (as recommended in the American Heart Association's guidelines) should be administered to patients with heart murmurs and/or artificial implants in order to prevent bacterial seeding of the heart or artificial implant.

Follow-up regarding squamous cell carcinoma

Patients with treated squamous cell carcinoma should be evaluated at regular intervals for the development of recurrence and/or metastasis.

In addition, patients with a history of squamous cell carcinoma are in general at increased risk for the presence and development of actinic keratoses and additional primary skin cancers and should therefore be evaluated and followed at intervals accordingly (22–38% of patients treated for skin cancer subsequently develop additional squamous cell carcinomas or basal cell carcinomas).

Also, since sun exposure has an etiological role in the development of skin cancer, patients should accordingly be told to avoid sun (and sunlamp) exposure, keep covered, wear a broad-brimmed hat and use a sunscreen with an SPF of 15 or greater when outdoors during the daytime.

Since alcohol ingestion and use of tobacco products can cause oral/ aerodigestive squamous cell carcinoma, patients using these products should discontinue their use.

MALIGNANT MELANOMA

Overview

Malignant melanoma is the most potentially dangerous of the commonly encountered skin cancers.

Histologically, malignant melanoma is characterized by the presence of atypical melanocytes in the epidermis and frequently in the dermis. (Normal melanocytes are pigment-producing cells that produce the pigment melanin and are typically found in the epidermis – the superficial cutaneous layer that is located immediately above the dermis.)

Etiological/risk factors regarding malignant melanoma

Personal history of malignant melanoma

Patients with a personal history of malignant melanoma are at increased risk for the development of additional, new primary malignant melanomas.

Sun exposure

History of sunburns and/or intermittent sun exposure may be of greater significance with regard to the development of malignant melanoma than is chronic, long-term, cumulative sun exposure, and adults who have sun-induced freckles have about a two-fold to six-fold increase in the risk for malignant melanoma.

Dr A. Bernard Ackerman does not feel that sunlight of itself causes malignant melanoma but instead feels that ultraviolet light is an inducer of malignant melanoma in persons who are genetically predisposed to malignant melanoma.

Precursor lesions

Overview   Certain lesions have an increased risk for the development of malignant melanoma within them, and these lesions are considered to be precursor lesions for malignant melanoma. (Malignant melanoma can also occur *de novo*, on normal integument without a precursor lesion).

Common melanocytic nevi   Malignant melanoma can develop within common melanocytic nevi (discussed in Chapter 24), and it has been felt that common melanocytic nevi have a slightly greater risk of malignant melanoma developing within them than does normal skin. However, it can be thought that the majority of malignant melanomas arise on normal skin and not within common melanocytic nevi. This can be accounted for by the idea that the risk of malignant melanoma developing within a given area of a common melanocytic nevus is slightly greater than is the risk of malignant melanoma developing within the same-size area of normal skin, but because the total surface area of normal skin is greater than the total amount of skin area occupied by common melanocytic nevi, it can be concluded that it would be more likely overall for malignant melanoma to develop on normal skin.

Common melanocytic nevi without change and without features (as described later in this chapter) suggestive of malignant melanoma are not prophylactically excised but are watched. However, if change or features suggestive of malignant melanoma are present or develop, complete excisional biopsy of the lesion is done (as discussed later in this chapter).

Congenital melanocytic nevi   It is not entirely clear as to the exact risk regarding small versus large congenital melanocytic nevi developing malignant melanoma within them, but it is reasonable to say that congenital melanocytic nevi (Chapter 24), especially large ones, have a risk of malignant melanoma developing within them (even deeply within them, in which case early detection may not be possible) that is greater than is the risk of malignant melanoma developing within common melanocytic nevi, and prophylactic excision versus observation of congenital melanocytic nevi is performed accordingly. Therefore, all patients with a congenital melanocytic nevus should be seen in conjunction with a dermatologist.

Cellular blue nevi   Malignant blue nevus, which may be a variant of malignant melanoma rather than a distinct entity, can develop within a cellular blue nevus (discussed in Chapter 24), so cellular blue nevi should generally be prophylactically excised. Malignant blue nevus can also develop *de novo* (i.e. unassociated with a precursor lesion).

If a lesion is a blue nodule that has suddenly appeared, if a pre-existing blue nodule is enlarging, if a blue nodule is congenital, or if a blue nodule or plaque is greater than 1 cm in diameter, complete excisional biopsy of the lesion should be performed, as discussed later in this chapter.

Dysplastic melanocytic nevi   In addition to being precursor lesions for malignant melanoma, dysplastic melanocytic nevi are felt to be marker lesions for malignant melanoma in that it is felt that the presence of dysplastic melanocytic nevi is a risk factor for the development of malignant melanoma at sites that are not necessarily within dysplastic melanocytic nevi, although there is disagreement among dermatologists regarding malignant melanoma risk associated with dysplastic melanocytic nevi. (The relationship of dysplastic melanocytic nevi to malignant melanoma is discussed below, and dysplastic melanocytic nevi are discussed in more detail in Chapter 24.)

Genetic factors

Members of certain families in particular have an increased risk for the development of malignant melanoma, and a family history of malignant melanoma (particularly in first-degree relatives, which are parents, siblings and children) is considered to be a risk factor for malignant melanoma.

Individuals with a family history of cutaneous malignant melanoma in a first-degree relative have been said to have an eight-fold increased risk for malignant melanoma in comparison to individuals who have no family history of cutaneous malignant melanoma in first-degree relatives, and patients with at least two first-degree relatives with malignant melanoma have been said to have a particularly high risk for malignant melanoma.

It has been said that patients who have dysplastic melanocytic nevi in addition to being in a familial melanoma family have a significantly increased risk for the development of malignant melanoma, while patients who have a personal history of malignant melanoma in addition to having dysplastic melanocytic nevi and being in a familial melanoma family have an even greater risk for the development of subsequent primary malignant melanoma, although, as noted below and in Chapter 24, there is disagreement among dermatologists regarding malignant melanoma risk associated with dysplastic melanocytic nevi.

It has been said that patients who have malignant melanoma and who are in a familial melanoma family have an increased risk for multiple primary malignant melanomas and for dysplastic melanocytic nevi in comparison to patients who have malignant melanoma and who are not in a familial melanoma family.

It should be noted that some dermatologists feel that the number of families with true familial melanoma is very small.

Dr A. Bernard Ackerman believes that persons who develop malignant melanoma do so because such persons have a genetic predisposition for malignant melanoma. He does not feel that sunlight of itself causes malignant melanoma but instead feels that ultraviolet light is an inducer of malignant melanoma in persons who are genetically predisposed to malignant melanoma.

Number of melanocytic nevi

Patients with a large number of melanocytic nevi are considered to have an increased risk for developing malignant melanoma. Therefore, patients with more than the average number of melanocytic nevi can be considered, with regard to this risk factor, to be at increased risk, relative to the average person in the population for which the average number of melanocytic nevi was determined, for the development of malignant melanoma. Regarding the average number of melanocytic nevi, Dr Arthur R. Rhodes referred to studies involving Europeans and Australians, in *Fitzpatrick's Dermatology in General Medicine*, 5th edn., 'In 432 European whites between the ages of 4 days and 96 years, nevi that were 3 mm in diameter or larger were detected in females and males, respectively, at a median number of 0 and 2 in the first decade, 16 and 10 in the second decade, 24 and 16 in the third decade, 19 and 10 in the fourth decade, 12 and 15 in the fifth decade, 12 and 4 in the sixth decade, and 3.5 and 2 from the seventh through the ninth decades. In a series of Australian whites, the average number of nevi per person peaked at 43 for males and 27 for females during the second and third decades, respectively, and decreased to very few in the sixth and seventh decades.'

Also, it has been said that patients with 50–99 small non-dysplastic melanocytic nevi or more than ten large non-dysplastic melanocytic nevi have a risk for the development of malignant melanoma that is twice the ordinary risk. As noted below and in Chapter 24, there is disagreement among dermatologists regarding malignant melanoma risk associated with dysplastic melanocytic nevi, but it is safe to say that the risks regarding dysplastic melanocytic nevi are at least as great as those regarding non-dysplastic melanocytic nevi.

Halo melanocytic nevi

Halo melanocytic nevi (see Chapter 24) may be associated with a personal or family history of cutaneous malignant melanoma and/or dysplastic melanocytic nevi, ocular malignant melanoma, vitiligo (see Chapter 7) and pernicious anemia.

If the nevus component of a patient's halo melanocytic nevus is benign appearing (i.e. there are no features that are suggestive of malignant melanoma – such features are discussed later in this chapter) and is positioned centrally within a depigmented halo component that is symmetrical, the lesion need not be removed for biopsy but should be watched, and if features that are suggestive of malignant melanoma develop in the nevus component, if asymmetry regarding the depigmented halo component develops, or if the nevus component becomes no longer centrally positioned within the depigmented halo component, complete excisional biopsy of the lesion (as discussed later in this chapter) should be performed.

On the other hand, if the patient first presents with a halo nevus in which the nevus component is not benign appearing or is not positioned centrally within a depigmented halo component that is symmetrical, complete excisional biopsy of the lesion should be performed at the time of the patient's first presentation.

As noted above, halo nevi may be associated with a personal or family history of cutaneous malignant melanoma and/or dysplastic melanocytic nevi. Therefore, if a patient has a halo nevus or halo nevi, it is advisable to find out whether he or she has a personal or family history of malignant melanoma or dysplastic melanocytic nevi. As noted previously in this chapter, personal history of malignant melanoma is a risk factor for developing additional, new primary malignant melanomas. Family history of malignant melanoma (particularly in first-degree relatives) is considered to be a risk factor for malignant melanoma. Dysplastic melanocytic nevi are felt to be risk factors for malignant melanoma, although, as discussed in more detail below, there is disagreement among dermatologists regarding this.

Lastly, since halo nevi may be associated with cutaneous malignant melanoma, dysplastic nevi and vitiligo, I perform total body examination in which I check for these conditions in patients with halo nevi.

Relationship of dysplatic melanocytic nevi to malignant melanoma

As alluded to above, there is disagreement among dermatologists regarding the extent to which dysplastic melanocytic nevi are precursor lesions for malignant melanoma (i.e. the extent to which there is an increased risk for the development of malignant melanoma within dysplastic melanocytic nevi) and the extent to which dysplastic melanocytic nevi are marker lesions for malignant melanoma (i.e. the extent to which the presence of dysplastic melanocytic nevi is a risk factor for the development of malignant melanoma at sites that are not necessarily within dysplastic melanocytic nevi).

Some dermatologists, who can be said to be in agreement with what one may call Dr Wallace H. Clark Jr's school of thought, feel that dysplastic melanocytic nevi are precursor and marker lesions for malignant melanoma to a greater extent than are common melanocytic nevi and *per se* significantly increase an individual's risk for malignant melanoma. Other dermatologists, who can be said to be in agreement with what one may call Dr A. Bernard Ackerman's school of thought, feel that so-called dysplastic melanocytic nevi are no different from so-called common melanocytic nevi with regard to being precursor and marker lesions for malignant melanoma and therefore are no more significant with regard to malignant melanoma risk than are so-called common melanocytic nevi. It should be noted that members of neither school of thought advocate prophylactic excision in general of so-called dysplastic melanocytic nevi that are without change and without features (as described below) suggestive of malignant melanoma; such lesions are in general watched instead of being prophylactically excised, and if change or if features or lesions suggestive of malignant melanoma develop, complete excisional biopsy is performed, as described below.

I feel that patients with what is clinically felt to be a dysplastic melanocytic nevus should be seen in conjunction with a dermatologist because a health-care provider with an untrained eye might mistakenly clinically diagnose what is in actuality a malignant melanoma as a dysplastic melanocytic nevus and also because there are dermatologists who feel that dysplastic melanocytic nevi are precursor and marker lesions for malignant melanoma and *per se* increase an individual's risk for malignant melanoma (although, as discussed above, there is disagreement among dermatologists regarding this). Also, patients with a histologically confirmed (i.e. biopsy-proven) dysplastic melanocytic nevus should also be seen in conjunction with a dermatologist, again because there are dermatologists who feel that dysplastic melanocytic nevi *per se* increase an individual's risk for malignant melanoma (although, again, as discussed above, there is disagreement among dermatologists regarding this).

Relative quantification of risk factors for malignant melanoma

According to Dr Arthur R. Rhodes in *Fitzpatrick's Dermatology in General Medicine*, 5th edn., individuals who have a new melanocytic nevus or a melanocytic nevus that has changed or is changing have a very high relative risk regarding the development of cutaneous malignant melanoma (where relative risk represents the degree of estimated increased risk for individuals who have the risk factor compared to individuals who do not have the risk factor and where a relative risk of 1 implies no increased risk). Regarding the development of cutaneous malignant melanoma: adults (more specifically, individuals 15 years of age and over) in comparison to children (individuals less than 15 years of age) have a relative risk of 88;   individuals who have a congenital melanocytic nevus have a relative risk of 2–21; individuals who have 50 melanocytic nevi that are ≥ 2 mm in diameter have a relative risk of 4–54; individuals who have 12 melanocytic nevi that are ≥ 5 mm in diameter have a relative risk of 41; individuals who have five melanocytic nevi that are ≥ 5 mm in diameter have a relative risk of 7–10; Whites in comparison to Blacks have a relative risk of 20; individuals with a personal history of cutaneous malignant melanoma have a relative risk of 9; individuals who have a first-degree relative with malignant melanoma have a relative risk of 8; individuals who have immunosuppression have a relative risk of 4; individuals who have marked sun-induced freckles have a relative risk of 4; individuals who have sun sensitivity have a relative risk of 3; individuals who have a history of excessive sun exposure have a relative risk of 3; individuals who have a dysplastic melanocytic nevus or dysplastic melanocytic nevi in addition to having a personal history of malignant melanoma and being in a familial melanoma family have a relative risk of 500; individuals who have a dysplastic melanocytic nevus or dysplastic melanocytic nevi in addition to being in a familial melanoma family but who do not have a personal history of malignant melanoma have a relative risk of 148; and patients who have a dysplastic melanocytic nevus or dysplastic melanocytic nevi, have no personal history of malignant melanoma and are not in a familial melanoma family have a relative risk of 7–27.

It should be noted that some dermatologists feel that the number of families with true familial melanoma is very small (see above). Also, as noted above and in Chapter 24, there is disagreement among dermatologists regarding malignant melanoma risk associated with dysplastic melanocytic nevi.

Prognostic factors for malignant melanoma without distant metastasis

Overview

The major prognostic factor for patients with malignant melanoma without distant metastases is the presence or absence of satellites, in-transit metastases and regional lymph node metastases. Distant metastases are metastases that are other than (i.e. that are beyond) satellites, in-transit metastases and regional lymph node metastases. Satellites are secondary cutaneous malignant melanoma lesions arising from tumor emboli within the dermal and subdermal lymphatics between the primary malignant melanoma lesion and the regional lymph nodes and are within 2 cm of the primary malignant melanoma lesion. In-transit metastases are secondary cutaneous malignant melanoma lesions arising from tumor emboli within the dermal and subdermal lymphatics between the primary malignant melanoma lesion and the regional lymph nodes and are more than 2 cm from the primary malignant melanoma lesion. Patients who do not have distant metastases but do have satellites, in-transit metastases and/or regional lymph node metastases have a worse prognosis than do patients who do not have distant metastases, satellites, in-transit metastases and regional lymph node metastases.

Clinical prognostic factors for malignant melanoma that is localized
(i.e without evidence of regional lymph node and distant metastasis)

Age of the patient   It has been shown that the prognosis tends to be worse for older patients.

Sex of the patient   It has been shown that men tend to have a prognosis that is worse than that for women.

Lesional site   It has been shown that patients with malignant melanoma on the extremities, excluding the hands and feet, tend to have a better prognosis than those with malignant melanoma on the head, neck, trunk, palms, soles, or subungual (i.e. nailbed) regions.

Histological prognostic factors pertaining to the primary malignant
melanoma lesion for malignant melanoma that is localized (i.e without
evidence of regional lymph node and distant metastasis)

Tumor thickness   This variable is of fundamental prognostic importance, with prognosis worsening as the tumor thickness increases. For patients with malignant melanoma that is localized, tumor thickness that is less than 0.85 mm has corresponded to a 5-year survival rate of 99%; tumor thickness of 0.85–1.69 mm has corresponded to a 5-year survival rate of 94%; tumor thickness of 1.70–3.64 mm has corresponded to a 5-year survival rate of 78%; and tumor thickness that is ≥ 3.65 mm has corresponded to a 5-year survival rate of 42%.

Other data have shown that tumor thickness that is ≤ 0.75 mm has corresponded to a 5-year survival rate of 96%; tumor thickness of 0.76–1.49 mm has corresponded to a 5-year survival rate of 87%; tumor thickness of 1.50–2.49 mm has corresponded to a 5-year survival rate of 75%; tumor thickness of 2.50–3.99 mm has corresponded to a 5-year survival rate of 66%; and tumor thickness that is ≥ 4.00 mm has corresponded to a 5-year survival rate of 47%.

It should be noted that studies have shown that the optimal tumor thickness cut-off levels for staging purposes are < 1 mm, 1–2 mm, 2–4 mm and > 4 mm.

Presence of ulceration   This is a very important prognostic variable, with prognosis being worse if ulceration is present.

Presence of regression   Patients having tumors < 1 mm in thickness with marked tumor regression have an increased risk for metastasis.

Presence of microscopic satellites   Patients with tumors that have microscopic satellites have a worse prognosis and an increased risk for local, regional and distant recurrences.

Presence of vascular invasion   Prognosis is worse if vascular invasion is present.

Lymphoid response   Prognosis is worse if the lymphoid infiltrate is decreased.

Mitotic rate   The greater the mitotic rate, the worse the prognosis.

Tumor cell type   Patients with malignant melanomas that are composed of spindle-shaped malignant melanoma cells have a better prognosis than those with malignant melanomas that are composed of other malignant melanoma cell types.

Clark's level of invasion   Clark's level I refers to malignant melanoma *in situ*; Clark's level II refers to malignant melanoma that enters the papillary dermis; Clark's level III refers to malignant melanoma that fills the papillary dermis; Clark's level IV refers to malignant melanoma that enters the reticular dermis; and Clark's level V refers to malignant melanoma that is in the subcutaneous fat. (Malignant melanoma *in situ* is malignant melanoma that is confined to the epidermis, which is the superficial cutaneous layer that is located immediately above the dermis, which is the cutaneous layer that is located immediately above the subcutaneous fat.

The papillary derm refers to the superficial portion of the dermis. The reticular derm refers to the deep portion of the dermis.)

The deeper the Clark's level of invasion, the worse the prognosis: for patients with malignant melanoma that is localized, Clark's level I (i.e. malignant melanoma *in situ*) with adequate excisional treatment should theoretically correspond to a 5-year survival rate of 100%; Clark's level II has corresponded to a 5-year survival rate of 99%; Clark's level III has corresponded to a 5-year survival rate of 95%; Clark's level IV has corresponded to a 5-year survival rate of 75%; and Clark's level V has corresponded to a 5-year survival rate of 39%.

It should be noted that studies have shown that for staging purposes Clark's level of invasion adds little prognostic information to that derived from tumor thickness.

Prognostic factors for malignant melanoma with regional lymph node metastasis and without distant metastasis

The number of positive lymph nodes   This is the most important lymph node metastasis variable in terms of prognosis (and is more important than is the size of positive lymph nodes). The prognosis worsens with increasing number of positive lymph nodes.

Location of the primary malignant melanoma lesion   It has been shown that patients who have their primary malignant melanoma lesion on an extremity and who have regional lymph node metastasis without distant metastasis have a better prognosis than do patients who have their primary malignant melanoma lesion on the head, neck, or trunk and who have regional lymph node metastasis without distant metastasis.

Age of the patient   Older patients who have malignant melanoma with regional lymph node metastasis without distant metastasis may have a worse prognosis than do younger patients who have malignant melanoma with regional lymph node metastasis without distant metastasis.

Survival rate   Patients with regional lymph node metastasis without distant metastasis have been shown to have an overall 5-year survival rate of about 37% and an overall 10-year survival rate of 32%.

Prognostic factors for malignant melanoma with distant metastasis

The number of metastatic sites   The greater the number of metastatic sites, the worse the prognosis.

The resectability of the metastasis   A patient with, for example, a solitary lung, brain, or bowel metastasis that is resectable can have a prolonged survival time.

The site of metastasis   Metastatic sites such as the liver, brain, bone, or lung are associated with a worse prognosis than are sites such as distant lymph nodes, skin, or subcutaneous tissue.

The length of time of remission preceding metastasis   The prognosis is worse for patients with a shorter length of time of remission preceding metastasis.

Sex of the patient (possible factor)   Some studies have shown a worse prognosis for males.

Serum lactate dehydrogenase level   Elevated serum lactate dehydrogenase level has been associated with a worse prognosis.

Survival time and survival rate   Patients with malignant melanoma with distant metastasis have been shown to have an overall median survival time of about 6 months once metastasis to distant sites has developed, and the overall 5-year survival rate for patients with malignant melanoma with distant metastasis has been shown to be 5%.

Clinical features suggestive of malignant melanoma

Clinical features that are suggestive of malignant melanoma can be remembered by thinking of 'A, B, C and D'.
'A' stands for asymmetry – malignant melanomas tend to be asymmetrical.
'B' stands for border – malignant melanomas tend to have borders that are irregular and/or poorly demarcated or poorly circumscribed. (Irregular borders are borders that are jagged, scalloped and/or notched. Poorly demarcated or poorly circumscribed borders are borders at which the pigment of the lesion trails off, fades, or leaches into the surrounding normal skin instead of stopping sharply and abruptly at the surrounding normal skin.)
'C' stands for color – malignant melanomas tend to have irregular pigmentation and may have within them red coloration, white coloration, blue coloration and/or gray coloration. Irregular pigmentation is pigmentation that is characterized by different tan and/or brown shades that are present irregularly or haphazardly within the lesion. Red coloration can be a manifestation of inflammation, which can occur in malignant melanomas. White coloration can be a manifestation of lesional regression, which can occur in

malignant melanomas and is considered to be a sign of poorer prognosis when seen in malignant melanomas. With regard to blue coloration, melanin, which is brown in color, can be located deeply in the dermis in malignant melanomas (this can also occur in some benign lesions), and when such deeply located melanin is seen through the dermis overlying it, it is seen as blue in color as the result of an optical effect. Mention should be made of amelanotic malignant melanoma, which is uncommon; presents without tan, brown, blue, gray and black pigmentation (i.e. it is amelanotic); and is generally reddish in color.

'D' stands for diameter – when combined with other clinical features of malignant melanoma, a lesional size ≥ 5 mm (roughly the size of a pencil's eraser head) is suggestive of malignant melanoma. (This characteristic can be considered to reflect the size of malignant melanomas at the time of diagnosis, and one must be aware that malignant melanoma starts out tiny and grows from there.)

'D' can also stand for dark – the presence of very dark brown or black coloration can be suggestive of malignant melanoma. Very dark brown and black are unusual colors for common acquired melanocytic nevi in individuals who have lightly pigmented skin, although dark pigmentation is not unusual for common acquired melanocytic nevi in individuals with darkly pigmented skin. However, regardless of an individual's skin color, one should be suspicious of very dark brown or black in lesions that are located on peripheral sites (e.g. hands or feet) or on mucous membranes.

Common acquired melanocytic nevi normally tend to grow in accordance with the growth of their anatomic location, and all melanocytic nevi within the area of anatomic growth should be growing similarly. The growth of a lesion without the associated similar growth of other melanocytic nevi in the area should make one suspicious of the differently growing lesion.

Any change in color, shape, border, etc. of an individual pre-existing lesion should make one suspicious of the changing lesion.

Special considerations regarding malignant melanoma

It is important to remember that malignant melanoma as well as benign melanocytic nevi and lentigo simplex lesions (see Chapter 24) can involve mucous membranes and nail beds.

Pigmented nail streaks and malignant melanoma

Malignant melanoma as well as benign melanocytic nevi and lentigo simplex lesions can be present in the nail matrix and as a result can produce pigmented nail streaks, which are typically brown streaks that are oriented longitudinally in the nail plate and extend from the proximal nail fold to the distal edge of the nail. (The nail matrix is located under the proximal nail fold and produces the nail plate. The proximal nail fold is the skin fold that is located at the proximal edge of the nail plate.)

Pigmented nail streaks can also be caused by drugs (e.g. minocycline (Minocin®)), can be solitary or multiple, and can involve a single nail or multiple nails.

Benign pigmented nail streaks are seen not uncommonly in Black individuals, who nonetheless can have pigmented nail streaks due to malignant melanoma in the nail matrix.

Pigmented nail streak features that should make one especially suspicious of the presence of malignant melanoma in the nail matrix include a solitary streak (if there are multiple streaks, they are not likely to be due to malignant melanoma, because it is not likely for a patient to have multiple malignant melanomas in multiple nail matrices at one time); a streak in a White patient; a streak that is irregular in any patient (e.g. a streak that has different shades of color and/or has edges that are not sharply demarcated in that the pigment trails off, fades, or leaches into the adjacent normal nail and does not stop sharply and abruptly at the juncture with the adjacent normal nail); a streak that is changing in any patient; a streak that is very dark in any patient; a streak that is very wide in any patient; or a streak that is associated with pigment involving the skin of the proximal nail fold in any patient (this is called Hutchinson's sign and is a late finding of malignant melanoma involving the nail matrix).

Biopsy of suspect melanocytic lesions

Overview

If a patient has a lesion that has features (as described above) that make one suspect the possibility of malignant melanoma, the lesion optimally needs complete excisional biopsy, because if there is malignant melanoma present within the lesion, the entire lesion needs to be present in the biopsy specimen so that the maximum depth and thickness of the malignant melanoma can be determined histologically (i.e. microscopically) on the initial biopsy for staging purposes that determine prognosis and optimal treatment. In addition, complete excisional biopsy should be performed because the entire lesion should be present in the biopsy specimen so that the overall architecture of the entire lesion can be assessed histologically (e.g. to see whether the lesion is symmetrical) and because a narrow rim of normal skin surrounding the lesion should be present in the biopsy specimen so that the peripheral margins of the lesion can be assessed histologically (e.g. to see whether the peripheral margins of the lesion are well-demarcated). In difficult cases such assessments can be important in determining whether the lesion is a malignant melanoma or a benign melanocytic lesion. Complete excisional biopsy is also optimal because there is no risk of missing malignant melanoma developing within a melanocytic nevus, as a result of sampling error, which can occur if only a portion of the lesion is removed for biopsy. Therefore, unless one is skilled in performing the necessary complete excisional biopsy, the patient should be referred to a dermatologist. Also, if the lesion is too large for a complete excisional biopsy to be feasible, a dermatologist would be the optimal physician for determining the best way to biopsy a portion of the lesion so as to get the best specimen possible for obtaining the best histological information possible, short of complete excisional biopsy. When doing a biopsy of a lesion on a mucous membrane, appropriate systemic antibiotic prophylaxis (e.g. as recommended in the American Heart Association's guidelines) should be administered to patients with heart murmurs and/or artificial implants to prevent bacterial seeding of the heart or artificial implant.

Biopsy regarding pigmented nail streaks

If a patient has a pigmented nail streak that has features that make one suspect the presence of malignant melanoma involving the nail matrix (see above), the patient should be referred to a dermatologist for evaluation and consideration of performing a nail matrix biopsy to rule out the presence of malignant melanoma in the nail matrix. (Biopsy of the nail matrix involves temporarily reflecting back the proximal nail fold as a flap in order to gain access to the underlying nail matrix so the lesion can be biopsied.)

If there is any uncertainty at all as to the cause of a pigmented nail streak, the patient should be referred to a dermatologist.

Staging of malignant melanoma

If it is determined that a lesion is malignant melanoma, staging needs to be done in order to determine prognosis and optimal treatment.

Malignant melanomas with Clark's levels greater than I (i.e. malignant melanomas other than malignant melanoma *in situ*, which is malignant melanoma confined to the epidermis) have the potential for metastasis, with the potential for metastasis increasing as the histological thickness of the malignant melanoma increases.

Malignant melanomas with metastatic potential can metastasize locally in the form of satellites, in-transit metastases and regional lymph node metastases and can metastasize distantly to virtually any organ, but the most common sites of distant metastases are the non-visceral sites that include the skin, subcutaneous tissue and distant lymph nodes. The next most common sites include the lungs, liver, brain, bone and intestines. (See the discussion previously in this chapter regarding satellites and in-transit metastases. Regional metastases have been considered to include in-transit metastases and regional lymph node metastases. Distant metastases are metastases other than satellites, in-transit metastases and metastases to regional lymph nodes.)

A thorough history (including review of systems) and physical examination (including total body integumentary examination) need to be done, and any positive findings should be further evaluated accordingly. Patients with malignant melanoma are at increased risk for developing and therefore having additional primary malignant melanomas, which can be present anywhere on the integument, and malignant melanomas with the potential for metastasis (i.e. malignant melanomas other than malignant melanoma *in situ*) can metastasize to anywhere on the integument as well as to virtually any other organ. A baseline chest X-ray is appropriate.

If there are no palpable lymph nodes, sentinel lymph node biopsy, which has been considered to be the current standard of care for surgical staging of malignant melanoma patients who have no clinical evidence of regional or distant metastases, can be performed for patients whose malignant melanomas are greater or equal to 1.0 mm in thickness or whose malignant melanomas are less than 1 mm in thickness with Clark's level IV invasion or with ulceration histologically (or possibly with other poor risk factors such as axial location in males or histological regression) in order to determine whether there are subclinical microscopic metastases to the regional lymph nodes. Sentinel lymph node biopsy involves a technique in which labeling agents are injected at the site of the primary malignant melanoma (prior to its therapeutic wide local complete excision) in order to determine the regional lymph node basin to which the site drains and to locate the first lymph node or lymph nodes to which the site drains. Removal and histological examination of this lymph node or these lymph nodes – the so-called sentinel lymph node or nodes – are then performed. If there is no tumor within this lymph node or these lymph nodes, it can be assumed that the other lymph nodes in the basin are also negative. On the other hand, if tumor is found within the sentinel lymph node or sentinel lymph nodes, it is assumed that there may be tumor in other lymph nodes in the lymph node basin, so all of the other lymph nodes in that basin are removed and examined histologically so that the extent of the lymph node involvement can be determined and so that the risk of future metastasis from involved lymph nodes is reduced by virtue of the removal of the involved lymph nodes. (Extent of lymph node involvement is a prognostic factor in that the prognosis worsens as the number of involved lymph nodes increases.)

If lymph nodes are palpable, they are removed and examined histologically for metastatic malignant melanoma.

If it is determined that metastasis to lymph nodes has occurred, additional evaluation for distant metastases can include liver function tests, liver–spleen scans and imaging studies of the chest and abdomen.

Lastly, relatives and family history should be taken into account regarding malignant melanoma in order to identify relatives and patients who are at increased risk regarding malignant melanoma and therefore should be followed accordingly.

Treatment of malignant melanoma

Treatment of malignant melanoma involves wide local complete excision of the primary tumor with clear margins of a width that should be determined by a dermatologist, surgeon, or oncologist.(When doing an excision of a lesion on a mucous membrane, appropriate systemic antibiotic prophylaxis – e.g. as recommended in the American Heart Association's guidelines – should be administered to patients with heart murmurs and/or artificial implants to prevent bacterial seeding of the heart or artificial implant.)

In addition to the surgeon's or the dermatologist's therapeutic wide local complete excision of the primary tumor, an oncologist can provide adjuvant therapy to prevent relapse in patients in whom all visible tumor has been removed but in whom there is a high risk for relapse.

Known metastatic disease is treated by an oncologist, sometimes in conjunction with a surgeon if resection of metastatic involvement is appropriate.

An algorithmic approach to newly diagnosed malignant melanoma

An approach to patients with newly diagnosed malignant melanoma based on the algorithm elucidated by Dr Jan H. Wong in the pamphlet *Melanoma News: Highlights from the 24th Annual Hawaii Dermatology Seminar* first involves histological staging of the primary tumor with regard to histological primary tumor variables discussed above.

If the patient has clinically positive (i.e. palpable) lymph nodes, these are removed and histologically examined for metastatic tumor.

If the patient has no clinically positive lymph nodes and if the primary tumor is greater or equal to 1 mm in thickness or if the primary tumor is less than 1 mm in thickness with Clark's level IV invasion or with primary tumor ulceration histologically (or possibly with other poor risk factors such as axial location in males or histological regression), sentinel lymph node biopsy is performed as discussed above.

If the patient is histologically lymph node negative, wide local complete excision of the primary tumor is performed, and the patient is observed and followed as discussed below.

If the patient is histologically lymph node positive, wide local complete excision of the primary tumor, a regional lymph node dissection, and metastatic evaluation (e.g. magnetic resonance imaging of the brain and computed tomography of the chest and abdomen) are performed.

If no distant metastases are found, the patient is given adjuvant therapy as discussed above and followed as discussed below.

If distant metastases are found, the patient is given appropriate therapy for the metastases as discussed above and followed as discussed below.

Follow-up regarding malignant melanoma

Follow-up for patients with malignant melanoma is geared toward detecting tumor relapse. This includes detecting local recurrence at the site of the excision of the primary tumor as well as detecting local and distant metastases in patients whose tumors have metastatic potential. Malignant melanomas other than malignant melanoma *in situ* have metastatic potential. Malignant melanomas with metastatic potential can metastasize locally in the form of satellites, in-transit metastases and regional lymph node metastases. They can metastasize distantly to virtually any organ, but the most common sites of distant metastases are the non-visceral sites that include the skin, subcutaneous tissue and distant lymph nodes, and the next most common sites include the lungs, liver, brain, bone and intestines. (See discussion previously in this chapter regarding satellites and in-transit metastases. Regional metastases have been considered to include in-transit metastases and regional lymph node metastases. Distant metastases are metastases other than satellites, in-transit metastases and metastases to regional lymph nodes.)

Follow-up for patients with malignant melanoma also involves detecting the development of new primary malignant melanomas. (Patients with malignant melanoma have an increased risk for the development of new primary malignant melanomas.)

In general, follow-up should be performed in conjunction with, and according to the recommendations of, a dermatologist and, if indicated, an oncologist and should include a thorough history (including review of symptoms) and physical examination (including total body integumentary examination), with any positive findings being evaluated accordingly. Malignant melanoma can metastasize to anywhere on the integument as well as to virtually any other organ, and, as just noted, patients with malignant melanoma have an increased risk for the development of new primary malignant melanomas, which can develop anywhere on the integument. Also, a chest X-ray should generally be done annually for patients with high-risk malignant melanomas.

Since about 1–6.75% (probably about 3%) of patients with malignant melanoma have a recurrence 10 or more years following initial diagnosis and treatment, since malignant melanomas have recurred at least 19 years following initial diagnosis and treatment and since patients with malignant melanoma have an increased risk for developing new primary malignant melanomas, it is reasonable to follow patients with malignant melanoma for life.

Metastatic malignant melanoma and potential malignant melanoma metastasis/relapse are treated and followed accordingly by an oncologist, with a surgeon resecting metastatic lesions for which resection is appropriate, as described previously.

Patients who do not have, but are at risk for developing, malignant melanoma

Patients who do not have malignant melanoma but are at risk for developing malignant melanoma should in general be followed in conjunction with a dermatologist, and patients who are at particularly high risk for developing malignant melanoma (e.g. patients with high-risk factors or many risk factors for developing malignant melanoma) should be followed at frequent intervals, as determined by the dermatologist.

SPECIAL CONSIDERATIONS REGARDING SKIN CANCER

In discussing skin cancers, it should be mentioned that I have seen cases of ecthymatous (see Chapter 17) involvement of skin cancer (e.g. basal cell carcinoma) in which patients presented clinically with a crusted ulcer with *Staphylococcus aureus* infection of the ulcer confirmed by bacterial culture. However, in these cases, the lesions did not resolve with appropriate ecthyma treatment, and subsequent skin biopsy revealed skin cancer (e.g. basal cell carcinoma).

RECOMMENDATIONS REGARDING EARLY DETECTION OF SKIN CANCERS

In order to detect skin cancers early, a total body integumentary examination should in general be performed routinely by the patient's primary care physician or dermatologist yearly. Also, enquiries about a family history of malignant melanoma should be done in order to identify individuals who are at increased risk for malignant melanoma and therefore should be followed accordingly.

Total body integumentary examination should be carried out more frequently for patients who have an increased risk (as described above) for skin cancer, with the examination frequency being determined by each patient's situation.

In general, patients who have an increased risk for skin cancer should be followed in conjunction with a dermatologist unless the patient's primary care physician has particular skill, knowledge and confidence in diagnosing, treating and following patients regarding skin cancer, but patients who have an increased risk for developing malignant melanoma in particular should in general always be followed in conjunction with a dermatologist.

A total body integumentary examination should be performed because, as discussed above, skin cancer can occur virtually anywhere on the integument. A total body integumentary examination consists of examination, in good lighting, of the scalp (including the hairy and any bald portions of the scalp), face, lips, mouth, ears, the areas around and behind the ears, neck, hands (including finger webs, sides of the fingers, nail beds, nails and palms), arms, trunk (including the axillae), legs, feet (including the toe webs, the sides of the toes, nail beds, nails and soles), buttocks, the area between the buttocks, pubic region, groins and anogenital region.

Ideally, all patients (but especially patients at increased risk, as discussed above, for skin cancer) should be told what to look for regarding skin cancers (as discussed above) and should carry out self-examination of the above-described total body sites monthly, which can be considered to be analogous to women doing monthly self-examinations of the breast. The use of two mirrors (e.g. a hand mirror and a full length mirror) and/or the assistance of the same person each month can facilitate the patient's total body integumentary self-examinations.

SKIN CANCER PREVENTION

In order to prevent skin cancer, all patients should be told to avoid sun exposure, keep covered, wear a broad-brimmed hat and use a sunscreen with an SPF of 15 or greater when outdoors during the daytime.

A METHOD OF PERFORMING SHAVE BIOPSIES AND RECOMMENDATIONS REGARDING SHAVE BIOPSY FOLLOW-UP CARE

Overview

Except for lesions clinically suspected of being malignant melanoma or keratoacanthoma (for both of which, complete excisional biopsy is the optimal type of biopsy, as discussed above), shave biopsy is probably in general the best type of biopsy to perform in order to confirm histologically a clinically suspected skin cancer's diagnosis, because a shave biopsy is minimally invasive, leaves a minimal scar when performed properly, is relatively easy to perform and is such that it allows for the most treatment options if the lesion turns out to be a skin cancer. (However, when the diagnosis is not obvious or when tumor is suspected within scar tissue, a punch biopsy is preferable to a shave biopsy. If the health-care provider is not trained in doing punch biopsies, the patient can be referred to a dermatologist for the punch biopsy.)

When performing biopsies of lesions on mucous membranes, appropriate systemic antibiotic prophylaxis (as recommended in the American Heart Association's guidelines) should be administered to patients with heart murmurs and/or artificial implants in order to prevent bacterial seeding of the heart or artificial implant.

A shave biopsy is billed as 'skin biopsy'.

Performing a shave biopsy

I perform a shave biopsy as follows: I draw up 1% lidocaine with or without epinephrine into a 3-ml syringe using a large-bore needle, such as a 21-gauge needle. (Epinephrine decreases bleeding and prolongs the local anesthetic effect via vasoconstriction. However, I do not use epinephrine on such sites as the fingers, toes and penis – some dermatologists recommend not using epinephrine on the nose and ear lobes also – because epinephrine can cause excessively decreased arterial blood flow at such sites, and this can result in tissue necrosis.) I then replace the large-bore needle with a small-bore needle, such as a 30-gauge needle.

I clean the skin of the area to be biopsied with an alcohol swab and then dry with sterile gauze, after which I provide local anesthesia by injecting the lidocaine intradermally so that it infiltrates the lesional skin and the skin around the lesion, with each injection beginning in the previously injected site and then extending beyond, because injecting local anesthetic in this way is less painful. (Injecting the local anesthetic slowly into the skin also lessens the pain of the injection.) In order to prevent accidental intravascular injection of anesthetic, aspiration (pulling back on the syringe's plunger) should be performed immediately prior to each time the anesthetic is injected.

The shave biopsy can then be performed using a no. 15 scalpel to remove the lesion to be biopsied flush to the surface of the skin, with the scalpel blade being oriented parallel to the surface of the skin and cutting horizontally. (If necessary, the lesional skin can be pulled or stretched tautly by a finger or fingers of the free hand during the time the shave biopsy is being performed.) Alternatively, particularly if the lesion to be biopsied is flat, the path of the no. 15 scalpel blade can curve slightly below the surface of the skin during the course of the biopsy procedure, but one must bear in mind that the deeper the scalpel blade curves below the surface of the skin, the more prominent is the scarring that can potentially result. One must be aware that if the tissue removed during the biopsy is inadequate, the skin cancer, if indeed one is present, can be missed (in which case this would be called 'sampling error'). Therefore, unless the physician is skilled in performing the appropriate biopsy, the patient should see a dermatologist because the biopsy can be inadequate and can miss the skin cancer, if one is present, due to sampling error, in which case the biopsy might merely show benign inflammation and/or actinic keratosis and miss the skin cancer.

It should be noted that some dermatologists use a double-edged 'blue blade' (i.e. a Gillette Blue Blade® double-edged safety razor blade) in place of the no. 15 scalpel when performing shave biopsies. In this case, when it is still wrapped in its individual paper packaging, the 'blue blade' is bent along the midline of its long axis (i.e. along the midline that runs parallel to the two sharp edges of the blade) until the blade snaps into two pieces, with each piece consisting of a half blade with one sharp edge. One of these half blades is then removed from the paper packaging and held at both ends by the thumb and index finger so that the sharp edge runs between the thumb and index finger. The thumb and index finger should be squeezed together slightly so that a curvature of the sharp edge of the blade occurs. The sharp edge of the blade is then used to perform the shave biopsy as described above for a no. 15 scalpel. It should be noted that when a 'blue blade' is used in this way for a shave biopsy, the above-described curvature of the sharp, cutting edge causes the shave biopsy path to curve a little more deeply than it does when a no. 15 scalpel is used.

After the shave biopsy is performed and the biopsy specimen is placed in the formalin bottle to be sent to the pathology department for histological examination, blood overlying the wound is dried using sterile gauze, and a Drysol® (aluminum chloride 20%) solution-soaked cotton-tipped applicator is applied to the wound in order to provide hemostasis. (The aluminum chloride solution acts as a cauterant.) Fresh, Drysol-soaked cotton-tipped applicators may need to be applied repeatedly to the wound in order to achieve complete hemostasis, but for the Drysol to be effective in providing hemostasis, the wound must be dried by being dabbed with sterile gauze immediately prior to each application of the Drysol-soaked cotton-tipped applicators to the wound. To slow brisk oozing of blood before application of the Drysol-soaked cotton-tipped applicators, steady pressure can be applied to the briskly oozing area with sterile gauze for at least 15–20 min without peeking. This may not only slow brisk oozing of blood to facilitate application of the Drysol-soaked cotton-tipped applicators, but it may also sometimes provide complete hemostasis without the need for using the Drysol-soaked cotton-tipped applicators.

Dressing the wound

After complete hemostasis is achieved, the wound is cleaned with an alcohol swab and then dried with sterile gauze. I then apply Polysporin Ointment® (polymyxin B sulfate/ bacitracin zinc) to the wound with a sterile cotton-tipped applicator and then cover the wound with a sterile piece of non-stick Telfa® pad cut to size so that it just covers the wound. The Telfa pad is held in place by the application of paper tape.

Wound care

Beginning the next day, the patient removes the dressing, cleans the wound using hydrogen peroxide and a sterile cotton-tipped applicator, dries the area with sterile gauze, applies the antibiotic ointment with a fresh sterile cotton-tipped applicator and then covers the wound with a fresh sterile piece of non-stick Telfa pad cut to size so that it just covers the wound, with the Telfa pad being held in place by the application of paper tape. The patient performs this wound care twice daily until the wound heals completely. I tell the patient to avoid water contact with the wound (especially soaking the wound with water) until the wound heals.

How to handle suspected wound infection

If subsequent development of bacterial infection of the wound is suspected (e.g. if increased erythema, increased tenderness, increased pain, swelling and/or pus subsequently develop), a bacterial culture and sensitivities (C&S) of the wound should be obtained, and the patient should be started empirically on a course of an oral antibiotic such as cephalexin (Keflex®)

250–500 mg every 6 h (or, if the patient cannot take cephalexin, erythromycin 250–500 mg every 6 h) for adults, if not otherwise unadvisable, with the antibiotic being modified according to patient response and C&S results. Pediatric dosage is as described in the package inserts.

Allergy to topical antibiotic

Allergy to Polysporin Ointment, or to any other topical preparation, can be manifested by the development of increased inflammation or by nonhealing of a wound without associated increased inflammation.

If a patient is allergic to Polysporin Ointment and not allergic to iodine, I have the patient use brown Betadine Ointment® (povidone-iodine) instead of Polysporin Ointment. Clear Betadine Ointment should not be used in this situation, because it contains the same active ingredients that Polysporin Ointment contains.

It should be noted that the clinical findings (i.e. increased inflammation) of an allergic reaction to the topical antibiotic being used for wound care can mimic some of the clinical findings of bacterial infection (although, in general, an allergic reaction to the topical antiobiotic would tend to be itchy, whereas a bacterial infection of the wound would tend to be painful and/or tender, and pus may be present). Therefore, when a bacterial infection of a wound is suspected, an allergic reaction to the topical antibiotic being used should also be considered.

ACCURACY OF PATIENT HISTORIES REGARDING SKIN CANCERS

Lastly, it is important to remember when taking a personal or family history regarding skin cancer that, in my experience, it is not uncommon for patients to say that they or relatives had malignant melanoma when in actuality they or the relatives had basal cell carcinoma or squamous cell carcinoma. This is probably because patients think of *malignant* melanoma when they are told that they have a *malignant* skin growth and because patients not uncommonly confuse the term *melanoma* with the term *carcinoma*, because these two terms sound alike. Distinguishing between malignant melanoma and basal cell carcinoma or squamous cell carcinoma is obviously important, because of the differences regarding the relative seriousness of these different types of skin cancer.

27

Secondary syphilis

Secondary syphilis is mentioned many times in the differential diagnoses of skin conditions discussed in this book, because secondary syphilis has been considered to be one of the two 'great mimickers' (along with drug eruption – see Chapter 3); the cutaneous eruption of secondary syphilis can simulate the appearance of the cutaneous manifestations of virtually any skin condition. For this reason, secondary syphilis should be ruled out whenever indicated according to the clinical situation. (As noted previously in this book, a negative rapid plasma reagin or Venereal Disease Research Laboratories test will rule out secondary syphilis.) However, since in my opinion actual cases of secondary syphilis are relatively rarely encountered in many clinical practices at this time, I have decided not to discuss it further other than to say that detailed guidelines pertaining to the evaluation, treatment and follow-up of syphilis and other sexually transmitted diseases have been published by the Centers for Disease Control, from which these guidelines can be readily obtained.

Glossary of commonly used dermatological terms

Abscess – A pus-filled cavity.

Actinic – Solar.

Bulla (plural: bullae) – A large, clear, colorless or yellowish fluid (serum)-filled blister that is greater than 1 cm in diameter.

Comedo (plural: comedones) – A hair follicle blocked by a keratin plug. (See *Keratin* in this glossary.) A closed comedo (also known as a white head) has a narrow, or undilated, follicular orifice (i.e. follicular opening) on the skin surface, whereas an open comedo (also known as a black head; the black coloration is due to melanin pigmentation of the comedo's keratin plug) has a wide, or dilated, follicular orifice on the skin surface.

Crust – Dried serum with variable numbers of red and/or white blood cells; lay persons refer to crusts as scabs.

Cutaneous horn – A digitate lesion composed of keratin, under which such lesions as an actinic (solar) keratosis, Bowen's disease (squamous cell carcinoma *in situ*), invasive squamous cell carcinoma, verruca (wart), or seborrheic keratosis may be present. See *Keratin* in this glossary. For discussion of actinic (solar) keratosis, see Chapter 25. For discussion of Bowen's disease (squamous cell carcinoma *in situ*) and invasive squamous cell carcinoma, see Chapter 26. For discussion of verruca (wart) and seborrheic keratosis, see Chapter 23.

Dermis – The cutaneous layer that is located immediately below the epidermis. (See *Epidermis* in this glossary.)

Ecchymosis (plural: ecchymoses) – A large area of purpura. (See *Purpura* in this glossary.)

Epidermis – The superficial cutaneous layer that is located immediately above the dermis. (See *Dermis* in this glossary.)

Erosion – A lesion in which all or part of the epidermis is lost without loss of the dermis. (See *Epidermis* and *Dermis* in this glossary.) *Erosion* is distinguished from ulcer. (See *Ulcer* in this glossary.)

Erythema – An increased amount of blood in cutaneous blood vessels such that a reddish coloration of the skin is produced. Areas of *erythema* blanch (i.e. the reddish coloration disappears) when pressure is applied. This is in contrast to *purpura*. (See *Purpura* in this glossary.)

Hyperkeratosis – Thickening of the stratum corneum. (See *Stratum corneum* in this glossary.)

Keratin – The protein of which the stratum corneum, hair and nails are composed. (See *Stratum corneum* in this glossary.)

Keratinocytes – The cells that comprise the bulk of the epidermis and produce the protein keratin. (See *Epidermis* and *Keratin* in this glossary.)

Keratosis (plural: keratoses) – A lesion made up of keratinocytes and containing the protein keratin. (See *Keratinocytes* and *Keratin* in this glossary.)

Keratotic – Having features of a keratosis. *Keratotic* refers to a lesion made up of keratinocytes and containing the protein keratin. (See *Keratosis, Keratinocytes* and *Keratin* in this glossary.)

Lichenification – Thickening of the skin with increased prominence of surface skin lines due to frequent scratching, rubbing and/or picking.

Macule – A small, non-raised, non-palpable lesion that is less than 1 cm in diameter and that is essentially an area in which the color is different from that of the normal surrounding skin.

Nodule – A large, solid bump that is greater than 1 cm in diameter.

Pain – A discomfort that hurts and that is spontaneously present without being elicited by application of pressure. *Pain* is distinguished from *tenderness*. (See *Tenderness* in this glossary.)

Papule – A small, solid bump that is less than 1 cm in diameter.

Patch – A large, non-raised, non-palpable lesion that is greater than 1 cm in diameter and that is essentially an area in which the color is different from that of the normal surrounding skin.

Petechiae – Pinpoint lesions of purpura. (See *Purpura* in this glossary.)

Plaque – A large, broad, raised, solid lesion.

Purpura – Cutaneous extravasated red blood cells that produce a reddish or purplish coloration of the skin. (Extravasated red blood cells are red blood cells that are present outside blood vessels.) Areas of purpura do not blanch (i.e. the reddish or purplish coloration does not disappear) when pressure is applied. This is in contrast to *erythema*. (See *Erythema* in this glossary.)

Pus – An exudate containing white blood cells.

Pustule – A cloudy, yellowish or whitish, circumscribed elevated skin lesion consisting of a collection of pus. (See *Pus* in this glossary.)

Scale/scaling/scaly – Flake/flaking/flaky.

Stratum corneum – The dead, horny, most superficial layer of the epidermis. (See *Epidermis* in this glossary.) The *stratum corneum* is composed of the protein keratin. (See *Keratin* in this glossary.)

Subcutaneous tissue – The tissue that is located immediately below the dermis. (See *Dermis* in this glossary.)

Telangiectasia – See *Telangiectasis* in this glossary.

Telangiectasis (*plural: telangiectases*) – a dilated, small, superficial cutaneous blood vessel, clinically manifested as a fine red line, which may or may not blanch (i.e. disappear) on application of pressure.

Tenderness – A discomfort that hurts and that is not spontaneously present but is elicited by application of pressure. *Tenderness* is distinguished from pain. (See *Pain* in this glossary.)

Tumor – A very large, solid bump that is greater than 2 cm in diameter. Tumor can also mean a neoplastic lesion.

Ulcer – A lesion in which the epidermis and deeper tissue are lost. (See *Epidermis* in this glossary.) *Ulcer* is distinguished from *erosion*. (See *Erosion* in this glossary.)

Verrucous – Warty.

Vesicle – A small, clear, colorless or yellowish fluid (serum)-filled blister that is less than 1 cm in diameter.

Bibliography

Freedberg I, ed. *Fitzpatrick's Dermatology in General Medicine*, 5th edn. New York: McGraw-Hill Education, 1999

Arndt K, Le Boit P, *et al.*, eds. *Cutaneous Medicine and Surgery: An Integrated Program in Dermatology*. Philadelphia: WB Saunders, 1996

Lever WF, Schaumburg-Lever G. *Histopathology of the Skin*, 7th edn. Philadelphia: JB Lippincott, 1990

Provost TT, Farmer E, eds. *Current Therapy in Dermatology*, – 2. Toronto: BC Decker, 1988

Bennett R. *Fundamentals of Cutaneous Surgery*. St Louis: CV Mosby, 1988

Fisher A. *Contact Dermatitis*, 3rd edn. Philadelphia: Lea & Febiger, 1986

Melanoma News: Highlights from the 24th Annual Hawaii Dermatology Seminar. Schering, 2000

Highlights from the 58th Annual Meeting of the American Academy of Dermatology: Focus on Hormonal Therapy. New York: Highlights, 2000

Index